HEALING THE FRACTURED MIND

HEALING THE FRACTURED MIND
A Revolutionary Method for Treating Addiction and Other Disorders

Felicity de Zulueta
with
Monique Notice, Jayshree Unadkat, and
Leonor de Escoriaza

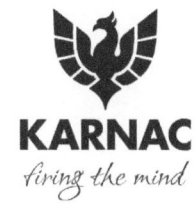

KARNAC
firing the mind

First published in 2025 by
Karnac Books Limited
62 Bucknell Road
Bicester
Oxfordshire OX26 2DS

British Library Cataloguing in Publication Data

A C.I.P. for this book is available from the British Library

ISBN: 978-1-91349-471-1 (paperback)
ISBN: 978-1-91349-492-6 (e-book)

Typeset by vPrompt eServices Pvt Ltd, India

Printed in the United Kingdom

www.firingthemind.com

To

Dr Bessel van der Kolk

*for his extraordinary inspiration and guidance in making sense
of the role of attachment in human vulnerability*

Contents

Acknowledgements

Working in the field of severe trauma or complex PTSD is challenging and requires patience and imagination to help those who suffer from its extensive and, at times, terrifying effects. Though my colleagues and I in the Traumatic Stress Service at the Maudsley Hospital did manage to help many of the men and women to reach a state of well-being in which they could resume a fairly normal life, it was not easy and often not achievable. For this reason, I was always on the lookout for a new therapeutic approach that would enable us to achieve better results and more fulfilled patients.

Dr Bob Johnson's work with prisoners finally revealed a different way of thinking about these mental disorders and enabled me to develop the Traumatic Attachment Induction Procedure and share its use with my psychotherapeutic colleagues. It is because of the enthusiasm of Pamela Lawson, Danièle Wichené, and Josefine Speyer who joined our clinical research group and their clients' amazing results that the four of us finally found the courage to share our findings with the world, with the support of my ex-patient Chloe, my friend Eve Lawino Abe, and my close family and friends.

However, it is not easy to share a new and potentially important discovery with professional colleagues. I was helped in this task by Professor Giovanni Liotti's enthusiastic support and that of Professor Giuseppe Craparo in Italy, as well as that of Dr Sandra Bloom in the United States, who is a wonderful example of courage in the face of loss and negativity. In the UK, Professor Joan Raphael-Leff encouraged us to pursue this work and it was Christina Wipf Perry, my first editor, who helped me overcome many obstacles and provided us with our first publishing contract, whilst the young psychologist Eleanor Arendt came to my rescue with last-minute assistance. However, without the patient editing and advice from my dear and modest friend Judy Larkin, a specialist in risk communication and contingency planning and a research fellow at King's College, London, as well as a Fellow of the Royal Institution and Royal Society of Arts, and a board member of the Issue Management Council in Washington DC, I would not have been able to write this book. I am so grateful to all of you!

About the authors

Dr Felicity de Zulueta is an Emeritus Consultant Psychiatrist in Psychotherapy at the South London and Maudsley NHS Trust and an Honorary Senior Lecturer in Traumatic Studies at Kings College London. She developed and headed both the Department of Psychotherapy at Charing Cross Hospital, linked to the Cassel Hospital, and, later, the Traumatic Stress Service in the Maudsley as a specialised service for survivors of childhood abuse, domestic violence and refugees suffering from severe complex PTSD and other dissociative disorders.

She has published papers on the subject of bilingualism, post-traumatic stress disorder, and other trauma induced disorders from an attachment perspective and is the author of *From Pain to Violence: The Traumatic Roots of Destructiveness* (Wiley-Blackwell, 2nd edition, 2006). She is a founder member of the International Attachment Network and the recipient of the Sándor Ferenczi Award 2020 for the "for the best published work in the realm of psychoanalysis related to trauma and dissociation in adults and/or children".

She lectures worldwide on the origins and treatment of complex PTSD and violence, has been a consultant to UNICEF and to the Singaporean army, and promotes the use of a video-based therapy called Video Interaction Guidance for the treatment of traumatised families in the UK, Italy, (Milan and Torino), Mexico, Ecuador, Ireland, and Tanzania. She works as a freelance consultant psychotherapist with training in psychoanalytic psychotherapy, systemic family therapy, group analysis, EMDR, and Lifespan Integration. She developed a new therapeutic procedure called the Traumatic Attachment Induction Procedure (TAIP) and is currently carrying out clinical research on the traumatic attachment, its different manifestations, and its theoretical and therapeutic implications. This book is based upon that research.

Leonor de Escoriaza is a clinical psychologist in private practice in Madrid. Her initial training in both France and Spain was the foundation for her integrative and transcultural approach. Leonor is a certified Lifespan Integration therapist, working mainly with adults with complex trauma and attachment issues. Whilst in the UK, Leonor worked with several charities focusing on expatriate, refugees, victims of abuse, and adults with intellectual and learning disabilities. She is also interested in equine therapy and therapy with the help of animals. She joined the TAIP research group in 2018.

Monique Notice, MA, MBACP (Accred), is a psychotherapist in private practice with a very diverse demographic for short- or long-term psychotherapy. She has a background in nursing (RGN) and completed her master's degree in psychodynamic therapy in 2012. In 2013, she became an accredited member of the BACP. She previously worked in an alcohol and drug agency that provides one-to-one and group therapy to people struggling with addictions. She joined the TAIP research group in 2012.

Jayshree Unadkat, MBACP (Accred), is a psychotherapist in private practice working with culturally diverse individuals and couples, and also works in NHS mental health services. She completed her master's degree in contemporary psychodynamic counselling/psychotherapy in 2013. She previously worked as a counsellor with adults struggling with addictions and also with young and older carers. She joined the TAIP research group in 2012.

Preface

Valerie Sinason

Felicity de Zulueta is deservedly a seminal figure in the field of traumatic attachment both nationally and internationally. A female psychiatrist, group analyst, and psychoanalytic psychotherapist, she managed to be a unique therapeutic voice in a leading hospital where, historically, biology, males, and the quantitative were often privileged over the qualitative. However, she is also a thoughtful biologist who cares deeply about research as well. Her multicultural upbringing and awareness of the refugee experience of parents and grandparents gives her a capacity to speak several languages, literally and symbolically. She has managed to be a bridge between different forms of treatment, with trainings in group psychoanalysis, psychoanalytic psychotherapy, systemic family therapy, EMDR, and Lifespan Integration.

She was born in Colombia, in 1948, the granddaughter of a Spanish political refugee and daughter of a refugee when her father had to flee "la Violenza". She was brought up learning four languages in Borneo, Switzerland, Uganda, and Lebanon where she took the French Baccalaureate in Philosophy. She speaks English, French, Spanish, and Italian. In 1966 she came to England and obtained a degree in Biology at the University of East Anglia followed by a medical degree in Cambridge and Sheffield before specialising in psychiatry and psychotherapy at the Maudsley Hospital in London.

At the Maudsley she created and developed a specialised service for survivors of childhood abuse, domestic violence, and refugees suffering from severe complex PTSD and other dissociative disorders. It became internationally known with referrals from across the UK and abroad. She trained mental health staff in Singapore, Kosovo, and Ecuador and has a TEDx talk on *Pain to Violence*, her first seminal book.

As a consultant at the leading psychiatric teaching and treatment hospital in the UK, the Maudsley, her work has been profoundly influential and her relational attachment-based research on trauma continues to spread influence.

She retired from her clinical work in the NHS in 2011 and is now an Emeritus Consultant Psychiatrist in the South London and Maudsley NHS Trust, an Honorary Senior Lecturer in Traumatic Studies at the Institute of Psychiatry and Kings College London, a founding member of WAVE, the International Attachment Network and received the 2020 Sándor Ferenczi Award from the International Society for the Study of Trauma and Dissociation (ISSTD). She was a founder member of the London Aces hub, writes, and lectures. She is married and has one son and two grandchildren.

For the last forty-five years, Dr de Zulueta, as a British group analyst, psychiatrist, and psychotherapist, has aided victims of trauma and dissociation through her teaching, writing, treatment programmes, and research. However, it was her seminal first book *From Pain to Violence: The Traumatic Roots of Destructiveness* (published in two editions in 1993 and 2006), that cemented her international reputation and brought her further acclaim in providing the scientific rationale behind the need for a more humanitarian justice system and therapeutic approaches to violence. Showing how hurt produces hurting (rather like Daniel Defoe understanding "Give me not poverty lest I steal"), produces profound polarised reactions. Such researched humane concepts can evoke fear and a desire to threaten. Obviously, I am in the group who were profoundly nourished by this work.

Indeed, *From Pain to Violence* is on my list as one the most significant books I have ever read in the field of trauma and has remained there ever since I read the first edition thirty years ago.

It has not been bearable politically or historically to look at the cause of violence and address it and perhaps it never will be. The populist answer of punitive responses, austerity, overcrowding in prisons, lack of support for forensic psychotherapy tends to win. However, Felicity's work reminds us that the protection of parents and babies to achieve the best possible attachment is the most significant long-term answer.

In highlighting the significance of the nature of early attachment trauma in providing the roots of violence she emphasises the importance of early mother/parent–child interactions. This is because the brain is essentially being "programmed" in those early years and "children learn unconsciously and biologically to modulate feelings of all kinds". In addition to discussing the four main types of attachment, how they are formed, and how they affect individuals throughout their lives, she also provided hope and help in describing effective treatments for both violence and trauma. Some of the greater international awareness on trauma, dissociation, and attachment is thanks to Felicity's work. *From Pain to Violence* is notable for providing a detailed overview of the role of trauma in violent behaviour with a psychological, biological, psychotherapeutic research underpinning.

It was when creating and developing the new Department of Psychotherapy at Charing Cross Hospital and the Cassel Hospital, which preceded her Maudsley post, that she found most of her patients showed violence as a long-term after effect of childhood trauma. She wrote: "My early experiences in South America and later in Africa and in the Middle East had made me wonder how it could be that so much kindness could so easily turn to so much hate and bloodshed".

She took a year's sabbatical to research this subject, knowing she did not agree with the Kleinian hypothesis of innate human destructiveness. Through her research she realised the significance of John Bowlby, had a memorable meeting with him, and was encouraged to write and research these issues further. This led to *From Pain to Violence*, her watershed book, as a result of which she was personally invited to work at the Maudsley by the forensic specialist, Professor Gunn.

As a result of her investigations, she emphasised that the current high level of violence may well be linked to the effects of childhood and adult trauma which were far more widespread than had hitherto been acknowledged. She also made major links with another hero of mine, Professor Bob Johnson, who showed that if violent prisoners were listened to in a particular way in therapy, their disclosures of past trauma in relation to their main attachment figure emerged, and then a reduction in their violence followed.

The Traumatic Attachment Induction Procedure or TAIP

On asking Felicity about the consequences of her connection with Professor Johnson, she replied:

> It was seeing Bob working with a prisoner on television that inspired me to try and work out how he achieved such amazing changes in the way his patient thought and behaved. I realised he was using an imaginary separation reaction, much like Ainsworth carried out with her Strange Situation, which led me to develop a a simplified version of the Strange Situation to be used with adults who had suffered traumas in their early life. We began using it in the Maudsley with marked success and it is then that I realised that what we were dealing with was the outcome of the "traumatic attachment" so well described by Allan Schore.

> Following my retirement I was able to recruit my current group of psychotherapists interested in using this procedure which led to the further discoveries described in this book.

> This work completed my research into the traumatic origin of violence: it lies in the split self, resulting from the early traumatic attachment and is also found in other so-called "difficult-to-treat conditions".

Felicity's own words from her conclusion in Chapter 6 do the best job of clarifying her findings:

> My use of the TAIP with forensic patients has finally brought to light the missing link that I was looking for when I wrote my book *From Pain to Violence: The Traumatic Roots of Destructiveness*. I concluded then that "violence is not an innate biological instinct: it is the manifestation of both our disrupted attachment bonds and our shattered self" (Zulueta, 2006,

p. 344). I never imagined that, by developing the TAIP and using it to explore the minds of homicidal patients, I would be able to locate the cause of their disrupted attachments and their shattered or divided Self, both due to the development of the *traumatic attachment* in their early childhoods.

So, in the decades which have followed since her seminal book, Felicity has come up with another major theoretical advance. The TAIP has confirmed the existence of the divided Self which is due to the *traumatic attachment* and is the cornerstone of dissociation. This, amazingly, makes the condition reversible.

Patients who have undergone this process have ended up feeling healed and normal

Obviously, this procedure needs careful research if it is to be applied to people with more severe dissociative disorders, such as dissociative identity disorder, for example, and with some patients with intellectual disability where we have found the nature of traumatic attachment is so severe that it represents a concrete internalised death-wish and an infanticidal attachment (Sinason, 1992; Brett Kahr, 2007). Felicity remains open to extending her research, in a careful way, with other clinical groups.

When I organised the Association of Child Psychotherapy's eightieth birthday conference for John Bowlby, I asked him what the best thing about being eighty was. With a wicked grin he replied immediately: "It is having your old enemies have to admit you were right!"

Felicity has gracefully watched as, Cassandra-like, she is only believed after the event. She has learned, despite the emotional cost, how to withstand the familiar pushback that comes to all pioneers with something to say that disrupts societal dissociation. "I feel I keep being shut up and hitting a brick wall."

Echoing the words from Bowlby's paper ("On knowing what you are not supposed to know and feeling what you are not supposed to feel", 1979), Felicity's brave work keeps pushing at boundaries.

Bowlby found the study of other animals helpful in understanding our species. In the era of Attenborough's documentaries and an international interest in attachment in all animals, this new book, thirty years in labour, appropriately begins with an elephant in the room—the real elephant!

Felicity factually states:

> I was invited to join a *National Geographic* team making a film aimed at exploring the causes of elephants' destructive behaviour in Africa. This experience was to confirm my view, also held by those who work with these animals, that elephants can suffer from the effects of trauma in a very similar way as humans do.

Her multicultural lived experience, which included animal experiences too, informs Felicity de Zulueta's work. She stays with the surprising and disturbing data her work provides until she has an answer and then she provides it in a language suitable for the general public and professionals alike.

In addition to the usual mixed response that comes to pioneers, work with babies and small children in our culture is valued less than work with adults. As a nursery teacher, I earned less and had less status than as an adult lecturer. As a child psychotherapist, status is lower than that of an adult psychotherapist. Accepting the crucial task of providing the most enriching environment for the little ones and their family is the golden route to reducing mental illness and addiction in adult life.

Elephants have almost the longest gestation of any animal and Felicity's two books have had long gestations in order to produce something substantial. Congratulations to Felicity and her team of psychotherapists on this seminal work!

Valerie Sinason, *PhD*
Poet, writer, child and adolescent psychoanalytic psychotherapist (retired) and adult psychoanalyst
Founder and patron for the Clinic of Dissociative Studies UK

Introduction

This book is written at the request of one of my patients, Chloe. She was diagnosed as suffering from "borderline personality disorder", a controversial diagnosis. Our therapeutic four-year-long journey was a challenging one but ended twenty-five years ago in a totally unexpected way: she finally felt like a "normal" person. At the end of her last therapeutic session, she stood up to face me and said: "It is now my turn to tell you something that you need to do: you must write about the way you enabled me to live as a normal person."

Most of my psychiatric colleagues do not believe that this disorder is curable and yet twenty-five years later, Chloe continues to "live her life in the real world" without ever reverting back to the terrible and terrifying self-destructive states of her past life. She is present in this book. We both hope that other people who suffer as she did will benefit from the therapeutic use of this new procedure called the Traumatic Attachment Induction Procedure (TAIP) that enables psychotherapists to elicit the underlying cause of not only "borderline personality disorder" but also addictions, unresolved grief, complex PTSD, and violent behaviour.

My three co-authors, Monique Notice, Jayshree Unadkat, and Leonor de Escoriaza, who each approached me after hearing me talk, have been and continue to be an essential part of this clinical research project. They have each written a chapter to describe how they discovered the TAIP and what it has been for them and for their clients. By seeing people with different diagnoses, we are finding that this new approach is particularly effective with so-called "difficult-to-treat disorders", now that we have discovered the underlying reason for why people suffer from these distressing emotions and accompanying urges.

We also hope that more psychotherapists will be interested in taking up the short online training in the use of the Traumatic Attachment Induction Procedure (or TAIP) that we offer, whether they are trained in psychoanalytic psychotherapy, EMDR, schema therapy, or Lifespan Integration. It is a rewarding journey for both therapist and client and hopefully will be available for many more people in the future.

CHAPTER 1

The elephant in the room

Delinquent elephants

One day, many years ago, whilst working in the Traumatic Stress Service (TSS) at the Maudsley Hospital, I had an unusual phone call from a journalist called Charles Siebert from the *New York Times*. He asked me: "Doctor, do you think that elephants can suffer from post-traumatic stress disorder?"

This disorder, referred to very often as PTSD, is what my work is all about. We were treating adults who had been traumatised in many different ways. Half of these men and women were refugees from different parts of the world, who suffered emotionally and physically from the terrible effects of war, torture, and often terrifying journeys to reach safety. The other half were people currently living in the UK, who had been brought up in often horrifying circumstances as children and who now suffered from the effects of these overwhelming experiences. When talking with these men and women we would often refer to their symptoms as "wounds of the mind". This made more sense to them.

The idea that human beings can suffer from experiences of abuse or neglect at the hands of their parents or other people is often dismissed, even today. So, when faced with the possibility that elephants might be suffering from a similar condition, I must confess that it took me a few minutes to respond. Could those magnificent gentle giants that I had seen as a teenager, wandering about in the savannahs of Uganda in the early 1960s, suffer from the same symptoms as the people we treated in the TSS?

And then, I remembered how, during that period of my life, my parents had found themselves in charge of a very small elephant which had survived the killing of its mother. The journalist wanted to know more, so I told him how well my mother Gillian had cared for this little animal—so well that he settled down happily into his new home. He was fed with large bottles of strengthened milk and wandered about our garden in the company of a young Ugandan kob which my mother had adopted a few months earlier. Come the night, our little "tembo", as elephants are called in Swahili, would settle down in our garage with the antelope and our black Labrador by his side. He appeared safe in their company.

Unfortunately, it did not take very long for my parents to realise that their delightful little elephant would soon require the milk of two cows to feed it and that he would soon be too large to fit into our garage. We did not have the amenities for a growing young African elephant since we lived in small colonial settlement of typical English houses and small gardens in the town of Kabale, up in the Kigezi hills, miles away from the game park where he came from. It was painfully obvious that we would have to find another home for him. The zoo in the capital, Entebbe, seemed the best place to send him to. However, I told the journalist, although the zoo gave him the right food and attended to all his physical needs, what they could not give him was the loving care he had had from Gillian. "He was a lonely little elephant and he died. He had no attachment" (Siebert, 2006).

As I spoke, I remembered the work of John Bowlby, the twentieth-century British developmental psychologist and psychiatrist who spent his life studying what goes on between mothers and their babies. During the Second World War, many women in the UK were required to work in the munitions factories. This meant that they had to leave their infants in the care of specialised nurseries set up for this purpose. Bowlby noted that many of their infants became ill, and even died, despite the good physical care that they received. Like our little elephant, they needed something more, something specific that goes on between mothers and their infants.

What maternal ingredients were these infants missing, Bowlby wondered? To resolve this mystery he turned to ethology, the study of animal behaviour. This is when he got in touch with Harlow, who was studying infant rhesus monkeys separated from their mothers (Harlow & Mears, 1979, pp. 88–89). They were given, instead, a surrogate cloth mother and a surrogate wire mother which had a nursing bottle of milk attached to it. It soon became clear that they much preferred to cuddle up to their "cloth mother" where they spent most of their time and they only went to the wire mother when hungry. When placed in a strange environment, these young monkeys would often return to hug their cloth mother for reassurance before exploring their surroundings (Harlow & Mears, 1979, pp. 88–89). This led Bowlby to refer to the behaviour seen between the primate mother and her offspring as "attachment behaviour" which he defined initially as:

> Any form of behaviour that results in a person attaining or maintaining proximity to some other closely defined individual who is conceived as better able to cope with the world. (Bowlby, 1988, pp. 26–27)

From an evolutionary perspective, its most obvious function was the protection of human and other mammalian infants. A complementary form of attachment behaviour has also evolved in the infants' parents.

As these recollections whizzed through my mind, I realised that elephants, like humans, have a very long childhood, during which time they are also totally dependent on their mothers and aunties. I felt that our little elephant suffered the same fate as the babies who died in the war-time nurseries. He had managed to survive the loss of his original mother by *attaching* himself to Gillian who provided him with the sensitive loving care that he needed. Her loss was too much for him and precipitated his end.

Well before the concept of PTSD had been developed, Erich Lindemann defined trauma as the "sudden uncontrollable disruption of our affiliative bonds" (1944). The term "affiliative" refers to our need to be with others: I felt that this is what our little elephant suffered from, as did the infants in the nurseries during the war. This definition made a lot of sense in our work in the TSS.

Following my phone conversation with Charles Siebert, I was invited to join a *National Geographic* team making a film aimed at exploring the causes of elephants' destructive behaviour in Africa. This experience was to confirm my view, also held by those who work with these animals, that elephants can suffer from the effects of trauma in a very similar way as humans do (Sheldrick, Moss, Bradshaw, & Schore, 2005).

The film was made because of the increasing levels of abnormally violent elephant behaviour that had been reported in Africa and Asia, leading to the deaths of hundreds of people. This was taking place in parallel with a marked decline in the elephant population from 10 million in early 1913 to around 415,000 in 2015.

The film begins in Pilanesberg National Park in South Africa, set up in the early 1990s as a safe haven for wildlife and tourism. It is 1996; the manager of the park, Gus van Dyk, is very worried because forty-nine of his white rhinos have been killed. Poachers are clearly not responsible as their bodies have all been found with their valuable horns intact. We see that the carcasses have large gaping wounds in their flanks.

Elephants still had the reputation of being peaceful giants who were very rarely violent; this is probably why it took quite some time for Van Dyk to work out that the killers were, in fact, the young male elephants who were living in the park.

However, they could behave very aggressively when in musth (during the period of musth, male elephants announce a state of heightened aggression and intention to fight with glandular secretions and by urine-marking and vocalising), as I discovered as a young teenager.

One day, when we were driving through the bush, exploring the Murchison Falls Park in Uganda, a huge male elephant suddenly stepped in front of our campervan. He raised his trunk and emitting vigorous high-pitched trumpeting sounds, his huge ears flapping, he charged. It seemed to me that in a few seconds he would be upon us!

Fearing the worst, I tucked myself in the very narrow cupboard next to my seat. Fortunately, we had a skilled and experienced driver who was used to these male elephantine manifestations so that when I emerged, feeling rather sheepish, the terrifying animal had disappeared.

What was happening in Pilanesberg, however, was grotesque because the elephants were not only killing but also raping the white rhinos. This had never been known to happen before. The predictable question in everyone's mind was: why were these young males behaving in such a destructive manner? The answer was to be found, as it is with violent human delinquents, in their early-life experiences.

Ten years before these young male elephants started their killing rampage, they had been born to female elephants roaming in the Kruger Park in South Africa. This happened to be at a time when there were too many elephants and a quick solution had to be found to prevent the park's ecosystem from being destroyed.

Coincidentally, several farmers in the interior were turning their land into game parks to attract tourists. They naturally wanted elephants, but the adult animals were considered much too heavy to be transported over long distances. So, instead, the plan was to cull the females with young calves and to transfer their calves to new locations where they were be left to fend for themselves.

The film takes us through the scene that these young elephants must have experienced: the sound of shots and the sight of their huge mothers' bodies collapsing before them. What it did not show was even more gruesome as the distressed calves were then tied to the legs of their dead mothers so that they could not escape. Instead, they had to witness men chopping the carcasses into meat for the local market.

We will never know if these very young elephants retained actual memories of these terrifying scenes, but our work with survivors of trauma shows only too clearly how deep and long-lasting their effects are. My colleague, Bessel van der Kolk, who introduced me to this work put it so clearly:

> We have learned that trauma is not just an event that took place sometime in the past: it is also the imprint left by that experience on mind, brain and body. This imprint has ongoing consequences for how the human organism manages to survive the present. (Van der Kolk, 2014, p. 21)

The affected elephants in Pilanesberg, and increasingly elsewhere, show evidence of PTSD-like behaviour, such as an abnormal startle response indicating a high state of arousal, unpredictable aggression, and antisocial behaviour, much like their human counterparts with similarly traumatic backgrounds. We also know that infant elephants being treated in Carol Sheldrick's elephant orphanage in Kenya suffer from terrifying nightmares at night, no doubt reliving the horrific experiences of loss they suffered before their admission. This is a cardinal symptom of PTSD in humans and is one of many intrusive symptoms whereby emotions, sensations, and events from the past are experienced again and again in the present.

In the orphanage, one of many African keepers devoted to healing these calves spends the night with his charge and acts as a "surrogate matriarch", comforting and soothing the little animal back to sleep when it wakes up in a state of agitation and terror (Bradshaw, 2005; Sheldrick Wildlife Trust, 2021).

The normal life of elephants and the web of attachment

To better understand the effects of these early traumas and losses suffered by the young elephants in Pilanesberg National Park, let us have a look at the lives of elephants in an environment that is relatively undisturbed by destructive human activities. This is an environment that hardly exists now, the setting in which the elephant became the animal that it is now through natural selection over thousands of years. These one-time gentle giants used to play an important role in African communities and were attributed "with superintelligence and almost human feelings for its companions" (Moss, 1992).

They normally live into their seventies and are highly socialised, living most of the time as a close community. The females form a herd of mothers, aunties, and older experienced females, moving through the bush, feeding and attending to their calves under the leadership of their matriarch who makes most of the decisions. By the waterside, they drink and play amongst themselves, wallow in the mud, and spray each other. The elephant calf is constantly being touched, caressed, and helped to keep up with the herd. It is gently pushed up steep banks and, when in trouble, its mother and other females come to the rescue. Calves are so closely attached to their mothers that they rarely stray further than three metres away before the age of eight. The attachment bond between the mother and her calf is very deep. If it is ill, the mother will not leave her calf and she will do everything she can to nurse it back to health. Should the mother die, it will be raised by the aunties and grandmothers.

Moss, who spent many years studying elephants describes what happened to a calf named Ely who was born crippled with poorly articulated carpal joints. The herd stayed with him, helping him and caring for him. She goes on to describe Ely and two members of the herd:

> As the two elder elephants walked, they continually turned to look back at the calf that was shuffling along behind. Every few feet they stopped and waited for him to catch up before moving on. The progress was very slow, but they showed no impatience. It was a poignant sight and highlighted the incredible caring nature of these non-human animals. (Moss, 1992, p. 72)

Months later, Ely became capable of walking unassisted. Their loving care paid off. The calf's attachment interactions with its mother, aunties, and grandmothers is the first stage of socialisation (Bowlby, 1969). It enables its emotional and hormonal systems to become attuned to that of its elders and other calves. Simultaneously, its brain begins to absorb the complex social culture and communication system of the elephant group in which it grows up.

From about eight years onward, the calves' adolescence or second phase of socialisation sets in, during which puberty and sexual maturity take place. The young females join the older female network where they learn how to assist in deliveries and help with the raising of calves as well as gaining knowledge of the local area. If there are no older females, as happened in Pilanesberg Park, their absence at this stage of the young elephants' development can lead to sexual reproduction at a much earlier age, as well as maternal neglect and high levels of stress.

At the same stage, the young males are seen to leave their original family to participate in older all-male groups under the influence of mature adult males. Through these new relationships, they learn how to navigate the complex interactions that take place between each other: this involves further regulation of their emotional and hormonal systems so as to develop an appropriate way of behaving in the herd as they become adults. It is also a time when these young ones meet other males of a similar age with whom they can spar and thereby establish themselves in the social hierarchy. They travel with the older males, learning where to forage and find water (Bradshaw & Schore, 2007). Elephant survival is strongly affected by access to the social and ecological knowledge that older elephants hold: where to go, what to eat, how to avoid danger.

The Pilanesberg calves who suffered from the effects of not having their time with the adult mature males during their adolescence appeared more affected than the females who were also deprived of the support of older mature females. It has been suggested that developmental disruptions in mammals may be more pronounced in males than females because their brain development is slower (Schore, 1994).

The adult male elephants differ from most other mammals by not competing over territory. Throughout the year, they alternate moving together or apart, joining the herd of females from time to time.

It is now well documented that elephants have a complex communication system: "two or more elephants can rely on and utilize a myriad combination of trunk waving, positioning of head and bodies, tail and feet, and vocalizations" (Bradshaw, 2004).

African elephants have also been found to use subsonic patterns, well below the range of the human ear, to communicate over long distances, which they use to broadcast the death of a member of the herd or to announce a sudden change (Payne, 1998).

The importance of intimate contact and group bonding amongst elephants cannot be overemphasised and its importance becomes very apparent when they experience a death in their community. Mothers have often been seen standing for days close to the body of their calf, often caressing and touching it as if trying to bring it back to life or saying goodbye.

The death of a matriarch is particularly difficult for elephants as their entire community is affected. The death of one called Emily is described by Cynthia Moss (1992, p. 30). The group participated in several "mourning rituals" around her body and then around her bones over months and years, every time they visited her remains:

> The animals stopped and reached their trunks out. They stepped closer and very gently began
> to touch her remains with the tips of their trunks, first light taps, smelling and feeling, then

strokes around and along the longer bones … Emily's daughter and granddaughter pushed through and began to examine the bones. And soon after, another daughter arrived with her two daughters. All elephants were quiet now and there was a palpable tension among them. One daughter concentrated on Emily's skull, caressing the smooth cranium and slipping her trunk into the hollows in the skull. The other was feeling the lower jaw running her trunk along the teeth—the area used in greeting when elephants place their trunks in each other's mouth. The younger animals were picking up the smaller bones and placing them in their mouths before dropping them again. (Moss, 1992, p. 61)

Mourning seems to be intrinsic to the natural equilibrium of the elephant community, as I found out when I read that a group of elephants in an American zoo suddenly became aggressive and difficult following the death of one of their members. The reason for their disturbed behaviour was found to be due to the fact that the body had been removed before they could mourn its loss. "When the skull of the deceased was brought back to the elephant group, the elephants immediately gathered around it and began the ritual of touching and caressing as described by Moss. After this, they resumed their previous 'normal behaviour'" (Bradshaw, 2004).

Do we need to mourn as much as elephants do, I ask myself, as we face a tidal wave of socially unmourned deaths from Covid-19? The mourning ritual used to be part of the social fabric of Britain until the First World War, when, faced with the loss of 750,000 British young men, leaving behind them as many as 248,000 widows and 381,000 children, patriotic stoicism was encouraged, and pre-war funerals and mourning customs were abandoned. The psychological need for the British "stiff upper lip" and the more material need for civilian employment both mitigated against such "morbid practices". This attitude persisted into the Second World War, and to this day (Zulueta, 2006a, p. 56). Could we be paying the price, I wonder, as I look at the very high levels of depression and anxiety so many are now suffering from?

The healing power of attachment

We can now see what an abnormal life the young Pilanesberg elephants had been through, having suffered the terror of losing their mothers and the resulting premature weaning and neglect they had to endure as calves when they did not have any mature female to care for them. We do know that the company of other siblings and young ones can provide some form of attachment that probably enabled these calves to survive.

Anna Freud and Sophie Dann provide a very moving account of how important such peer attachment can be even for very small children. They studied six three-year-old German-Jewish orphans who were rescued from the concentration camps in 1945. They spent a year being rehabilitated in the UK before being sent to the United States to be fostered. This took place in a country house where they were looked after by nurses trained in the Hampstead War Nurseries (Freud & Dann, 1951). Four of these children had lost their mother at birth, one boy lost his before the age of twelve months, and another boy at an unspecified date.

They had always lived in a group setting and had formed very close attachments to one another. Their caregivers noticed that right from the beginning these children would not form any attachments with adults:

> The children's positive feelings were centered exclusively on their own group. It was evident they cared greatly for each other and not for anybody or anything else. They had no other wish than to be together and became upset when separated from each other even for short moments … The children's unusual dependence on each other was borne out further by the almost complete absence of jealousy, rivalry and competition, such as normally develops between brothers and sisters or in a group of contemporaries who come from normal families … They were extremely considerate of each other's feelings. (Freud & Dann, 1951, pp. 131, 133–134)

They shared everything with each other. On walks they were concerned for each other's safety in the traffic. When playing, they assisted each other and admired each other's productions. At mealtime, handing food to their neighbour was more important than feeding themselves. There was no sign of envy. "Behaviour like this was the rule and not the exception" (ibid., p. 34).

It appears that the children safeguarded their relationships by expressing their anger against the adult staff. The authors of the study make the point that in English society, the child's relations to his/her brothers or sisters is subordinated to his/her relationship to his/her parents so that their mutual relations are often marked by jealousy, envy, and competition.

The way these orphans behaved towards each other shows that such negative behaviour is not inherited. It is the result of a particular form of upbringing. Strangely enough, it also shows what very small children left to themselves can survive even if surrounded by a culture of destruction such as the one in which they lived in the concentration camps. By attending strictly to their own need for a caring attachment and rejecting the intervention of grown-ups (except for accepting food and water) they survived as three-year-olds. However, would they have maintained this kind of social behaviour into adolescence?

The staff looking after them were very surprised by their cooperative behaviour as there was a belief among professionals at the time that every disturbance of the mother–child relationship was always pathogenic (ibid., p. 168). Freud and Dann point out that these six children "were neither deficient, delinquent, nor psychotic". Not only did they master many of their anxieties, but they also developed "social attitudes" and were even able to learn a new language—English—despite all the upheavals they had endured during their short lives. After a year's rehabilitation in 1946, they were sent to the United States to be fostered.

Returning to our orphaned elephants in the Pilanesberg National Park, we can see how the attachments they formed with one another provided them with enough support to survive. What was now missing were the mature older elephants to deal with the male youngsters' uncontrolled sexual and aggressive behaviour in their teenage years.

This is probably what was going through Van Dyck's mind as he realised that he would lose all his rhinos if he did not shoot their killers. By this stage, however, he had found that all these young male elephants were in musth, and that this was happening many years too early and far too frequently. Also, by measuring the testosterone levels in their dung he had found that they were much higher than normal, which explained the volume of secretions streaming from their temporal glands and their hypersexual behaviour. This could perhaps account for why they tried to mount the young female elephants who rejected them, before they started raping the rhinos.

Van Dyck was very reluctant to kill these young elephants, so he decided to introduce two older bull elephants into the park. He felt that it was a risk worth taking. We see in the film how these two massive animals, weighing nearly eight tonnes each, had to be adequately sedated to be safely transported in huge lorries. They survived the journey and, after emerging from their trucks, we witness them meeting the young "delinquent" elephants. It does not take long for the elders to assert their senior position and, as they do so, the young ones' behaviour calms down. Over a short period of time, Van Dyck reports that their testosterone levels are coming down and that the once extended musth is suppressed.

But, best of all is the delight on the park manager's face as he announces that there are no more dead rhinos! Their contribution was enough in this case to stop the killings and the abnormally early musth cycles (Bradshaw, 2015). A similar result was apparently achieved in another game park, but this approach was not always so successful (Slotow & Van Dyck, 2001; Bradshaw & Schore, 2007).

What does this surprisingly positive outcome mean for both elephants and humans?

Elephants, like us, are born to attach to their mother and other parental figures, not only for protection but also to ensure that they develop into adults that fit in with the complex social dynamics of the herd.

As I suggested earlier, these attachments between infants and their mothers and other caregivers have many attributes which will become apparent in the next few chapters. We have learnt that it is through the attachment interactions that take place between infants and their parents that their emotions and behaviour are moulded to adjust to the social life of their elephant community.

This complex network of attachments could be defined as a "living web" that connects each member of the herd to every other member via their different intimate emotional interactions and levels of communications. It is a source of life energy, comfort, "joy", and "affection" that elephants share with each other.

Cynthia Moss describes the meeting of two related groups of elephants, one led by an old female she had named Teresia, and the other led by a younger female called Slit Ear. They have been calling each other for some time and have begun to run as they get closer and closer.

> Suddenly ahead of them was a group of elephants running out of the trees and coming straight for them. Teresia stopped for a moment in alarm, then recognized Slit Ear, and both groups ran, rumbling, screaming and trumpeting toward each other. The younger animals had moved ahead of Teresia but when the groups came together, Slit Ear ignored the others

and pushed through to reach Teresia and greet her. Both elephants raised their heads up into the air and clicked their tusks together, wound their trunks around each other's whilst rumbling loudly, and holding and flapping their ears in the greeting posture. They whirled around and leaned and rubbed on one another. Meanwhile all the other members were greeting each other with much spinning, backing, urinating, ear flapping, entwining of trunks, and clicking of tusks. All the elephants were producing so much temporal-gland secretion that it dribbled down along their chins and into their mouths. Above all, the sounds of their greeting rent the air as over and over again they gave forth rich rumbles and piercing trumpets of joy. (Moss, 1988, pp. 124–125)

She stressed that this elephantine joy plays a very important part in their whole social system, which she points out is very complex: "Both male and female elephants' relationships radiate well beyond the family group through a multi-tiered network of relationships encompassing the whole population."

The close bonds between individuals are constantly being reinforced by tactile interactions and vocal communication. Family members often make physical contact, rubbing one another, touching each other with their trunks, leaning against each other when resting. The younger animals are often playing, and the older ones spend a lot of time taking care of the younger calves. In this way, bonds between different age groups develop early on. The best indicator of the strength of the bonds between elephants is the greeting ceremony.

I am well aware that, although elephantine joy resembles human joy, their experience is somewhat different from ours, especially as we don't own a trunk! However, we do have arms and humans can express their loving joy in many different ways, some a lot more expressively perhaps than the rather muted English hug.

It is perhaps not surprising that, as we share so many of the emotions displayed by the elephants, their attitude to death is also strangely reminiscent of ours, as we saw earlier on. Whilst being a source of strength, and joy, the living web of attachments that connects all members to each other is also a source of sadness, as death leads to the loss of a valued and loved member of the community.

Elephants' attachment to one another can be so deep that it does appear to extend beyond the end of life. For instance, the more important the member of the herd, the more important the ritual. By touching the bones and remains of their lost companion, they may well remember their times together and thereby acknowledge their loss.

Moss concludes: "The network of relationships is the fiber that makes elephant society. These relationships range from the strongest bond of all, that of the mother and infant, to mere acquaintanceship between animals whose ranges rarely overlap" (Moss, 1988, p. 125).

This network is also their source of strength and resilience in stressful times.

For humans too, our attachment relationships have a similar lifegiving function but can also become a source of vulnerability in traumatic circumstances, as we have seen with the elephants.

The destructive power of trauma for elephants and humans

Unfortunately, we are currently witnessing the destruction of the elephant's way of life in Africa and in Asia. This is taking place through culling, hunting, poaching, and the encroachment of human habitations and farming on the land the elephant herds once used to migrate upon.

The plight of the young calves in South Africa is but one example of the many difficulties elephants are now facing. In another park, 90 per cent of male deaths were caused by other male elephants, compared to 6 per cent in stable communities.

In many parts of Africa and Southeast Asia, elephants deprived of their natural environment have been striking out against villages, crops, vehicles, and humans. In some areas, as a result of widespread trauma in these reduced herds, the mourning rituals, so closely linked to their attachments to each other, are also disappearing (Shannon et al., 2013).

In these shrunken and transformed landscapes, the elephants' complex social attachment system is being destroyed: the absence of mature maternal care results in immature females becoming mothers who are often unable to give their calves the "good enough" maternal care that they will need to live in equilibrium with the rest of the herd.

The similarity between elephants and the humans that live near them is a subject close to Dr Lawino Abe's heart as I found out when we were both involved in the making of the film taking place in Pilanesberg National Park. An animal ethologist and wildlife-management consultant living in London, she was born and grew up in the Acholi community of Northern Uganda, where her father was a highly respected teacher and a conservationist working in the parks. During her childhood, her family was forced to flee from Uganda on two occasions because of the violent attacks on the Acholi community carried out first by Idi Amin in the 1960s, and then during the subsequent twenty-year civil war that developed between the government's National Resistance Army (NRA) and the rebel Lord's Resistance Army (LRA) in Northern Uganda. Her family was forced to flee when her parents' home was raided and property on their farm was burnt down by the NRA.

Despite these traumatic moves and all that goes with refugee life, she joined Uganda's Makerere University as an undergraduate in 1982 and later obtained her doctorate from Cambridge University in 1994. It was when she was studying in Uganda that Abe chose to study the elephants in the Queen Elizabeth Park. When she first arrived, there were fewer than 150 elephants left from a population of nearly 4,000. Most of the killings had taken place during the war with Tanzania that led to Amin's overthrow. The soldiers of both armies wanted as much lucrative ivory as they could obtain.

In her interview with Charles Siebert, she said: "[T]his was war. They'd just throw hand grenades at the elephants, bringing whole families down and then cutting out the ivory. I call that mass destruction" (Siebert, 2006). She then described how the last survivors of the park

> never left one another's side. They kept in a tight bunch, moving as one. Only one elderly female remained, and Abe estimated her age to be at least 62. It was this matriarch who first

gathered the survivors together from their various hideouts on the park's forested fringes and then led them back out as one group into the open savanna. Until her death in the early 90's, the old female held the group together, the population all the while slowly beginning to rebound. (ibid., 2006)

Lawino Abe named the park's matriarchal saviour Lady Irene, after her own mother whom she describes as an Acholi matriarch. "'It took that core group of survivors in the park about five or six years … before I started seeing whole new family units emerge and begin to split off and go their own way'" (Siebert, 2006).

It was when working in the Queen Elizabeth Park that Abe began to realise that there was an "absolute coincidence" between what had happened to the elephants she was studying and what had happened among the Acholi. This became the subject of her thesis, where she details the parallels she saw between the plight of the orphaned male elephants and the young Acholi children (Abe, 1994).

These youngsters had survived Amin's attacks and the prolonged civil war between the NRA and the LRA. During that time, 90 per cent of the inhabitants were displaced into concentration camps supposedly "for their own protection", where they suffered from disease and the effects of the endless violence inflicted upon them. Many died as a result. Their elders, who "held" the culture of the group, were systematically killed. All the surviving children who were not kidnapped by the LRA to fight for them, have grown up without parents. Although the camps were finally disbanded in 2012, this huge and lengthy displacement has destroyed the cultural foundations of Acholi society: farming, education, and family and community relations have been broken, leaving the proud and previously self-sufficient Acholi dependent on the UN World Food Programme.

As Abe told Charles Siebert:

> They don't go to school. They have no schools, no hospitals. No infrastructure. They form these roaming, violent, destructive bands. It's the same thing that happens with the elephants. Just like the male war orphaned calves, they are wild, completely lost. (Siebert, 2006)

It so happened that one of these young men was being treated in the TSS where I worked. This young Acholi was an orphan who had lost all the members of his family except for two older brothers. One of these brothers had been serving in the Ugandan army when his unit captured the rebel battalion of the LRA in which his younger brother was forced to fight. He was able to rescue his younger sibling and they eventually made their way to London. The younger brother was in his second year of therapy for the terrible experiences he had been through, and was gradually gaining a sense of belonging through the shared traditions and language of his people living in London.

It is interesting that one of the big issues these two brothers were struggling with at the time was how to deal with the death in London of one of their relatives. The Acholi tradition required

THE ELEPHANT IN THE ROOM   13

them and their relative's body to be flown back to the land where he came from; however, the financial cost of this was far too high for the two young men. For the Acholi, it is very important to be buried in their own land. Like the elephants and many human communities across the world, mourning rituals needed to be respected for the well-being of the community. Fortunately, technology came to the rescue of the ritual as the body was flown to the Acholi tribal lands and the two brothers were able to follow the funeral online.

"The elephant in the room"

The reader may well wonder what elephants have to do with *our* lives?

By choosing to share aspects of elephant community life in their natural environment, I hope to illustrate the importance of attachment relationships from the moment we are born to the moment we die. The greatest care is given to the little calf by its female caregivers so that it has the greatest possibility of developing into an elephant which can fulfil its needs by cooperating with the other members of its community. During adolescence, as sexual maturity begins, more experienced adult females and males take over and guide the young elephants in developing their future roles as adult females and males and how to live in equilibrium, within and beyond the herd.

By sharing their experience, we have an idea of what attachment bonds—the subject of this book—are all about in mammals like us. These relational experiences are involved in the nurturing of the young, the upbringing of the "teenagers", the effects of separation, of reunion, of loss, death, and the capacity to achieve an emotional and physical equilibrium when their internal world is thrown "out of sync" due to neglect or loss, as we saw with the teenage calves once they were in the company of the older adult males.

What these social animals highlight is the importance of providing a safe and caring community environment in the earliest years of life, built through a living network of specialised relationships, that enables infants to take up their adult role in the life of the herd. Without this experience, elephant interaction with one another and with their environment can be severely affected, leading to violence and even death.

Human infants also thrive when they are brought up in a sensitive, interactive, secure, and loving environment with their mothers and "alloparents" or other parental figures, which in many human communities include males. Interactions with siblings and other children are also as important for children's social development as they are for elephant calves, which is partly why so many have been negatively affected by the constraints of Covid-19 lockdowns.

Moving into adolescence, between puberty and adulthood, when the second major reorganisation of the brain takes place, both elephants and humans undergo major hormonal and behavioural changes. The example of the mature male elephants' role may be useful in reminding parents that they are still very much needed during this phase of development when their children's brains can be rewired for a better future by forming positive and creative relationships. What are the "magic" ingredients provided by these close bonds between these animals and between humans which seem to be so important in their early years?

This is the very question that came up in Bowlby's mind when he witnessed the infants separated from their mothers in the war-time nurseries becoming ill or dying (Ainsworth & Bowlby, 1954). He was made even more aware of the importance of the attachment bond between mothers and their children when he published in 1944 a paper entitled: "Forty-four juvenile thieves: Their characters and home-life". He noted how, over several years, over half of the people convicted for theft were under the age of twenty-one, and the thirteen-year-old teenage group appeared most frequently in court. His main interest was to find out more about the importance of the mother–child relationship in determining a child's emotional and social development.

His discussions with many of the mothers revealed strong feelings of dislike and rejection towards their children. It was also discovered that most of the children had spent a lot of time away from home. He found that a large proportion of children who steal persistently were of the "Affectionless character", resulting from long separations from mother or foster mother in childhood and other emotional traumas during the first decade of life. In his conclusion, he notes the importance of attending to the early life of children in relation to character development and the need for a better economic and social environment (Bowlby, 1944).

In 1951, when requested by the World Health Organization (WHO) to write a report on the mental health of homeless children in post-war Europe, Bowlby sought the view of many concerned at the time with the effects of maternal separation. One of his conclusions was that to grow up mentally healthy, "the infant and young child should experience a warm, intimate, and continuous relationship with his mother (or permanent mother-substitute) in which both find satisfaction and enjoyment" (Bowlby, 1951, p. 11).

Bretherton (1992) says that later academic summaries often leave out the reference to the "partners' mutual 'enjoyment'. They also neglect Bowlby's emphasis on the role of social networks and economic as well as health factors in the development of well-functioning mother-child relationships" (p. 765). She points out that Bowlby's earlier call to society to provide support for parents was still not being heeded in 1992 and, in my view, it remains so today in the United States and the UK:

> Just as children are absolutely dependent on their parents for sustenance, so in all but the most primitive communities, are parents, especially their mothers, dependent on a greater society for economic provision. If a community values its children, it must cherish its parents. (Bowlby, 1951, p. 84)

I have also been made aware of the fact that the British government, at the time when Bowlby's report was published, not only ignored the need to support parents looking after their children, but used it to justify forcing women to relinquish the jobs that had given them new experiences and freedoms when the men were at war, and to return to their domestic chores. This is one reason why women of that generation and many feminists are critical of Bowlby.

However, his interest in the nature of relationships between parents and children has led to an extraordinary amount of research on the nature of our attachment relations which, if applied to our communities, could lead to a marked improvement both in the nature of our relationships with our children, and towards each other.

Indeed, where there is a will, there is a way! For example, Finland is "the only country in the developed world where fathers spend more time with school-aged children than mothers, to the tune of eight minutes a day" (*Guardian*, 2017).

According to an OECD Global Gender Gap report for 2023 (OECD, 2023), Finland is the second most equal country in the world after Iceland. *The Economist* claims that it is also the third best country in which to be a working mother. The reason for all these impressive achievements is that rather than focus on gender equality, their public policy focuses on what is good for children and on the right for a child to spend time with both parents. This goes hand in hand with the view that fathers play a crucial role in child development: so, in Finland, they receive nine weeks paternity leave during which time they are paid 70 per cent of their salary. Such a way of life is possible, but it requires different priorities from those under which we live in most Western countries.

Many authors are highlighting the destructive effects of our current system, in relation to both our mental health and our physical health, particularly in relation to children's first years of life. The resulting high levels of abuse and neglect in so many families are creating generations of individuals who suffer from the effects of addiction, violence, mental and physical illnesses, and premature death which could be avoided.

Conclusion

What we are discovering is that the human infant is born so early that it is the most vulnerable of primate infants: this gives humans the advantage of being very adaptable in different environmental and social contexts. However, being so totally dependent on mother and other caregivers for its development requires making sure that human babies are brought up in a safe environment with attuned and loving caregivers.

If neglected or abused, the infant brain develops an alternative developmental mode referred to as the *traumatic attachment* leading to different ways of perceiving, feeling, and behaving. In the field of adult mental health, these people suffer from the effects of addiction, unresolved grief, domestic and other forms of violence, borderline personality disorder (BPD), developmental or complex trauma, and other "disorders".

Thanks to the use of a recently developed procedure—we have named it the Traumatic Attachment Induction Procedure (TAIP), derived from the work of Professor Bob Johnson—I and my co-authors, together with a few of our patients and clients, will share our therapeutic experience in gaining access to the hitherto unconscious or implicit *traumatic attachment* and its internal working models (IWMs).

This is an account of these different journeys with our clients or patients from a past of chronic suffering to the discovery of their normal "selves" with the freedom to realise their long-hidden potential, free from addiction or other soul-destroying ways of life. Our work has made us aware of the extraordinary negative impact the *traumatic attachment* has had and continues to have in the world, a developmental outcome that John Bowlby predicted, with his remarkable prescience, would have consequences that are "vital to the survival of the species".

CHAPTER 2

Born to love and cooperate

Strange as it may seem, in our individualistic and competitive Western world, humans, like elephants, are born to attach to others, to love, to be loved, and to belong to a community. We now know that it is humanity's amazing ability to cooperate in large numbers that led to its dominant position in the world. Many scientists, like the biologist Theodosius Dobzhansky, have stressed the importance of mammals' capacity to connect as the reason for their evolutionary success, not their physical strength. He challenged the popular belief in the survival of the fittest by remarking that "the fittest may also be the gentlest, because survival often requires mutual help and cooperation" (Dobzhansky, 1962). Such a point of view may well lead us to question its validity when we find our species facing its own self-inflicted destruction due to a failure to cooperate in the face of the dangerous social and environmental crises we are confronted with.

Part of the answer to this paradox may lie in what happens to humans in the first years of life when faced with the terror of losing the mother on whom they totally depend. This may not be as outlandish an idea as it first appears. When, in 1993, I wrote my book *From Pain to Violence*, on the origins of human violence, it became very clear to me that the origin of human violent behaviour arises from damage to our attachment system, particularly when exposed to adverse early experiences in infancy. My hypothesis was supported by John Bowlby whom I met over tea by the fire in his sitting room. As I left, he said, "Please don't be too harsh in relation to the army. I owe some of my best friendships to the war." This made me smile as he was not the first English person to praise the war for the warm social interactions that took place during that time. Indeed, when I first arrived in the UK at the age of eighteen to study biology at the University of East Anglia, the landladies in my university accommodation would say,

"It is such a shame you were not here during the war; that is when we were at our best!" I must confess that at the time I was shocked and thought this was very strange, but it makes sense now as it was a time when the powerful English class divisions no longer mattered, and people were brought together through the war effort; it was a time of great camaraderie and of mutual support which may have made it possible to create the NHS in 1948.

It is in this context that Bowlby began to carry out his work on child and maternal health care as a director of child and family health department at the Tavistock Clinic in London. Sadly, for me, by the time my book was published, John Bowlby had died, but his work and his influence continues to inspire me and so many others, as will become evident in the following pages.

My other source of inspiration comes from the multiplicity of people I have met as patients during my forty years of working in the NHS, initially as a trainee and then as a consultant psychiatrist in psychotherapy. I had the privilege of listening to so many men and women sharing with me how they suffered, directly or indirectly, from the terrible effects of early childhood terror. However, I soon found psychiatry rather limited in its approach since it did not accept, at the time, that people's symptoms could be the result of what they had experienced or were experiencing in their lives. Their disorders were usually believed to be genetically induced, and they were given whatever diagnosis best fitted their symptoms and behaviour. As for their treatment, it was usually limited to taking the latest advertised medication, although, in some cases, group therapy and occupational therapy on the wards were also provided.

This was not what I expected as a medical student, following my three-week introduction to psychiatry. I was offered an elective period in the Emergency Clinic of the Maudsley Hospital in South London which, in those days, took place in the Outpatient Department. (It is now in the bowels of the hospital with metal bars and alarm systems to protect the staff because of the increasing levels of violence in the community.)

The Emergency Clinic was run at that time by a charming Irish consultant psychiatrist called Dr Anthony Clare, who was soon to become famous with his TV series on the BBC, *In the Psychiatrist's Chair* (Clare, 1992). In his obituary, following his premature death, he was described as the "the most brilliant and multi-talented psychiatrist of his generation … who did more than anyone else to improve the public understanding of psychiatry in Britain and Ireland" (Murray, 2007). I was, of course, unaware of his reputation, but what he said to me as I was about to see my first patient is etched in my mind: "Forget everything you have read and just listen to your patient." This advice made a lot of sense, and I have tried to follow it throughout my career, especially during my training on "Ward 1".

This was a very unusual ward for a psychiatric hospital, because it was run by a remarkable psychoanalyst called Dr Murray Jackson. His psychoanalytic approach opened my eyes to different ways of understanding what psychotic patients were saying and doing. He had a hypnotic way of speaking to these men and women which made the hairs on the back of my neck stand up as I listened to him. He could actually talk schizophrenic patients out of their catatonic fixed immobility and make sense of their behaviour. They loved him because they felt understood. This experience led me to specialise in psychotherapy, much to Dr Clare's chagrin as he had little time for the psychoanalysts in the hospital. He was right, as it turned out later, but I told him that it gave me the time to listen to my patients with an open mind and to be more myself, by sharing with them my thoughts, therapeutic approaches, and ideas which I hoped would be more meaningful for them than simply being prescribed medication.

Of course, it was much more demanding than I realised, and I certainly made mistakes, but at least I could apologise if I did! It is crucial to acknowledge that, although medication is often overused in psychiatry, it has an important role to play when people are too depressed to talk or are in a state of psychotic terror and it often enabled a psychotherapeutic dialogue to take place which otherwise would have been impossible.

It is through these repeated encounters with the reality of so many people's distressing and often terrifying experiences that I became aware of how vulnerable humans can be during their early lives. I also realised how many never had the dedicated family love and community support that is so necessary for humans to be able to communicate and interact with others in meaningful ways.

Perhaps, I was also more influenced than I realised by my experience as a four- to seven-year-old girl in the 1950s, when we moved to Sarawak, a British Crown Colony in north Borneo. My father was a malaria doctor working for the WHO, whose job it was to eradicate the offending mosquitoes and treat the sick of the Dayak tribes located in the longhouses in the interior of the island.

My sister and I were the only "white" children living in a small community of English men and women next to a Chinese and a Malay Kampong or village, surrounded by dense tropical jungle. The big, muddy-brown Baram River was our only connection with the outside world. The Dayaks lived upstream in longhouses made of wood and bamboo on stilts, high above the muddy banks of the river. Each longhouse contained many families living side by side and sharing the communal terrace outside their doors where they gathered to work, prepare food, look after their children, and gossip. The walls of the longhouse we regularly visited were beautifully decorated in red, yellow, white, and black, representing a circular medley of dragons, birds, fish, and plants. The Dayaks loved celebrating, so my father's arrival was always a pretext for a great party with dancing, singing, and drinking. They made a great fuss of us children as were the first white children they had ever seen. We would stay there a few nights while my father carried out his work and my mother took care of my baby sister.

I was looked after by these kind people who soon made me feel safe and at ease because the Dayaks were devoted to their children and spent most of their time with them. A Dayak child is never alone; day and night, they are in the care of mother, father, grandparents, and other relatives, including older siblings. The children shared community events and celebrations and gradually learnt to prepare meals, plant and harvest, look after others, swim safely in the crocodile infested rivers, and acquire hunting and fishing skills.

Men and women may have different social roles, but one sex did not dominate the other. When the chief in the longhouse we regularly visited died, his daughter took over his role. These indigenous tribes are rightly described as intensely community-driven people who value family and kinship as well as their deep spiritual connection with nature. I imagine that our ancestors of long ago may have lived in rather similar communities, a life for which our attachment system seems well prepared.

The Dayak men used to be head-hunters but Rajah Brooke (Sir James Brooke, a British soldier and adventurer who founded and ruled the Raj of Sarawak from 1841) made a deal with them to abandon head-hunting so as to restore peace amongst the tribes. He channelled their competitive spirits into boat-racing regattas down their foaming rock-studded rivers; their colourful dragon painted canoes were a wonderful sight to see.

Although I had been brought up speaking Spanish, when we arrived in Borneo, having fled the civil war in Colombia, I was soon speaking Malay, which was the *lingua franca*. During those few years, I think that I must have absorbed quite a lot of their way of life and thinking which differs so much from what I was to learn later during my time in "civilised" Europe. This early influence has become apparent to me from time to time. Perhaps it has been reflected in my interest in the nature of the magical ingredients within the attachments that bind us and our fellow mammals to each other and which can also tear us apart.

The importance of primate mothers and the development of the traumatic attachment

Bowlby turned to ethology, the science of animal behaviour, for a better understanding of the mother–infant attachment behaviour and met with Harry Harlow in 1958. This American psychologist was carrying out experiments on infant rhesus monkeys separated from their mothers. Paradoxically, studying attachment involves separation, and Harlow's experiments would not have received ethical approval today because of the suffering they caused to their subjects. However, at least the monkeys' painful experiences have taught us how damaging separation from mothers can be for primate infants, including humans, and made Harlow one of the most influential psychologists in the United States.

Harlow was a believer in the importance of love, which he defined as "the affectional feelings we have for others", and he was shocked to find out that there was practically no research on this crucial subject. In his book *Learning to Love* (1974), he identified at least five different loves, ranging from maternal love for the child, the child's love for mother, peer love, sexual love, and paternal love, to which we add the child's love for his or her father. For Harlow, "the maternal and infant affectional systems prepare the child for the perplexing problem of peer adjustment by providing him or her with the basic feelings of security and trust".

He strongly believed that "age-mate" (of similar age) experience is fundamental to the development of what he called sexual love. He wrote that in all primates the heterosexual affectional system is hopelessly inept and inadequate unless it has been preceded by "effective peer partnership and age-mate activities" (1974, p. 3). To demonstrate the importance of these different relationships, Harlow took rhesus monkey babies and isolated them from birth. Their cages were lit, and they were regularly fed but did not interact with any other monkeys.

By dividing them up into four groups, he was able to isolate them for differing periods of time for up to a year (Harlow & Mears, 1979). He found that the younger and longer they were isolated, the worse the developmental damage. The infants that were isolated for only three months and then placed in a nurturing social environment appeared to behave normally whilst those isolated for twelve months showed a devastating loss of social competence. The monkeys isolated for the first six months developed an abnormal pattern of behaviours such as sucking their digits or, in males, sucking their penises. This behaviour has been attributed to making up for the absence of the mother's nipple. They would also clasp different parts of their bodies with their hands and feet in the absence of a mother to cling to and rock themselves compulsively, a distressing sight which reminds us of the behaviour of the severely neglected children in the Romanian orphanages between the 1960s and the 1980s.

In another experiment, Harlow and his team provided eight separated infants with two surrogate "mothers", one made of metal that provided milk through an artificial nipple whilst the other was covered with a soft terry towelling material. The metal surrogate that only provided milk stood for "cupboard love": the belief in academic and psychoanalytic circles at that time was that babies would attach to whoever fed them. These infants were studied for 165 days, and Harlow found that all the monkeys spent more time with the cloth mother. The infants would only go to the wire mother when hungry. Once fed, an infant would return to the cloth mother for most of the day. If a frightening object was placed in the cage, the infant took refuge with the cloth mother, which had become its secure base. This surrogate mother was surprisingly effective in calming the youngster's fears: the infant would explore more when "she" was present. If "she" was absent, they simply lay on the floor, semi-paralysed, rocking back and forth, sucking their thumbs (Harlow, Dodsworth, & Harlow, 1965).

These findings support the evolutionary theory of attachment, in that it is the sensitive response and security imparted by the caregiver which is so important for the well-being of the infant, not just the feeding. Harlow and his team carried out various other experiments which highlighted what natural mothers do with their infants, such as rocking them, warming them, training them to communicate with others, playing, and encouraging separation—all of which go towards developing good peer interaction and, later on, sexual relationships.

Subsequent studies by Harlow and Suomi (1971) focused on rhesus monkeys reared in isolation for six months and then tested daily in a social playroom with pairs of socially competent age-mates.

> The "isolates" were found to show less object exploration and would not make social contact, play or show aggressive displays although they were often targets of unprovoked aggression.

However, by the fifth to the eighth month, these monkeys began to play more with the other social isolates and communicate with their threat display more frequently with each other. This meant that they showed some capacity for recovery after six months of isolation.

The females who had reached sexual maturity after total isolation were completely disinterested in mating with sexually eager breeding-stock males. So, they were artificially inseminated and called the "motherless mothers". (ibid., 1535)

Harlow and colleagues describe their behaviour in the most vivid terms. Their reaction to their newborn infants was to either completely ignore them or abuse them,

> by crushing the infant's face to the floor, chewing off the infant's feet and fingers, and, in one case, by putting the infant's head in her mouth and crushing it like an eggshell. Not even in our most devious dreams could we have designed a surrogate as evil as these real monkey mothers. (Harlow, Harlow, & Suomi, 1971, p. 545)

> However, unless the mothers actually killed their infants—and several did—the babies struggled for maternal contact day after day, week after week, month after month. The infants would cling to the mothers' backs, continually attempting to achieve ventral and breast contact despite efforts by the mothers to displace them. To our surprise, maternal brutality and indifference gradually decreased. From the fourth month onwards, the persistent babies that were finally able to obtain physically intimate contact with their mothers were actually punished less and permitted nipple contact more than the offspring of normal mothers. (Harlow & Suomi, 1971, p. 1535)

Since then, many of these "motherless mothers" have had second and even third babies and proved to be adequate or good mothers to their subsequent infants. However, as this improvement only involved maternal behaviour, they needed to be repeatedly artificially inseminated.

The importance to us of this piece of research lies in the way the infants respond to their mother's abuse: rather than escaping in fear, which would have led to their death, by attaching themselves even more to their rejecting parent they had a chance of surviving, and, in this case, their persistence actually altered their mother's behaviour which may well be why this behaviour has been selected throughout evolution since it ensured the infants' survival.

This paradoxical response of infants towards their rejecting mothers can develop in many other mammalian species, including human infants, where it is referred to as the *traumatic attachment*. It turns out to be extremely important in understanding how early developmental experiences can lead to human psychopathology and destructive behaviour. While this may well ensure children's survival, it is often at a great cost to them and their families.

The importance of social support

Having witnessed the therapeutic effect of infants on a few motherless mothers who turned into caring mothers, Suomi, Harlow, and Novak decided to investigate if infant monkeys could act as therapists for the previously separated infants. They chose three-month-old normal infants that had not yet developed the aggressive behaviour seen in older monkeys. When the "isolates" were introduced to these young "therapists", they huddled into a corner. The "therapists" responded by approaching their "clients" and clinging to them. The previously isolated monkeys were soon responding in kind and, as their "therapists" developed their social interactions amongst themselves, their "clients" copied and reciprocated these behaviours (Suomi, Harlow, & Novak, 1974).

By the age of one, both "isolates" and "therapists" were scarcely distinguishable in their social contact and interactive play and their abnormal earlier behaviour had disappeared. The researchers were delighted and concluded that social rehabilitation of monkeys could be attained. However, despite appearances, latent vulnerabilities remained that were exposed when these social "isolates" faced stressful situations or tasks requiring complex social discrimination (Anderson & Mason, 1978).

The results of Harlow's experiments suggest, yet again, that the mother or "primary caregiver's" role was not limited to satisfying their infant's primary drives such as the need for food. She also provided "comfort" and a secure base that enabled the infants to explore surrounding objects and cope with frightening sounds. These findings led Bowlby to propose that human infants have a strong need to form an attachment to a maternal caregiver in order to survive and develop socially appropriate behaviour (1988).

Many other separation studies have been carried out on other primates which are very relevant to our understanding of the importance of the attachment bond between mother and infant. Coe, Wiener, Rosenberg, and Levine (1985, pp. 64–65) studied infant squirrel monkeys' response to even temporary separations from their mother and found high levels of the stress hormone cortisol, indicating how stressful this experience was for this species. The accompanying response of the adrenal glands led, in the long term, to varying degrees of suppression of their immune system which may go some way to explaining the origin of the illnesses and deaths of the human babies in war-time nurseries. Providing the separated infants with social support when separated from their mothers not only reduces their levels of distress but also reduced the levels of suppression of their immune system.

It is interesting to note that bonnet macaque monkeys have a social structure whereby their infants spend a lot more time with other members of the group and the general behaviour of the group members is more permissive and responsive than it is in many other primate species. As a result, when separated from their mothers, the bonnet infants are adopted by the other females in the group and, after a period of searching and protesting, they settle down and show no signs of depression (Kaufman & Rosenblum, 1967). This is an example of how being brought up with multiple caregivers, as happens with many indigenous tribes, can be beneficial for humans too.

On the other hand, the pigtail macaques' mothers are quite possessive of their infants and will ignore or even attack unrelated members of the group. During these aggressive encounters to assert her dominance, the pigtail mother can occasionally injure her young. When separated from their mothers, these infants become severely depressed (ibid.).

The environment in which they live can alter the pigtail monkey's response to her infant. For instance, in a "rich" laboratory environment where toys and interesting objects were provided for the infants to interact with, they responded to their mothers' aggression by keeping their distance, whereas in the "poor" environment they responded by clinging to their mothers (Jenson, Bobbit, & Gordon, 1968). This tendency to cling to their mothers when they are punished is very much part of pigtail infant life and makes them more dependent on their mothers than the bonnet macaques.

The result is that the pigtail macaque's social structure is one of exclusive matrilines based on permanent mother–infant ties whilst the bonnet macaques live in a community with little social differentiation. However, if the bonnet macaques are experimentally deprived of their alternative relationships in early development, then they also end up showing a much stronger depressive response to separation from their mothers.

These various experiments show us how important the biological and social environment can be in both reinforcing or diluting genetic differences between or within primate species because of the adaptability of the attachment system (Plimpton & Rosenblum, 1983).

They also illustrate how different rearing practices clearly play an important role in the attachment behaviour of primates and in their subsequent development.

The fact that we share the same attachment system as our primate cousins means that humans share quite a few similar vulnerabilities when their social context is modified, both culturally and accidentally, as will become apparent in subsequent chapters. Human adaptive flexibility is readily apparent when we look at how different cultures have developed an enormously rich variety of social systems across the planet (Zulueta, 2006a, pp. 238–263).

One important child-rearing custom that comes to mind is how most indigenous tribes never leave their infants alone at night and are often very critical of the Western way of putting our babies to sleep in another room. Having experienced, both as a mother and grandmother, how difficult it can be to enable our little ones to feel safe enough to sleep in their solitary cots, I often wonder if tribal parents aren't onto something that we are missing because of our current way of life.

Paradoxically, could it be that relationship changes within the family system could alter the social structures within which we live? This may have been Bowlby's mission. Born in 1907, he was raised by a nanny in the conventional British fashion of his social class. She was his primary caregiver but left the family when he was four. He later described this as his greatest loss. He was then sent to boarding school at the age of seven where he really missed being with his parents. This background probably contributed to his passionate interest in finding out about the role of parents, and particularly the role of the mother, in the development of the child. Perhaps, by producing the evidence needed for improving the way children were raised, he hoped to change family life for others facing the pain that he endured by losing his nanny and then being sent to boarding school.

By 1969, Bowlby had produced the first volume of his trilogy on attachment. He concluded that it is a motivational system that we share with other mammals. Its biological function is to ensure the care and protection of the young. The relatively long period of infantile dependence and the lack of fixed predetermined action patterns in humans provide our species with the capacity for flexibility and learning which ensures a great adaptability to a wide range of environments.

He viewed the development of infants in terms of pathways wherein change is possible although, he emphasised, the degree and direction of change will depend very much on what took place beforehand. In so doing, Bowlby reminds us that human diversity and success as a species is highly dependent on the quality of an infant's early upbringing in terms of what kind of human behaviour we produce in our different societies.

It is because of his awareness of the importance of the early years in relation to our future behaviour that he stressed the importance of the attachment system:

> a system developed over time to ensure that any threat to the infant's sense of security will translate into the activation of its attachment system in order to elicit a protective caring response from its parents. In this way, the inherent vulnerability of the human infant can be transformed into its opposite, a socially integrated and fulfilled member of the social community in which he or she lives. (Bowlby, 1951)

Biologic regulators

Having defined the importance of the attachment bond, Bowlby ascribed the infants' behaviour following separation from their mothers to the loss of this important bond. Hofer, however, was not convinced that this was the whole story since his research on infant rats separated from their mothers at two months proved that what was taking place was much more complex. He was also very interested in finding out the components of the attachment bond and what it is that makes a maternal separation so stressful for infants.

The psychiatrist Professor Myron Hofer was struck by the similarities between infant–mother separation reactions and bereavement reactions. He emphasised that in adult bereavement there are two forms of disturbance:

1. The acute recurrent waves of distress, which last only minutes.
2. The chronic slowly developing background disturbances seen over weeks and months.

The human infant's grief is similar, except that acute distress precedes the slower chronic changes.

Both the adult and the infant go through a *protest phase* characterised by similar behaviours such as crying, which in infants is referred to as *separation cry*, agitation, aimless activity, and inactivity. Bowlby interpreted this behaviour as attempts to find the missing parent. The body itself undergoes physiological changes in both children and adults such as tearfulness, sighing, and muscular weakness as well as the hormonal and other physiological changes we mentioned in relation to the monkeys separated from their mothers. This acute phase is followed by a chronic phase in humans or a *phase of despair* in infants, during which they look sad and keep to themselves, hardly interacting or playing. They will rock back and forth and put their hands in their mouth and often refuse food. They can become emotionally and behaviourally hyper-responsive or hypo-responsive when interacting with people. The body also undergoes physiological changes: sleep is disturbed, there is often weight loss and cardiovascular changes, as well as muscle weaknesses in both adults and children. The latter also show a reduced body temperature and changes in oxygen consumption.

Hofer and his team of researchers were using rats at the time and were surprised to find that they showed a similar biphasic protest–despair response to maternal separation as well as a number of other unexpected responses. Their study involved providing two-month-old rat pups with different components of their maternal attachment to see what happened following their separation from their mother.

> For example, we found that providing one of the components such as warmth, to a separated pup prevented the slow decline in its general activity level [a response similar to Bowlby's *despair* phase] … but this had no effect on responses in other systems. The pup's cardiac rate continued to fall by 40%, regardless of whether supplemental heat or tactile stimulation was provided. (Hofer, 2006)

However, they then found that the cardiac rate in separated pups could, in fact, be maintained by a continuous infusion of milk to the stomach and the amount of nutrient could be used to regulate the pup's heart rate if the quantities were changed. This result was due to an effect of specific nutrients on receptors in the lining of stomach that are connected to the brain.

> We concluded from these surprising results that warmth provided by mother normally maintained the pup's activity levels and that her milk maintained her pup's heart rate. (Hofer, 2006, p. 86)

They subsequently found that graded levels of tactile stimulation during separation provided graded levels of quieting in the pups. Other maternal regulatory effects were found by Hofer's team and others (Hofer, 1994). He concluded that the chronic phase of grief is the result of an assemblage of different regulatory processes taking place between the mother and infant which are all deactivated by the loss of the mother–infant relationship.

> These *biologic regulators* may constitute an early stage in the development of what we believe to be *psychologic regulators* within early social interactions, as infants get older and species evolve. (Hofer, 1984, p. 187, original emphasis)

Thinking about the implications of these findings for human infants, Hofer hypothesised that similar simple maternal regulators would be found early in the baby's postnatal period, and he stressed that these "regulatory interactions such as touch, warmth and smell may well continue to be important for humans (as well as other animals), in adult life, with implications for human grief" (Hofer, 2006, p. 86).

This proved to be the case for a charming elderly woman whom I met travelling in Italy in the 1960s. The compartments in those days were designed to fit six passengers seated in two opposite rows, which made it easy for people to talk to one another, an excellent way of passing the time in Mediterranean countries. I used to enjoy these journeys, during my teens, because of the lively discussions that always took place. Thoughts and feelings on everything from the Pope to the most recent pasta recipe were openly shared. On one occasion though, death became the subject of conversation. It was at this point that the grey-haired woman all in black spoke up. She was obviously still grieving the loss of her husband. "Do you know what I miss most," she said. "It is the way he kept my feet warm in bed by wrapping his feet round my feet … Now they feel so cold!"

This simple experience touched us all and silence descended in the compartment for a short while. It has stayed with me. She summed up so well what it means to lose someone who has become an intimate part of one's life, taking us back to those early moments in life when a gentle touch or a warm embrace from a parent would restore peace in our troubled young minds.

Not surprisingly, Hofer's next concern was to establish how these early relationships can have such long-lasting effects. Having established that multiple hidden regulators exist within the mother–infant interaction, was it possible that parent–infant interactions could affect the course of the offspring's future development? His team looked at the effect of early weaning in rat pups at different times of their lives and found that several physiological and behavioural systems are altered in their developmental paths and in relation to each other, thereby changing the pups' vulnerability during their life span.

Hofer's work on *biologic* and *psychologic regulators* makes us realise that primate and human interactions have a regulatory function affecting our minds and bodies throughout our lives. Variations in the qualities of mother–infant relationships among humans thus appear to have deep biological roots in the form of their capacity to shape children's psychological and biological responses to their environment—effects that tend to extend into adulthood. This conclusion is particularly pertinent to our interest in the *traumatic attachment* which we have seen enacted by certain monkeys rejected by their mothers (Harlow & Suomi, 1971).

We will be returning to the formation of *psychologic regulators* in the formation of IWMs when looking at early human development.

Relationships as regulators

Reite and Capitanio introduced the idea that attachment behaviour is actually a form of psycho-biological synchronisation, a matching of rhythms in physical or physiological activities that take place between individuals:

> Converging evidence from a number of studies supports the notion that certainly one, if not the major, component of mother–infant bonding is the development of rhythmicity in the infant and the development of synchrony between the mother and the infants rhythms. (1985, p. 239)

Stern describes the process of *attunement* between mother and infant as "affect attunement", a state of mother–infant interplay where the mother mirrors her infant behaviour either directly or by using a different sensory modality. For example, a baby playing with her mother, may jiggle excitedly and the mother may respond by making exciting jiggling sounds which match the child's movement. Stern describes this synchronised behaviour as a matching of inner states between mother and infant, a form of attunement at an emotional level (1985, pp. 140–142).

Studies on peer interactions in kindergarten children show that they develop synchronous circadian rhythms between each other and that these change to their parents' cycle when the children are at home at weekends or on holidays. This demonstrates that when children interact frequently, they also become attuned to each other's behaviours and physiological rhythms (Field, 1985, p. 445).

Adults can also become attuned to each other in relation to bodily functions. For example, women sharing a room, or women spending a considerable amount of time together due to a close friendship, showed a synchronisation of their menstrual cycles. Hormonal signals seem to account for this mechanism, since exposing a group of women to the smell of a donor woman's armpit led to a shift of menstrual cycle timing in the recipient females' menstrual cycle so to conform with that of the donor female (Russell, Switz, & Thompson, 1980). This study supports the hypothesis that the time of menstrual onset may be modified by olfactory cues.

Field also notes that the disorganising effects of separation are not limited to mother–infant dyads. They also occur when monkey infants and children are separated from their peers, even though their behaviour is very different to that seen between a mother and her infant. Following separation, young monkeys do not cry or cling to one another when reunited but the physical and physiological effects are the same as those seen in infants separated from their mothers (Field, 1985, p. 425).

These observations, including Anna Freud's study on the children rescued from the concentration camps in our first chapter, led Field to conclude that:

> Attachment is basically a relationship that develops between two or more organisms as their behavioural and physiological systems become attuned to each other. *Each partner in the relationship provides for the other a source of stimulation and arousal modulation.* Loss or

separation from the partner or a change in the relationship would then lead understandably to behavioural and physiological disorganisation. (1985, p. 431, my emphasis)

Field adds that "separation may simply be an extreme example of the attached pair being unable to provide for each other optimal levels of stimulation" (ibid.).

Arousal modulation refers to how the mother can modify or control her infant's behaviour by soothing or stimulating his emotions; for instance, when the infant feels safe enough in mother's presence, he may start exploring the room they are in. However, every so often, he will make contact with his mother to reduce any anxiety he may be feeling before resuming his exploration.

This attuned synchronicity between human minds and bodies is also being explored by neuroscientists. Matthew Lieberman, one of the principal researchers in this field, states without reservation that the human brain is a social brain: "Just as we have a basic need for food and shelter, we have a basic need to belong to a group and form relationships" (Lieberman, 2013).

One of Lieberman's first studies, carried out with his wife Naomi Eisenberger, focused on the emotional pain caused by rejection. Most of us know how painful it feels when we break up a relationship or lose a close person in our lives. But are we aware that even a simple experience of rejection can really hurt? This is what the research subjects in a study carried out by Lieberman and his wife Naomi were to find out (Eisenberger, Lieberman, & Williams, 2003).

Each subject was put in a brain scanner to play an internet video game called Cyberball, where three people throw a ball around to each other. The research participants were led to believe that the other two people in game were also part of the study but they were, in fact, two pre-programmed avatars. At first all three players throw the ball to each other in turn. But then, at a certain point, the avatars stop throwing the ball to the research participants who then began to feel rejected; the more rejected the research subjects felt, the more activity was recorded in the part of the brain that records physical pain. Even after they came out of the scanner, the participants kept on talking to the researchers about how upset they were even though the study only involved a game (Lieberman, 2013). As Lieberman wrote: "We use the language of pain to express our emotions around loss such as 'he hurt my feelings' or a 'broken heart'" which can feel as bad as a broken leg.

Social pain is as real as physical pain, and it is a sign that something is wrong and a way of communicating this to others and getting help. Social pain signals that we are alone and that we are vulnerable.

From the beginning of human life, a baby's distress cry calls the mother to reunite with her child and tend to his or her needs. In studies of other mammals like rats, if the mothers don't respond to their pups' distress calls, they die within two days of birth.

Various studies involving brain scans have been developed to illustrate the importance of the human need for a loving response when in physical pain. One of the first was carried out by Goldstein, Weissman-Fogel, Dumas, and Shamay-Tsoory (2018), who set up a fascinating study on the impact of hand-holding when a partner is in pain. The researchers state that "Hand-holding is a feel-good gesture that is of far greater importance than mere contact between palms and digits would suggest". In fact, the move creates a connection between brains that can measurably reduce the physical pain being endured by one of the parties. The study shows that "pain can be modulated by touch".

The researchers studied twenty men and women in a long-term romantic relationship under four different scenarios, with each couple being subjected to all four of the scenarios. In the first scenario, the women were subjected to pain through a device on their arm that delivered high heat, while their partner was asked to sit beside them without touching. Next, the women were not subjected to any pain, while their partner was asked to sit beside them without touching. In the third scenario, partners were asked to hold hands when no pain was being inflicted upon the women and, in the fourth scenario, the women were subjected to pain while their partners held their hands.

In all these scenarios, the researchers used a new type of electroencephalogram (EEG) technology that allowed them to measure electrical brain activity in both partners simultaneously to assess if there was any correlation between them. They then asked the women to rate the level of pain in each scenario according to a ranking table they provided. Their findings indicated that hand-holding when pain was being administered increases the mutual connection between the two brains which the researchers called "brain coupling": this involved the central regions of the brain of the person suffering from the pain and the emotional right hemisphere of their partner. In other words, the degree of pain relief the woman experienced when her partner held her hand was closely related to the degree of *empathy* her partner felt for her during the experiment. The role of empathic attunement in stressful situations is so important as it can prevent traumatisation.

The researchers found that the level of pain experienced by the women was lower in the hand-holding condition and that the couples' brainwaves were synchronised during hand-holding.

This is but one of many experiments demonstrating how brain activity can be seen to synchronise between individuals who have close intimate relationships (Sahi et al., 2021). "Attachment can provide both an attunement experience and the potential to repair the damage brought about by the stressful experiences" (Schore, 1996).

These studies are so important, not only because they show the significance of attunement-based communication through the attachment bond, but also because they highlight that emotional pain is every bit as real as physical pain because, as Lieberman stated, our sense of experiencing separation is intrinsic to who we are.

It makes sense when we take on board how important relationships are for our well-being, both physical and mental. This is why bullying can have such a powerful negative effect on people. Lieberman sees it as the most pervasive form of rejection at a societal level: between the ages of ten and sixteen, 10 per cent of students in the United States have been found to be bullied regularly and are seven times more likely to be depressed compared to other children.

A 1989 Finnish study was carried out on 5,000 students who had been victimised at the age of eight: they found that these individuals were six times more likely to have taken their own lives by the age of twenty-five (Klomek et al., 2009).

Neuroscientists have been able to show that, just as rejection can hurt, being socially valued and fairly treated activates the human brain's reward system, the same brain areas that are activated by loving the taste of chocolate. These interpersonal experiences are rewarding because they make humans feel that they matter and that they belong.

One of the most interesting findings to come out of Lieberman's research using brain scans is discovering that, when his subjects finish doing some kind of non-social task, the network for social thinking is switched on almost instantly. This area of the brain, called the default network, engages in social cognitions such as thinking about other people, oneself, and relationships or "making sense of other people and ourselves". This is another feature of the human brain that reveals the importance of social relationships.

Newborns show this default network activity almost from birth. According to Liebermann, it is the brain's preferred state of being, thereby priming the human infant for his or her future social life based on understanding, empathy, and cooperation when good enough parental care makes this possible.

The development of the secure self

The importance of good, supported maternal care is so important when we look at how the human infant develops from infancy to adulthood. We have had a glimpse of how separation and other adverse social experiences can affect the development of primates and how long-lasting these effects can be. Hundreds of books have been written about complex achievements of the human brain but they usually fail to take into account the price that humans can pay for this achievement. It is because of the protection provided by our acutely sensitive attachment system between infant and mother and other caregivers that humans can develop so early outside the womb and thereby adapt so well to different environments, both natural and cultural. However, it is also because of this acutely sensitive attachment system that human beings suffer the possibility of real pain every time they form a relationship with another human being who has the power to leave or reject them. This is so dramatically important during the first two to three years of human life because of its implications in adulthood.

This book focuses on just how powerfully human infants can be affected by such experiences and how this knowledge can provide us with the tools to prevent endless infant tragedies and the resulting destructive minds in adulthood through which individual survival is achieved but at the expense of love and cooperation. The short account of human development that now follows helps to illustrate why and how brains do differ as a result of what takes place between the infant and his or her mother and what effects this has on a person's mind and behaviour.

Allan Schore's description of the developmental role of the attachment system is succinct: "Attachment can be defined as the interactive regulation of biological synchronicity between organisms" (Schore, 2000).

The sculpting of the infant's right hemisphere through brain-to-brain regulation

From the moment a human infant is propelled out of the safety of the womb and emerges relatively unscathed from the birth canal, she can often find herself on the receiving end of countless terrifying new sensations involving blinding lights, loud noise, and the pain of rough handling or metal forceps. At such terrifying moments the stress hormones are released until the mother's familiar smell and voice accompanied by her soothing touch come to the rescue.

This is the first of many future experiences for the infant when the terror of being alone, hungry, or in pain gives way to the relief of feeling safe and the bliss of feeling loved. As Perry puts it so well:

> In the arms of that caregiver, that is that magic moment literally weaving together the neurobiology of all these different systems. The biology of attachment is that a baby learns by thousands of good experiences that this stress is tolerable because it leads to reward, and this pleasurable outcome is cathexsized (bound up) to a person, Mom … Ultimately just seeing or hearing Mom makes you feel safe and pleasurable. (Perry, Pollard, Blakley, Baker, & Vigilante, 1995)

Bearing in mind the fact that human infants are born so early in their development, that they are extremely vulnerable and totally dependent on their "caregivers", it makes sense that any threat to their sense of security will translate into activation of their attachment system through piercing cries of distress. In favourable circumstances, this will elicit a protective caring response from a sensitive parent who will attend to their needs and ensure their safety.

The experience of birth and of later interactions between infants and their caregivers are made possible by the action of endogenous opiates and oxytocin. This small neuropeptide dates from about 100 million years ago and has evolved in parallel to the development of mammals, contributing in many ways to making them and us what we are now. According to Dr Sue Carter, who has spent her adult life studying this molecule, its original role was to help humans to be sociable and connect with others rather than to respond defensively (Carter, 2017).

This important first step involves developing a mother–infant attachment relationship that is safe enough for vulnerable immature infants to survive outside the womb thanks to mother's milk and her loving attuned, empathic responses. This is why oxytocin is often called the "love hormone". In human communities, oxytocin also evolved to enable mothers to form attachments with their partners, other family members, and the community. It does this by inducing a sense of safety, reducing the effect of stressors, blocking fear, and increasing trust.

Both sexes synthesise oxytocin, although oestrogen can increase sensitivity to its actions.

Over time, this adaptive molecule took on other roles. As Carter said: "You can understand it as a universal hardware, which our bodies can access with all different kinds of software" (2017).

It promotes healing and restoration and has antioxidant and anti-inflammatory properties as well as regulating the immune system. Last, but certainly not least, is the role of oxytocin in regulating the "mammalian vagus nerve", which is the most recently evolved branch of the autonomic nervous system (ANS).

How parents and infants communicate: the core principle of "serve and return"

Professor Trevarthen is of the opinion that babies are born communicators that come into the world ready to have a conversation (2011a). Following years of working on the early development of children in interaction with their parents, he states in a talk of his that:

> babies come into the world with their own self and with the sense of the difference between themselves and another person and with a complete set of emotions. The way they interact with people shows that they are ready to be part of an interaction, part of a couple doing things together and you couldn't do it if you are only concerned with yourself. You have to have what we now feel is a space in your mind for another person. (CDC video)

To illustrate his point, in the video, Trevarthen then comments on a wonderful recording of a communicative exchange between a father and a premature baby. The infant is strapped in his carrier to his father's chest and, almost hidden from view. We can hear a tiny voice emerge from the bag, a little "uh" sound. The father responds in kind with a somewhat louder and deeper "uh" sound. The observer, Trevarthen, comments on the timing:

> as you can hear the baby and the father alternating quickly and then you can hear long pauses between vocalisations, one in four seconds long, leaving a space for his father's reply. This means that the infant is making phrase length paused inside its mind without any support or from his father. I think babies come equipped with motives which are directed towards human contact and making conversational contacts with other people: they are trying to communicate. They've got a recognition of the human person in front of them and they want to interact. (CDC video)

The "serve and return" attuned interactive principle taking place in the infant–father interaction is now seen as central to caregivers' communication with children as it promotes healthy infant development. Experiencing the adult's focused attention helps build a secure attachment and the parent's response to the infant's "serves" strengthens the baby's confidence.

"Serve and return" interactions are also essential for healthy brain development. The repetition in the back-and-forth interactions reinforces pathways of synaptic connections, enabling them to become stronger and more complex.

> An older child is playing with his mother: he takes the *initiative* by pointing to a ball and looks back at his mother. She receives his initiative by looking at the child and then looks at the ball and says "ball". (CDC video)

She then responds with a new initiative by saying in an approving tone, looking from the ball to the child: "Yes, you can see the ball up high. I think you want it".

> She is naming what she is seeing, doing or feeling which is a way of making important language connections in the child's brain.
> The child receives her communication with a vigorous nod and returns by pulling her mother towards the ball and looks back at her expectantly.
> The mother gets the ball down for the child and gives it to her saying with a friendly look and tone: "There you are". (CDC video)

(Very helpful videos on "serve and return" and other developmental issues are on the website provided by the Centre of the Developing Child at Harvard University.)

Attachment, as a psychobiological interaction, fulfils many other functions through the infant–parent relationship, functions that are crucial to the infant's later developments and to how he or she relates to the world both in the present and in the future. For example, human infants are unable to regulate their hormones (Hofer, 1984), nor can they regulate their emotions, either positive or negative, which means that they cannot soothe or comfort themselves. It is through the development of their attachment bonds with their primary caregivers that babies' early physiological and hormonal systems gradually become regulated, functions that he or she will gradually acquire throughout development.

As Siegel put it in a lecture: "The brain is now seen as a self-organising system organised through mutual and rhythmic regulation of affect between mother and infant."

These attuned interactions result in the moulding of the infant's right brain over the first three years of life. At birth, the baby's brain has 50 trillion synapses and, by the age of three, there are 1,000 trillion, during which time new synapses have been formed and "hard wired", whilst unused ones have been pruned out of existence. Neural circuits develop across the brain. As Hebb put it so succinctly: "Neurons that fire together, wire together" (1949).

Mirror neurons, attunement, empathy, and mentalization

As we have seen in our earlier description of human interactions, humans are exquisitely adapted to interact since their survival depends on it. The mother's empathic responses to her infant's communications whilst she feeds, holds, caresses, talks, plays, and sings lead to a matching of inner states of attunement.

How does this happen?

Humans are basically social beings as we learnt from Lieberman and many others. Whenever we are not focused on a task, our brains switch to the default network which focuses on making sense of other people and ourselves. The capacity to understand or make sense of what others are doing is due to the presence of *mirror neurons* which were originally discovered in monkeys and are assumed to exist in humans because of brain-scan evidence of their actions. These specialised neurons (in the parieto-frontal cortical areas of the brain, just above our eyes) are activated when we do an action and when we observe someone else doing the same action. The sequence of actions leading to a goal enables the observer to understand what the action is about, the "why" of the action without any emotional involvement.

Mirror neurons in other areas are involved in processing subjective feelings, empathy, uncertainty, and developing a sense of Self and enable the observer to understand and to feel the emotions of others, to empathise with others. One such area is the insula, which is a small region of the cerebral cortex located deep within the a large fissure that separates the frontal and parietal lobes from the temporal lobe and facilitates our concept of self-awareness. This includes the awareness of our bodies and emotions, and how they interact to create our perception of the present moment.

As the reader may have noticed in the example of the attuned "serve and return", when the mother responds to the child's first initiative, by acknowledging that the child is seeing the ball and then, as she deduces that he wants it, she is in touch with what's going on in her child's mind: this empathic interaction results in a child who can attune with others and put himself/herself in the mind of another through the activation of the mirror neurons (Gallese, 2003; Gallese, Keysers, & Rizzolatti, 2004; Gallese & Singaglia, 2011).

Goleman refers to these attunement processes as "both low-road circuits and high-road circuits":

> "Primal empathy" which includes non-verbal synchrony, is an early subcortical emotional resonance between individuals. For instance, a baby cries in a nursery, and other babies start crying in response.
>
> "Empathic accuracy" requires activation of the prefrontal cortex as thought and feelings are joined in an understanding of the "other". (Goleman, 2006)

The first of these circuits is referred to as *emotional empathy* and involves a rather automatic implicit or unconscious processing of visible information about others. The second applies to Fonagy and Target's concept of "mentalization" which they described as developing in the infant when the parental figure gives meaning to the infant's experiences or shares and predicts his or her behaviour. It is what enables people to understand each other in terms of mental states, to interact successfully with others and is key to developing a sense of agency and continuity (Fonagy & Target, 1997). This definition of mentalization appears to be more of a cognitive process that involves the cortex and therefore fits in with Goleman's concept of "empathic accuracy". Fonagy has, in fact, renamed it the *cognitive mentalization system* (Fonagy & Luyten, 2009).

The formation of internal working models

In a secure child, these daily interactions involving the mirror neurons also end up providing the secure child with repeated comforting memories of interactions with his or her mother that the brain synthesises into IWMs (Bowlby, 1988, pp. 129–133). These are described as "mental representations" or templates of how the attachment figure is likely to respond when the infant is frightened or in need: the result is a sense of security in a child whose parent was responsive at such times.

These regulating experiences are equivalent to Hofer's *psychic regulators* referred to earlier on. They fulfil a regulatory emotional function through the integration of Hofer's *biologic and psychologic regulators* and allow for the expansion of the child's coping capacities as well as being protective in relation to later traumatic experiences (Schore, 1996, 2000). Infants also develop IWMs in relation to their fathers and other individuals involved in their regular care. These may be of a different attachment type than the mother's IWMs (Bowlby, 1982).

Attunement, empathy, and the autonomic nervous system

What enables mothers and other caregivers to respond in an attuned way to their offspring? They do so in the same way as other mammals do, through the activation of their specific emotional system called the *mammalian vagus* (otherwise referred to as "the ventral vagus complex" of the autonomic system by Porges). This historically more recent vagus system developed in mammals in order to enable parental figures to look after their young in an optimal manner for their development. When this system is turned on, the mammalian vagus stimulates the individual into an optimal state of arousal and thereby elicits in the caring mother a warm facial expression, loving eye contact, a soothing voice, and, last but not least, optimal brain function: this enables the parent to assess her infant's needs, make sense of his or her communications and keep an eye on the environment so as to maintain their joint safety (Porges, 1997).

These interactions between the infant and a "sensitive" caregiver form part of the process of attunement which is, as we now know, fundamental to the successful development of the young. At its simplest, it describes the process of harmonising, being on the same wavelength, but in the world of attachment, it is more specific. As Dan Siegel (2001) says: "Emotionally attuned communication, the sharing of non-verbal signals, allows for the child to 'feel felt' and to create a secure attachment with that connecting adult" (p. 84).

Without the capacity to attune, humans experience a void, cut off from the intimate interactions that supply us with the "emotional oxygen" of our existence and the capacity to attune and empathise. This emotional void is what traumatised individuals often refer to when they attempt to describe their internal world and is due, as will become apparent in the next chapter, to the splitting of the "Self" resulting from the *traumatic attachment*.

The role of emotions and Porges' polyvagal theory

We owe it to the neuroscientist Stephen Porges to have revealed the central importance of emotions in mammalian behaviour. He was studying the vagus nerve, which is a part of the ANS that controls our vital functions such as breathing, digestion, and heart rate, many of which we are not consciously aware of. His experiments led him to formulate the polyvagal theory where he describes the role of the three autonomic vagal subsystems that exist in humans (Porges, 2009, 2017). In tune with previously mentioned authors, he sees humans as a social species and explicitly emphasises that human survival is dependent on co-regulating our neurophysiological state via social interaction.

As we have seen, the human infant's dependence on mother provides us with the model of all future interactions, since the mother not only regulates the infant, but the infant reciprocally regulates the mother. This interactive co-regulation ensures reciprocity, connectedness, and trust between humans as well as physiological homeostasis: in other words, it ensure a neurobiological link between our mental health and our physical health.

Porges formulated the polyvagal theory based on his study of structures in the brain stem, called the nucleus ambiguous, that co-ordinates the striated muscles of the face and head with the viscera via the ANS (2009). He reminds us that the mammalian vagus, which enables us to bring up our infants in a safe and loving way, is, in fact, the most recent development of this system. However, it is important to be aware of the power of the earlier more primitive part of the ANS which is the reptilian system as it will be seen to play a crucial role in the development of the *traumatic attachment*.

The reptilian vagus—*fight–flight* or Yellow Zone

The reptilian system becomes active in people when they are frightened and face danger because humans, like all animals, are geared to survive in the face of danger. This requires the activation of what Porges refers to as the "mobilization system" or *ventral vagus complex* which depends on the sympathetic system of the ANS that promotes the *fight–flight–freeze* response. When action is needed, the sympathetic system triggers an active response by accelerating the heart rate, increasing the breathing rate, boosting blood flow to the muscles, activating sweat secretion, and dilating the pupils. When people find themselves in this state, they are usually either in a rage or in panic mode. The brain is focused on how to deal with the threat and is therefore not functioning at its best and is not in a cooperative mode. It is when humans are in this emotional state that they are most likely to commit destructive or violent actions. I refer to this emotional state as being in the Yellow Zone (see Figure 2.1 on p. 39).

The reptilian vagus—*freeze*/dissociate or Red Zone

If safety is not achieved through the *fight–flight* mode of the Yellow Zone, the endangered individual succumbs to the effects of what Porges refers to as the "immobilization system" involving the dorsal vagal complex (DVC). It is present in all vertebrates and depends on the primitive unmyelinated top side of the vagus nerve. It normally provides primary control of subdiaphragmatic visceral organs, such as the digestive tract and, under normal conditions, it regulates these digestive processes. However, under stress, as part of the old reptilian parasympathetic system, it promotes immobilisation or self-paralysis by slowing down the heart rate and breathing whilst the pupils constrict and, in certain cases, it can lead to loss of consciousness and death. I refer to this emotional state as being in the Red Zone (see Figure 2.1 on p. 39).

However, for mammals including humans, the *freeze* response can also be life-saving. Imagine a little fawn, peacefully grazing in a wood, suddenly becomes aware of a lion prowling between it and its mother. Were it to call her or run towards her, as its attachment system dictates when in danger, the lion would see it and kill it. Instead, the fawn freezes and thanks to the release of endorphins that accompanies this response, its vocal or speech area in the brain switches off. So long as it is downwind from the predator, it is likely to survive. Once the predator has gone, the fawn shakes off the effects of its *freeze* response, bleats, and runs towards its mother. Endangered human infants in the hands of a terrifying caregiver resort to a similar *freeze* response and survive, through disconnection or dissociation, as will be illustrated in the next chapter, but its effects are, unfortunately, harmful in the long run.

It is important to remember that the *freeze* response is accompanied by the release of endorphins, nature's anaesthetics, as the Scottish explorer David Livingstone found out when attacked by a lion. As he felt the animal's jaw clamp his shoulder. the shock of the attack produced what Livingstone described as a sort of dreaminess. "There was no sense of pain nor feeling of terror, though [I was] quite conscious of all that was happening," he said.

The mammalian vagus—Green Zone

The third and most recent autonomic subsystem that is present in mammals is the "social engagement system" and involves the ventral vagus system, which I referred to earlier as the *mammalian vagus.* It is dependent on the myelinated vagus nerve which lies in the lower part of the vagus nerve and promotes all the functions that are needed in forming an empathic and synchronised attuned interaction between parents and their infant: optimal emotional arousal, good eye contact, a warm facial expression, a soothing voice, and, interestingly, optimal brain function.

This "ventro vagal complex" or more simply described as the "mammalian vagus", regulated by oxytocin, connects the lower regions of the prefrontal cortex of the brain to the heart and lungs and controls the muscles of the face and head that we use to communicate emotions, feelings, and ideas. I refer to this emotional system as the Green Zone (see Figure 2.1 on p. 39).

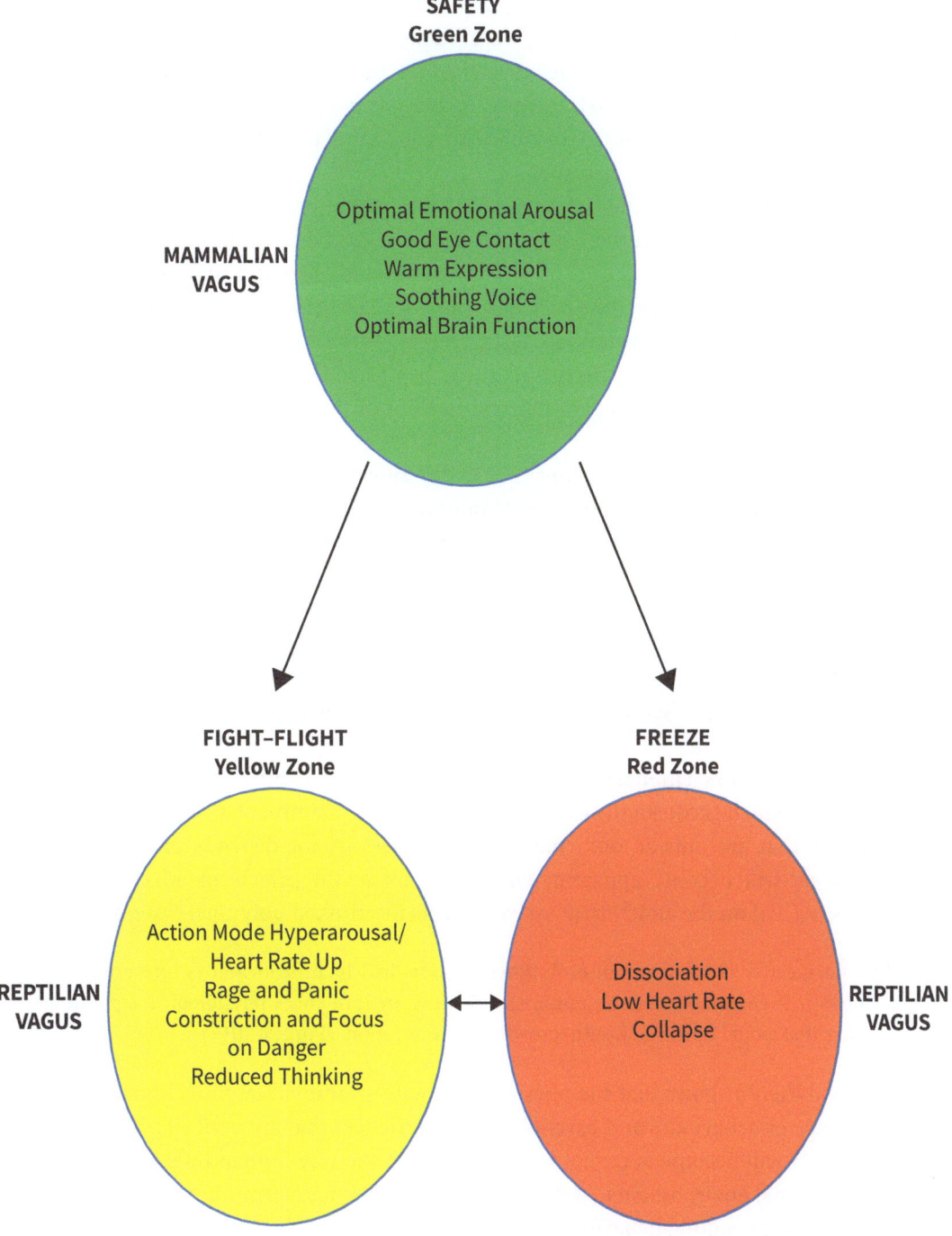

Figure 2.1 Simplified summary of the autonomic nervous system's functioning

This means that, as long as the "social engagement system" or Green Zone is functioning, the other two "mobilising" and "immobilising" vagal subsystems are kept in homeostatic balance or, to put it more simply, if the Green Zone is switched on, the Yellow and Red Zones are switched off. This is very important, because humans can voluntarily switch on their mammalian vagus by using breathing exercises, often inspired by yoga, and thereby control our *fight–flight* response as well as prevent a *freeze* response.

This is achieved thanks to the orbitofrontal or prefrontal cortex that sits over the eyes: it regulates emotional arousal via the ANS' mammalian vagus nerve and inhibits impulses from the amygdala which monitors all sensory stimuli, particularly fear and aggression.

Following Porges' polyvagal research and his wife Carter's studies on oxytocin, a new therapeutic approach has been developing in relation to healing the attachment wounds of the past: if a vulnerable child or insecure adult can be provided with a "safe" attuned oxytocin-inducing relational experience, reparation and healing of those early emotional wounds can begin to take place.

In the field of psychotherapy, Schore (2022) describes this as a right brain to right brain psychotherapy involving the interacting right brains of the therapist and his or her client. Beyond psychoanalytic psychotherapy, other therapeutic approaches have been developed that enhance attunement and access to the Green Zone; these are proving to be very effective therapeutically such as video interaction guidance (VIG) for parents and their children (described in more detail in Chapter 10) and equine therapy for complex trauma (described in more detail in Chapter 6). VIG therapists have to learn in detail how to attune their communication to their clients' needs, based on a "serve and return" model, which my psychotherapeutic colleagues might find helpful.

The polyvagal theory emphasises the importance of taking into account the state of our nervous system which is constantly evaluating risk in the environment, prioritising behaviours and decisions that are outside our conscious awareness. A lot depends on our earlier life experiences, as will become apparent when we look at the effects of adverse childhood experiences (ACEs) on the attachment system and its interlinked polyvagal system:

> This perspective is based on an evolutionary model in which behaviour is interpreted as adaptive if it enhances survival, minimizes distress, or influences physiological state in a manner that would optimize health, growth and restoration. (Porges, 2017)

The polyvagal theory shows that the physiological state an individual finds himself/herself in limits the range of behaviours and psychological experiences that are available. The important role of the ANS will become apparent when we look at the way human infants adapt to their different emotional environments, as it plays a crucial role in determining the nature of their emotions and their resulting behaviour. Damage due to ACEs leads to difficulties in developing appropriate social, and emotional communicative behaviours.

The polyvagal theory, the Covid-19 pandemic, and the role of racism

As part of this book was written during the Covid-19 pandemic, I could not help being aware of the effects that the lockdown was having on us all: to be shut off from human contact when what we need most is to be close to those we love; to be alone with one's worries and unable to connect brought out all our individual insecurities.

Porges encouraged people to use online video communication services to make contact with others and it certainly helped to some degree. However, for those who could not access the internet and for those living alone, it must have been soul destroying. Children banned from attending school suffered, too, as we have seen how much they rely on playing with each other and being supported by their teachers for their emotional regulation and cognitive development. In addition, any stress at home was only made worse through the social and economic circumstances many found themselves in as they struggled to keep their jobs and care for their families This contributed to a rise in domestic violence, with no place to escape to and no one to protect vulnerable adults and children, and greater inequality in the context of accessing support services.

One of the pandemic's main effects was to highlight the racial inequality that exists in our societies. Not only did people of colour and immigrants struggle more to make a living but they also suffered from the invisible, but all too real, deadly effects of the racism that exists in our societies. Whilst it is acknowledged in the United States, but still all too present, institutional racism has been officially denied by the government in the UK. However, the statistics relating to Covid-19 deaths speak loud and clear as to its destructive existence. A review by Public Health England, published in June 2020, promised to examine why people from ethnic minorities were more likely to contract and die from Covid-19 and to make recommendations for "further action that should be taken to reduce disparities in risk and outcomes from Covid-19 on the population" (Aldridge et al., 2020).

The review confirmed previous data showing that ethnic minority groups were the most likely to have the Covid-19 diagnosis and the death rates were highest amongst the different black and Asian ethnic groups: black and other multi-ethnic groups had a 10 to 50 per cent higher risk of death than white British people. However, there was no mention as to what could be done to reduce those disparities. In other words, not a thought has been given to how best to protect these vulnerable ethnic groups. Medical and race equality organisations are angry and frustrated that a review that set out to examine the disproportionate effect of Covid-19 on people from ethnic minority groups ended up making the problem worse by basically telling them "you are second rate, you matter less".

This is the central racist message that impacts these people's lives, many of whom in this case worked for the NHS. It confirms just how racist this system still is and demonstrates that racism is in itself a public health problem because it is a disease that kills people. Such a message in times of crisis makes people more fearful and insecure because they know that their lives are seen as dispensable. This insecurity leads to increased levels of chronic stress which we now know is accompanied by high levels of systemic inflammation, increased risk of disease, particularly cardiac illness, researchers have found that affected mothers give birth to lower-birth-weight children who also develop chronic stress. The critics of the public health review state that there is no stopping Covid-19 without stopping racism.

Secure and insecure attachments

Unfortunately, as we know only too well, not all infants have the benefit of an attuned attachment experience with their mother and other caregivers, which they need in order to thrive. These children can end up developing what Bowlby's co-researcher Mary Ainsworth called "insecure" attachments.

It was whilst in Uganda, where her husband worked for a few years, that she decided to study the quality of mother–infant interactions. She worked with mothers of twenty-six Ganda families with unweaned babies, observing their interactions for two hours every two weeks for nine months. The highly sensitive mothers gave her a lot of information about their children and proved to have securely attached infants who cried little and explored happily in their presence. The insecurely attached babies cried frequently, even when in mother's arms, and did not explore much. The not-yet-attached infants did not show any differential behaviour towards their mother (Ainsworth, 1967).

Once back in the United States, Ainsworth carried out a similar study with Baltimore families and then developed the "Strange Situation", a twenty-minute "miniature drama" with eight episodes to measure the nature of mother–infant attachment behaviours and styles of attachment. This is still used today.

The experiment is set up in a small room with one-way glass so the behaviour of the infant can be observed. Infants were aged between twelve and eighteen months. The sample comprised one hundred middle-class American families. The procedure was conducted by observing the behaviour of the infant in a series of eight episodes lasting approximately three minutes each:

1. Mother, baby, and experimenter (lasts less than one minute).
2. Mother and baby alone.
3. A stranger joins the mother and infant.
4. Mother leaves baby and stranger alone.
5. Mother returns and stranger leaves.
6. Mother leaves; infant left completely alone.
7. Stranger returns.
8. Mother returns and stranger leaves.

The Strange Situation classifications or attachment styles are based primarily on four interaction behaviours directed towards the mother in the two separation and reunion episodes (Episodes 5 and 8) (Ainsworth, Blehar, Waters, & Wall, 1978).

The infants were subdivided into three main groups (A, B, and C) depending on how they reacted following the two separations from their mother. These separation experiences act as stressors which reveal the underlying nature of their attachment relationship to their main caregiver.

The securely attached

The Group-B infants who comprised 63 per cent of the population of infants were classified as *securely attached* compared to their insecurely attached counterparts in Groups A and C. They were more positive and cooperative in their behaviour towards their mothers compared to the other groups and, at home, their mothers were seen to be sensitive to their infants' signals and tender in the way they handled their children. In the Strange Situation these infants used their mothers as a secure base from which to explore. They did not cry when mother left the room for the first time, but they did cry and protest when she left the second time. When finally reunited with their mother, they greet her with pleasure and extend their arms for a cuddle during which their body moulds into mother's and stays in contact for a couple of minutes before the attachment behaviour is deactivated. As toddlers, they are more flexible, curious, socially competent, and self-reliant than the insecure infants.

With parental empathy, the child "feels felt" and develops confidence in his or her experience and the trust that others can recognise their needs and the capacity to empathise and later mentalize (Siegel & Hartzell, 2003).

The individual sense of Self in the securely attached

Recent research confirms the sociologist George Mead's theory that if the individual possesses a sense of Self, it is only in relation to other selves; he saw the Self not as a structure, but as a process of interactions between organisms (Mead & Morris, 1934, p. 179), much as Siegel and Lieberman do in different ways. He sees the development of the Self taking place in two stages in individualistic Western societies:

1. *The individual sense of Self is* closely intertwined with the internal representation of the attachment figure as represented in the IWM. For example, infants who received sensitive loving care will view themselves as lovable: self-esteem and self-confidence are built on this interpersonal dance of attunement and empathy with the parents leading to a secure attachment and an expectation of being taken care of in times of trouble. Securely attached children will be capable of empathising with others and therefore able to form good attachments with others. This type of attachment, according to Schore (1996, 2000), becomes a primary defence against trauma induced psychopathology in later life.

2. *The social sense of Self* becomes much more important during adolescence in relation to the child's peer group attachments. According to Mead, the social context in which the

child is reared begins to impinge more directly on his or her sense of identity through the spoken language, culture and relationship to the outer world.

3. In many other societies, however, such as in parts of Africa, the Middle East, and Asia, a person is a person because of how other people see them. Shaming by social rejection is an extremely powerful method to make people comply, both at home and in the community. So, for example, whilst it is acceptable for young people in the West to challenge their parents' views as they grow up, this may not be allowed in more conservative/patriarchal cultures where parents (and grandparents) hold very important/authoritative positions.

Once we can see the Self as an organiser of inner and outer experiences that ensures a person's perceived sense of identity, we can understand how important it is to maintain this sense of identity and how disruptive and threatening it is to have it challenged (Guidano, 1987, p. 3). This means that even if people have been brought up in a secure environment at home, the experience of severe and repeated traumatisation elsewhere, through racism or bullying, for instance, may lead to feelings of helplessness and/or humiliation which can, in turn, lead to the loss of the capacity to empathise with others, and to violence.

The insecurely attached

Anything that interrupts the cycle of attunement affects the quality of the infant's attachment to a lesser or greater degree. Insecurely attached individuals suffer from the effects of not having had the parenting to enable them to feel safe in the company of others with the result that they can become either very anxious or very avoidant.

The "resistant or anxiously ambivalent" type or Group C comprised about 12 per cent of the population. Their mothers showed good attunement but were seen to be inconsistent at home because they were stressed, anxious, or exhausted, so their infants had to make their presence felt in order to be noticed: in the Strange Situation this leads to a clingy, angry behaviour when their mother returns from the separation. The children learn strategies to hold their parent's attention such as being disruptive. According to the long-term prospective Minnesota study, these children are likely to develop anxiety disorders in the future (Sroufe, 2005, p. 361).

The "avoidant type" or Group A comprised 20 to 25 per cent of the population. In the home situation, their mothers were often seen to be rejecting, particularly of close body contact, when their infants were frightened or in discomfort; they were also interfering and often neglectful. In the Strange Situation these avoidant infants appear indifferent to their mothers, attending to their toys and other things around them. Unlike the other infants, they showed no fear, distress, or anger when reunited with their mothers.

What is interesting is that their heart-rate measurements were very high during the separation and reunion episodes, which means that, despite appearances, their attachment behaviour was strongly activated. However, their apparent interest in playing with the toys provided a displacement activity that allowed them to stay near their mother without inviting her rejection: their behaviour is part of their defence against the pain of rejection.

At home, these avoidant infants manifested a lot more separation distress than the secure infants and, by twelve months, they often behaved aggressively towards their mothers and other children with whom they had negative interactions and would be hostile without provocation. In day care settings, these infants avoided their playmates and averted their gaze from them to the same degree as they avoided their mothers on reunion in the Strange Situation. These infants also showed less positive emotions than the other infants.

To achieve this state of detachment, these one-year-olds had learnt to deny and later denigrate the love and care they needed when faced with fear, helplessness, or loss. According to the Minnesota study, these children are likely to develop "conduct disorders" in childhood. This is a psychiatric label applied to patterns of antisocial behaviour where a child or young person repeatedly carries out aggressive acts that may cause them distress, social problems, and upset other people. In the same study, both the resistant and the avoidant infants often suffered from depression in later life (Sroufe, 2005, p. 361).

Troy and Sroufe (1987) studied nineteen pairs of children at play. In the pairs where one or both children were classed as "avoidant", there was victimisation. Five of these pairs had one partner who would regularly abuse his or her partner, both verbally or physically: in all of these couples, the abuser had an avoidant attachment and the victim had either an "anxious attachment" or an "avoidant attachment". This is an important finding as it shows that an avoidant child can be both abuser or victim which means that it is the relationship of the Self vs the Other that is internalised to form the template or IWM. The securely attached children were not victims nor did they abuse.

It is also important to remember that a child can develop different working models in relation to his or her caregiver: for instance, they can develop a secure attachment with one and an avoidant one with another.

The disorganised attachment type

A third category of insecure attachment was discovered by Main and Solomon in 1986 and named the *disorganised attachment* type or group D. These infants revealed the terrible impact of childhood abuse, neglect, or loss, which we will be addressing in our next chapter in relation to *the traumatic attachment* and its lifetime impact.

Conclusion: "It takes a village to grow a child"

Though most of us are brought up to believe that we are born predisposed to be independent and competitive as well as violent, what we are learning is what a few remaining indigenous people in the rain forests and deserts of the world know only too well: humans are born to cooperate, which is why we have become such a successful species.

In this chapter we reviewed the evidence indicating that the human brain is indeed a social brain. Securely attached individuals have a unique ability to read other people's minds and thereby cooperate effectively through attunement, empathy, and mentalization. They can, therefore, support one another, which is an effective way of reducing fear and other painful or destructive emotions. In fact, human relationships act as emotional regulators which is why the ending of a relationship can be so upsetting and painful and why the Covid-19 lockdowns had such disturbing effects on so many.

When not focused on performing a task, our brain automatically moves into the "default position", focusing on what is going on in our different relationships. However, for any of these positive relational experiences to take place a secure attachment is necessary, which means that we cannot underestimate the importance of providing parents, and particularly mothers or alternative parental figures, with a safe and supportive social context in which to bring up their children. This is especially important in the first three years of life and in adolescence, as will become clearer in the next chapter.

To become an adult human being who can benefit from and contribute to his or her community, a child needs caregivers who feel secure and who have access to loving care and the assistance of different family members and/or the surrounding community: these all play a crucial role in providing the developing infant with the social context that ensures the making of a securely attached child.

Or, as one of my patients put it when he was preparing for the arrival of his unborn child: "I must turn my home into a Green Zone with all the help I can get from outside and within"; this involved therapeutic and social support. He was aware, from his own violent childhood experiences, that both he and his partner needed to feel safe and supported; this would help them to provide the empathic attuned relationships that their infant would need to build the brain structures that enable infants to form secure relationships during their lifetime.

This approach is particularly important since we have discovered that the human infant is one of the most vulnerable mammalian infants because it is born so early: whilst this enables human infants to adapt remarkably well to the different communities, it can only happen if the parents can also provide them with the specific and appropriate care that they need. It is important to stress that meaningful interactions with more secure individuals or attuned therapy can reduce the individual's insecurity or even change their attachment style to a more secure attachment, particularly in adolescence: this is defined as "earned security".

Unfortunately, the use of our new Traumatic Attachment Induction Procedure (the TAIP) is revealing just how severe and far-reaching are the effects of the disorganised attachment and its associated *traumatic attachment*. This is the disorder that really highlights the case for protecting and supporting parents and their children during pregnancy and the first three years of the infant's life. Not only would these measures spare so much unnecessary suffering, but it would also make huge savings. This is the subject of our next two chapters.

CHAPTER 3

Nature's Stockholm syndrome

Abuse and emotional neglect by a mother suffering from a dissociative disorder

A mother of Turkish origin, Figen, was referred to me in the TSS by a child psychiatrist, because her eighteen-month-old son, Asen, who appeared emotionally frozen, showed signs of abuse.

Figen did not understand why she had been referred to be assessed nor did many of the staff involved in her care in the community. The social workers reported that she appeared to be functioning well and, when they visited her in her very tidy home she seemed to be caring towards her son.

I noticed that he was unusually quiet and stayed very close to his mother, showing little interest in the toys that I offered him. He seemed unhappy and very anxious. I understood why the referrer had described him as "frozen".

It was not until Figen had shared with me her childhood history of sexual abuse at the hands of male relatives in her native village, that she began to reveal what was going on between her and her son. She spoke of this, in a rather incoherent manner, as people who suffer from severe dissociation often do when speaking about their traumatic experiences.

When she had found out that she had a baby boy, she had asked for her pregnancy to be terminated because she was frightened of how she might react towards him. However, no one believed that this tidy, well-dressed, composed woman could possibly harm her child. Unfortunately, her fears were well founded as she revealed that she experienced him as her childhood abuser right from the moment he was born. Again, she asked for him to be adopted but to no avail, since she presented as a confident and well-organised mother.

It was the sight of his male genitalia that triggered horrifying memories of being abused and drove her to reject him. As he clung to her in terror, she found herself shouting and hitting him.

As the interview progressed, it became clear that Figen was not always aware of this abusive behaviour, which belonged to other dissociated states of her mind linked to the IWMs of her childhood traumatic experiences. Her levels of dissociation were very high, compatible with a diagnosis of dissociative identity disorder. As a result of our interview, Figen took up the offer of psychotherapy in relation to her childhood trauma and her son's well-being whilst he was temporarily fostered until his mother could take him back and look after him, ideally with the support of a family therapist specialised in working with traumatised children and their parents.

Many similar cases of severe child abuse are being missed, probably for the same reasons, since a parent's potential for dissociation and abuse would not be diagnosed in a standard psychiatric or social work interview; unfortunately, the effects of trauma-induced dissociation are still poorly taught and the existence of dissociation is still so often denied in the UK, even by my psychiatric colleagues. Having focused on the mother in my interview, we are left wondering what the effects of her rejection and abusive behaviour on her baby son were.

Fear-terror without solution: the origin of dissociation and the traumatic attachment

Beebe describes such an interaction between an infant and a disorganised mother so well that I will share her example from Schore's article:

> Each one escalates the ante and, as the infant builds up to a frantic distress, she may scream and, in this example, she finally throws up. In an escalating overarousal pattern, even after the extreme distress signals from her infant, such as a ninety-degree head aversion, arching away from the mother … or screaming, the mother keeps on going. (Beebe, 2000, p. 436)

Perry's description (https://www.childtrauma.org/trauma-ptsd) of the infant's distress as *fear-terror* recognises the extreme emotions that these infants experience during what is in fact a traumatic event in a developing child who is still totally dependent on her mother.

The mother of a securely attached child responds in a sensitive way and, through her attuned interactions during moments of joy or distress, she enables her infant to both regulate his emotions and establish an inner equilibrium: this enables him to gradually expand his coping capacities in relation to the outside world.

Beebe's infant has a mother who has a limited capacity to both attune and empathise with her child because she has been abused and/or neglected as a child and she has not had any therapeutic or loving help herself. Instead, she may perceive the child's behaviour as manipulative or even aggressive, as Figen did, and she is also unable to interactively repair the situation.

As a result, the infant's intense negative emotional states last for a very long time. The enduring effects of these repeated terrifying experiences is now well established through studies of emotionally neglected children:

> When infants are not in homeostatic balance or are emotionally out of control or dysregulated, they are at the mercy of these states. Until these states are brought under control, these infants must devote all their regulatory resources to reorganizing them. While infants do that, they can do nothing else. (Tronick & Weinberg, 1997, p. 56)

What these authors mean by "they can do nothing else" is that the infants do not have the resources to continue with their development and thereby miss out on important opportunities to learn and move on during critical periods of development. The reason for this is that a lot of neurobiological changes take place in the developing infant's brain and body during and after these terrifying experiences. Unfortunately, as we will discover, such experiences are not uncommon; many of the people who seek help from therapists have been through such disturbing experiences, which is why it is important to understand what is going on in their minds and bodies.

It isn't easy from the adult perspective to realise just how terrifying it is for infants to suddenly find themselves totally helpless in the face of what is, to them, the loss of their only source of loving comfort and life itself. They will finally respond, as most mammals do in the face of overwhelming danger, by "freezing" and escape by turning "inwards", thereby disconnecting from their terrifying mother. Interestingly, for most infants, this state of disconnection appears to enable a new connection to form, an imaginary helpful one to an idealised caring mother, one that enables these infants to survive. However, this happens at a heavy cost, as we will find out from those who survive and as our clinical research now shows.

In this chapter, we will try to understand what is going on in the minds and bodies of these infants because their reaction to these terrifying experiences with their main caregiver is what the *traumatic attachment* is all about and it is what gives significance to the unique responses that emerge when we use the TAIP. The origins of this procedure and its uses will be the subject of the rest of our book, described by therapists and some of the people they have worked with.

Main and Solomon's study of the disorganised attachment

In the 1980s, researchers in the field of attachment reported that the behaviour of many maltreated children they had studied using Ainsworth's Strange Situation did not fit in with the descriptions of either the *anxious ambivalent* or the *avoidant* insecure attachment behaviour that we described in our last chapter. Instead, these maltreated infants behaved in a conflicted, disorientated, and basically *disorganised* manner when reunited with their parent after brief separations.

Main and Solomon (1986) decided to study these infants by using the same Strange Situation, because it is designed to expose infants to the stress of two separations in order to reveal their underlying level of attachment insecurity.

Seventy per cent of their infants were at risk from emotional disorders and came from violent families while 15 per cent came from low-risk families where there was no evidence of abuse or neglect.

This combined group of infants also exhibited higher cortisol levels and higher heart rate levels than all the other attachment classifications, which indicates that they had all been through very stressful experiences.

During the Strange Situation, these infants displayed a variety of unpredictable disorganised responses when their parent returned to the room after a short period of separation. What Main and other researchers using this procedure describe is very different from what happened in the attachment experiments carried out on infant monkeys when they had been exposed to their mothers' frightening behaviours. Those primates did not flee, as could be expected; instead, they did everything they could to remain close to their mothers like the infants of the motherless mothers in Harlow's study.

Rat pups' behavioural and psychobiological response to maternal abuse

Subsequent studies carried out on rat pups by Sullivan's team show even more clearly how important it is for these infant mammals to remain attached to their mother, even when she abuses them: the following reference provides a very good summary of their work (Perry & Sullivan, 2014).

Perry and Sullivan set up three experimental studies using a rodent model of infant abuse to observe its effects on rat pups. Their findings also highlight the effects of abuse on the infants' subsequent neuro-development and behaviour as they grow up to become adults. The short lives of rats make them a very useful species to study the long-term effects of damage to the attachment system across the lifespan.

1. The first rodent model they used was a "naturally abusive" experiment where the mother rat is provided with insufficient bedding to build her nest. As a result, she keeps on trying to finish her task and, as she moves in and out of the nest, she tramples on her pups and handles them roughly, as well as providing them with less nursing time. What is remarkable is that, despite these multiple frightening and painful experiences, the rat pups continue to seek contact with their mother, or her smell, even when they are adults.

   As the authors point out, this context of social deprivation, which so many humans now face, is a stressful environmental risk for parents which can lead to infant maltreatment and the developmental damage that results from it. The human infants' utter dependency on their caregiver means that they owe their very existence to the parent who is looking after them, especially in the one- or two-parent family systems that characterise our fragmented Western societies. This puts an enormous responsibility on the parent, as we all know, especially when supportive social systems that once replaced, to some extent, the extended family, are being destroyed in the current political and economic environment.

2. In their second study, a classical conditioning paradigm was used whereby a painful electric shock, or a pinching of the rat pup's tail, is paired with a neutral smell so that they are attracted to and prefer that particular smell, even if it is accompanied by pain.

3. These researchers confirmed that abused rat pups seek contact with their abusing mother, much as Harlow's infant monkeys did. In addition, they found that to obtain this paradoxical response to mother and her smell, the experiment needed to be carried out within the first ten days of the pup's life; this is because the pup's neurobiological system only prevents it from learning to avoid smells associated with painful stimuli during the first ten days of their lives.

   Sullivan concludes that this as an evolutionary development, especially selected to prevent rat pups from avoiding their mother in those first days of life because brief painful experiences are usually part and parcel of typical early maternal care; this therefore ensures the rat pups' early attachment to their caregiver and hence their survival.

4. This led the research team to modify Ainsworth's Strange Situation, which they refer to as a Procedure (SSP), so as to use it with rat pups and expose their underlying type of attachment. They compared adversity-reared pups, like the ones mentioned above, with control-reared pups in their approach and interactions with their mother: although both groups interacted normally with their mother in the nest, the adversity-reared pups exhibited abnormal or atypical behaviours later during their development which were very similar to those shown by human children exposed to maltreatment (Opendak et al., 2020).

5. On closer examination, it was the pups' nervous system's response to their mother's nurturing behaviour, such as her licking, grooming, and milk ejection, that was blunted during the period when they were exposed to her abusive behaviour. The researchers conclude:

> Whilst attachment is preserved, its poor quality is associated with the pups aberrant processing of the sensory stimulation embedded in its interactions with its mother, including reduced regulation of the pup's brain and behaviour.

They further state that: "This information derived from animal models is critical for understanding the roots of pathology induced by early life maltreatment and is a causal link to later-life pathology in humans" (Opendak et al., 2020, p. 13).

These animal studies go a long way in supporting the current view that the "disorganised" attachment in children is the significant risk factor for later socio-emotional difficulties, including poor stress management and future psychopathology as well as changes in the way their nervous system functions (Opendak et al., 2020). This information makes me think of those "hidden biologic and psychic regulators" described by Hofer in Chapter 2 which we can now assume are integrated in the IWMs of these rat pups to exert their influence in later life (Hofer, 2014).

The human infant's dissociative response and the formation of the traumatic attachment

If so many mammals, like the monkeys and the rats we have described earlier, maintain their attachment to their abusive or neglectful mother through this paradoxical behaviour, what happens with human infants who have suffered abuse or neglect when they go through the Strange Situation?

Returning to Main and Solomon's study, they noted that a few infants showed clear signs of fear or terror when their mother appeared, but they did not find any obvious evidence of infants or toddlers who clung to their parental figure: instead, they displayed a variety of behaviours which appeared to the researchers as both unpredictable and *disorganised*. In other words, these infants did not appear to have an organised means of coping with the terror that they experienced when they faced their mother or other parental figures following their short separation (Main & Hesse, 1990). Whereas the insecurely attached *anxious ambivalent* or *avoidant infants* developed strategies to make sure that they could remain close to their mother and thereby continue to benefit from her protection and care, despite her failings, these *disorganised* infants did not appear to have evolved a behavioural system that enabled them to bypass their terror and maintain their close attachment to their mother to ensure their survival.

However, we do know that maltreated children end up developing a strong paradoxical attachment to their caregiver (Bowlby, 1965; Stronach et al., 2011). Abused children, even when they are adults, are usually very protective of their caregiver, often denying that they have been hurt or frightened. So, is there any evidence for this in the disorganised response of the infants in Main and Solomon's Strange Situation?

We know that these researchers were particularly struck by the behaviour of the infants who showed a simultaneous display of contradictory behaviour patterns lasting only ten to thirty seconds each: for instance, a few infants were seen as backing towards their mother, rather than approaching her face to face. Another sequential example of this behaviour is that of an infant who crawls towards his father, gets halfway there, stops, turns, and crawls into the wall, turns to face his father, and then puts his hands over his eyes (Main & Solomon, 1986).

> The impression in each case was that the approach movements were continuously being inhibited and held back through simultaneous activation of avoidant tendencies … Thus contradictory patterns were activated but were not mutually inhibited. (Main & Solomon, 1986, p. 117)

The authors make the interesting point that many of these infants simultaneously approach and avoid their caregiver without mutual inhibition which indicates that these two opposing behaviours appear to be independent of each other. The approach in many cases may be due to these infants initially responding to their inborn need to *attach* to their parent for safety, and then their *fight–flight–freeze* defence response kicks in, driving the children in the opposite direction. These two systems, the attachment and the defence systems, normally act in harmony as the infant mammal flees from the source of danger to find safety in the proximity of the caregiver. But the two systems clash whenever their caregiver, their normal source of safety, becomes terrifying: being repeatedly exposed to a parent who is either very frightening or very frightened motivates the infant to strive to be as close as possible and to run away at the same time.

Could it be that what Main and Solomon were witnessing, as they carried out the Strange Situation with these vulnerable infants was, in fact, the creation of the *traumatic attachment*?

They write: "the approach movements were continuously being completely inhibited and held back through the simultaneous activation of avoidant *tendencies*" due to the defence system, and then they note that this state of emotional "*dysregulation*" was "*being followed up in other infants by stilling and dissociation*" due to the final *freeze* response of the defence system (1986, p. 118, my emphasis).

According to Schore (2002), the psychobiological ANS response to trauma in *disorganised* infants involves two separate response patterns: hyperarousal and dissociation.

1. When an infant first begins to be frightened, the *sympathetic branch of her ANS* is switched on (and she is in what I refer to as the Yellow Zone). She cries and then screams in distress and the *fight–flight* response propels her into action by increasing her heart rate, blood pressure, temperature, breathing, and muscle tone as well as putting her on high alert. The thyroid hormone is released to stimulate the body's metabolism as is the stress hormone, cortisol, to release high levels of adrenaline and noradrenaline which triggers glutamate, a transmitter involved in sending signals between nerve cells in the limbic system. Symbolic processing into words is not possible in such states, with the result that these traumatic experiences are stored in sensory, somatic, behavioural, and affective states (Perry, Pollard, Blakley, Baker, & Vigilante, 1995). As Van der Kolk put it so well: "The body keeps the score" (2014).

2. If the *fight–flight* reaction is not possible, or does not achieve any change for the better, the *parasympathetic branch of the ANS* takes over and the infant is in what I refer to as the Red Zone. He or she "freezes", as mammals do in similar circumstances in order to conserve energy or feign death and thereby foster survival' (Nijenhuis, Spinhoven, Van Dyck, Van der Hart, & Vanderlinden, 1998). Vocalisation is often inhibited so as to protect the infant mammal from being heard by a potential predator. Many children become mute in such states, as do traumatised adults when triggered into reliving these terrifying moments.

3. In this state, numbing, avoidance, compliance, and restricted affect occurs: endogenous opiates are released to produce the numbing of pain as well as immobility. It is this parasympathetic mechanism that mediates the profound "detachment dissociation", a detachment from an unbearable situation. The infant is left staring into space with a glazed look. This is the infant's survival strategy when faced with terror without any other solution. It can, however, be dangerous because as the cortisol levels are elevated and there is a decrease in blood pressure, metabolic activity and heart rate collapse and even death can follow.

4. Finally, Schore describes how, in traumatic states of utter helplessness seen in children who are abused or neglected, both responses can be hyper-activated which results in the human infant experiencing "an inward flight" from the source of danger, in this case the threatening caregiver.

This process results in structural dissociation, a splitting of the Self which takes place for the infant to survive: children, and later adults will maintain their attachment to their desperately needed caregiver, by resorting to dissociation. In other words, they will develop an idealised attachment to their abuser by dissociating off their terrifying memories of being abused.

Bearing in mind that IWMs are internal representations of how the attachment figure is likely to respond to the child's attachment behaviour, two types of IWMs are created: that of an idealised attachment relation to mother and that of a "dysregulated Self in interaction with a miss-attuning frightening other" (Schore, 2001, p. 240). There may be many of the latter depending on what other terrifying experiences there have been between the child in relation to his or her terrifying or neglectful mother.

Could it be that some of the infants observed here, aged twelve to eighteen months, are, in fact, at different stages of developing this new way of coping with their terrifying situation?

An example in Main and Solomon's paper suggests to me that this may be the case:

> One infant hunched her upper body and shoulders at hearing her mother call, then broke into extravagant laugh-like screeches with an excited forward movement. Her braying laughter became a cry … And then suddenly she became silent, blank and dazed. (Main & Solomon, 1986, p. 119)

On hearing her mother's voice, this infant appears to be initially driven to move towards her and then she suddenly becomes silent, appearing blank and dazed: I think that Schore would agree that this is another example of freezing and dissociation. The ANS' parasympathetic defence system has taken over or "hijacked" the infant's attachment system to protect the helpless distressed infant, whose emotions are out of control: so she moves into a state of *dissociation*.

Whilst in that state, the development of the *traumatic attachment* and the two different types of IWMs could be taking place. According to Schore, the different dissociated states of the child in relation to the terrifying caregiver will develop around the fulcrum of the idealised attachment to that same caregiver. This results in the creation of different Self-states or different representations of themselves in relation to that same caregiver. By idealising their abusive mother, and "dissociating" all the past terrifying experiences with her, human infants can approach their mother when relational experiences would prevent any proximity to her, leading to the infant's certain death.

We have found these IWMs in those who suffer from fairly common disorders such as addictions or prolonged grief or from disorders with higher levels of dissociation resulting in a lack of Self-continuity in relation to the other, such as "borderline personality disorder" and other dissociative disorders, as we saw with Figen. All these individuals suffer to a varying degree from an inability to regulate their emotions, to empathise and mentalize. Bowlby referred to these as "segregated different states", achieved through a process of "defensive exclusion" we now call "dissociation" (1988, p. 70).

The idealised IWM of mother ensures traumatised infants' survival in early life

We can, therefore, hypothesise that the formation of the IWM of the idealised mother provides human infants with an invisible and unconscious way of maintaining their attachment to their abusive or neglectful mother in early life. Whilst rat pups and infant monkeys have developed a neurobiological system that enables them to behaviourally maintain their attachment to their mothers by clinging to her despite her abusive behaviour, human infants achieve the same result by creating an idealised unconscious traumatic attachment to their mother. They too will pay a price later in life.

The clinical evidence for this hypothesis will be presented in our therapeutic work with adult clients and patients, people who seek a way out of what they often feel is an unbearable existence.

The role of mother's face in relation to the genesis of disorganised attachment

Whilst Main focused her attention on studying infants who had suffered from abuse and neglect, she soon found out that many of these disorganised infants did not actually have abusing parents, at least not in the usual sense of the term. When she studied the parents' own attachment status using the Adult Attachment Interview that she developed (Main & Hesse, 1992) she found that many of these mothers suffered either from a recent loss or from the symptoms of PTSD at the time.

Their momentary blank faces would have betrayed moments of dissociation in relation to their past unresolved traumatic experiences or yet unmourned losses. Such experiences could affect their infants in the same way as the abusing mothers did because, when reliving a terrifying experience, during a flashback for instance, they could no longer connect with their child and their facial expression of fear or horror could have been terrifying to the child, leading to dissociation. Figen did not really see her baby once his male genitalia had triggered the memories of sexual abuse: he became the abuser of her past violating her in the present. This is very important because it explains why many of the infants who came from families where there was no evidence of abuse or neglect also developed a disorganised attachment (Main & Hesse, 1990).

Schore points out that mother's face is the most important visual stimulation in the child's world. Studies of attachment between mother and infant show that the mutual gaze that occurs between them triggers high levels of endogenous opiates in the child's growing brain. These are responsible for making the infant feel excited and happy in synchrony with their mother. Unfortunately, the opposite can also happen, as we saw in Main and Solomon's study.

During the phase of development between twelve and eighteen months, Mother's face is being encoded in the prefrontal-orbital area of the infant's right brain which specialises in encoding angry and fearful faces, both of which can lead to disorganised attachment behaviour (Schore, 2002). Indeed, the caregiver's face can be very frightening when the parent is angry and aggressive, but it can also be terrifying when a mother is "cut off" because she is dissociating.

Tronick's "still face" experiment (available on YouTube)

Professor Tronick at the University of Massachusetts Boston has worked for years to improve our understanding of infant mental life which, when he started his research in the 1970s, was almost non-existent. People did not believe that babies could engage in social interaction. This video is part of his study and it aims to show how infants are born ready to communicate and connect and how the way they are responded to by their caregiver matters enormously, with positive or negative lifelong consequences. Having just learnt that a parent's involuntary dissociation resulting from unmourned loss or unresolved trauma can be extremely damaging to their infant, we can see, from this video clip, just how sensitive a child is to changes in their parent's facial expressions.

It provides a very vivid example of how the lack of any expression on a mother's face can so easily precipitate emotional dysregulation which can lead to dissociation if the still face persists. I will be quoting Tronick's commentary from time to time as I describe what is happening in the video-recording of the "still face". This experiment involves a parent, in this case a mother, and a baby girl sitting facing each other.

> The mother starts by playing with her baby, who is about a year of age. She gives a greeting to the baby and the baby responds by giving a greeting back to her. Then the baby starts pointing to different places in the world whilst the mother is trying to engage with her. They are working to co-ordinate their emotions and their intentions, what they want to do in the world and that is really what the baby is used to.

And then, the researcher gets the mother to turn her face away from the baby and asks her not to respond to her baby as she faces her. "The baby very quickly notices this change and then she uses all of her abilities to try and get the mother back": she lifts an arm and looks at the ceiling, she smiles at the mother most invitingly and then she points because she is used to the mother looking at where she points, and makes a sound to go with it. She then puts both hands up in front of her and then leans back with a distressed face: she could be saying "what's happening here?" She claps her hands and, looking at the mother, she makes a screechy sound and could be saying "come on why aren't we doing this!" and then with an anguished look and clasping her hands together, she bites them.

Tronick points out that even in these *two minutes*, when babies don't receive a normal reaction, "they react with negative emotions, they turn away, they feel the stress of it and they actually lose control of their posture" as they twist about in their chair and cry because of the stress that they are experiencing.

At this point, the mother resumes her normal smiling behaviour and, leaning forward says "OK Becky, I'm here" in a very warm soothing voice, and she gently takes hold of her baby's arm and turns the child towards herself. The baby has regained her smile and looks straight at her mother who engages her by asking "and what are you doing?" and, as the baby lifts up her arms and leans forward with her arms outstretched, her mother responds by holding her daughter's hands in her hands and in this way they finish the downward movement of repair together.

Tronick then comments:

> It's a bit like the good, the bad, and the ugly. The good is that normal stuff that goes on and that we all do with our kids. The bad is when something bad happens but the infant can overcome it. When you stop the "still face", the mother and the baby start to play together again. The ugly is when you don't give the child any chance to get back to the good as happened with the parents of the disorganised infants in the Strange Situation.

This can happen for many reasons other than abuse or neglect or unresolved loss or trauma: a parent may be depressed or ill, or under the influence of drugs or alcohol. We have also developed a new relationship with a gadget that can so easily interfere with our parenting—the mobile phone: it rings and Mum picks it up to read a message, just as she was playing with her baby Jo. The message is interesting, and let's just see what else has come up. Meanwhile, baby Jo looks at Mum bemused and then tries to make contact to no avail. A minute later, we have a repeat of the "still face" experiment.

Other videos are available on YouTube that demonstrate how babies react just as strongly to their father's "still face". They behave in the same way in seeking connection with their fathers as they do with their mothers. It is important that fathers realise that they are very important in children's lives. Finnish fathers certainly know it and this kind of research reinforces one of the roles that fathers can have in their baby's life; they can have conversations, as we saw with Trevarthen's video in Chapter 2.

It is hardly surprising that infants are so affected by the "still face" because, in the natural environment in which we evolved, a still face could mean that the parent, be it mother or father, is either very ill, unconscious, or even dead. The infant's desperate attempts to bring her parent to life, and her final screams, are all attempts to ensure her own survival and a summons to the family or community to come to the rescue.

Sometimes, I feel that researchers in the field of disorganised attachment tend to minimise the emotional response of the infants they study by referring to their emotional experience as "fear". In my view "fear" relates more to how infants felt when they developed an avoidant attachment behaviour. The disorganised attachment is what follows when the attachment system is aroused to its most extreme level. It develops when a helpless infant or child feels the innate terror of either losing, physically or emotionally, the person they depend on entirely for their survival, or, of being threatened with death by the very being who is biologically there to enable them to live, a predicament for which there is no viable way out!

Liotti (2011) points out that "a fright without solution, even when devoid of violence or abuse, is akin to a traumatic event" (p. 57). These are *traumatic* experiences, which, using Lindemann's definition referred to earlier, are defined as "the sudden uncontrollable disruption of our attachment bonds" (1944). Now that we have seen how important our attachment bonds are for our well-being, providing us with the "emotional oxygen" of life, through attunement and empathy, we can begin to understand what such an experience means, especially to an infant whose development depends entirely on those magical interactions we saw so clearly in the elephant community and in these videos.

The importance of Tronick's 1975 video is that it also shows how a well an attuned sensitive mother can prevent dissociation taking place by regulating her distraught child's emotions back to the safety of their secure attachment relationship. It is well worth looking at, as it provides an example of the importance of *rupture and repair* in all human relations, and particularly in the therapeutic relationships.

One of my most severely traumatised patients, whose parents started neglecting and abusing her when she was still a premature infant, told me that she had often "gone blank" when psychotherapists simply sat in silence. She needed to feel connected to exist. Her parents' failure to attend to her terror left her with no solution but to dissociate in relation to any threat she experienced, however, mild it might seem to an outsider.

The "moral defence", toxic shame, and resistance to change

Returning to our understanding of disorganised infants and children, we have come to realise that, unfortunately, by idealising their mother and believing that their parent is a "good" parent, infants must also believe that they are to blame for their suffering and punishments. For some, who suffered from the effects of a disorganised attachment, life feels very bleak: many describe having this "pervasive belief" that they are "deeply and irredeemably flawed and unworthy which brings with it terrible feelings of shame". Their daily experience can be one of self-loathing and despair.

With reference to the moral defence, a recent study carried out in a psychiatric intensive acute-care setting of a hospital programme revealed preliminary findings which were consistent with the staff's clinical experience: a significant minority of their patients were found not to believe that they deserved to feel better. These particular patients were younger, diagnosed with more psychiatric disorders, and more likely to drop out of treatment or take longer to treat if they did not drop out.

> Patients with borderline personality disorder and posttraumatic stress disorder were significantly less likely to assert that they deserved to feel better. Patients with these disorders have frequently experienced abuse, bullying, assaults, and other forms of aggression in childhood and as adults. (Zimmerman & Becker, 2022a)

Ronald Fairbairn, a British psychiatrist and a psychoanalyst, named this self-belief the "moral defence": he pointed out that it has the advantage of giving disorganised children some sense of control over their future as well as the hope that, one day, especially if they are "good", they will finally obtain the loving care that they never had and still yearn for (1952).

This resulting sense of guilt and culpability also reinforces in their minds their identification with their abusing parents which, strangely enough, can rescue them from the terrifying state of disorganisation that they experience whenever they face their abuser. By being the one to blame for their terrible treatment they take control of their future, not their parent nor fate.

In this way, the "moral defence" can be *a powerful source of resistance to change in therapy* and may also be at the origin of disorganised controlling strategies adopted by many of these disorganised children from the age of four onwards.

Attachment disorganisation and the controlling strategies

As we learnt through Main's work with disorganised infants, their attachment system will be activated by terror or pain caused by their caregiver's neglect or abuse with the result that multiple fragmented representations of the Self are created around the fulcrum of the idealised attachment. These phenomena are very much in evidence in individuals who suffer from conditions with high levels of dissociation. They have no sense of self continuity as their Self is split into different representations of themselves in relation to their caregiver.

However, as Liotti pointed out, most of the children who develop a disorganised attachment do not suffer from its effects as they grow older. From about the age of four onwards "these disorganised children have developed an organised behavioural and attentional strategy towards their caregivers" (2011), which protects them from the distressing experiences of their past lives.

> Research data shows that they achieve such an organisation by exerting active control on their parents' attention and behaviour, either through caregiving or domineering-punitive

strategies. Controlling-caregiving strategies in children are identified by solicitous, overbright caring behaviour directed towards the caregiver. Controlling punitive strategies are identified by attempts to punish or embarrass the caregiver through harsh criticism. (Liotti, 2011, p. 237)

He notes that:

When disorganised Internal Working Models (IWMs) dominate their life since infancy, there is a good reason to inhibit the activities of the attachment system as often as possible throughout development: it protects both the child and their relationship with their parent's unbearably chaotic experience of disorganisation. (Liotti, 2011, p. 238)

These controlling strategies can collapse, however, when these children's attachment systems are strongly activated. For example, six-year-old *controlling* children appear to be well-oriented and organised in the way they think, behave, and seek attention, until they are shown pictures which remind them of their distressing past experiences of being neglected or abandoned, experiences that directly involve their attachment system.

One such picture shows parents leaving a child alone. The six-year-olds were asked what they thought the child in the picture would do, and how the child might feel in response to this experience of separation? These children, who had been judged as *disorganised* in the Strange Situation when they were one-year-old infants, responded by showing signs of "being inexplicably afraid and unable to do anything about it" (Kaplan, 1987, p. 109). One of the children said that the child in the picture felt "afraid!" and when asked why she was afraid, she said that "her dad might die and then she'll be by herself". And in response to being asked why she was afraid of that, she replies: "Because her mom died, she thinks her dad might die too".

This reaction seems "inexplicable" to the researcher because the little girl had not suffered any personal losses. However, knowing just how powerfully maternal separation affects these disorganised infants and how distressing they found the Strange Situation, her reaction makes more sense. This child is conveying to the researcher how terrifying her early disorganised experiences were for her: by equating them with death, she is showing how terrifying it is to be totally dependent on someone or something. It can kill one. Another boy's response to "What do you think the child will do?" replies: "Probably lock himself up." "Lock himself up?" the researcher asks. "Yeah, probably in his closet." "Then what will he do?" "Probably kill himself."

These responses reveal that the six-year-olds' disorganised attachments remained but were inhibited by the children's' subsequent controlling behaviours. For this reason, many studies and reviews on the role of the disorganised attachment suggest that it is present in many other conditions but may have been hidden by controlling strategies or be present in the body as somatic dissociative symptoms which are rarely picked up.

These findings suggest that at least three different developmental pathways are possible for these disorganised children:

1. For those children who have developed successful controlling strategies with their caregiver and who have not been exposed to any further strong or prolonged activation of their attachment system through further traumatic experiences, there is no theoretical reason why they should manifest any dissociative features linked with memories of fear without solution, especially if they are also attached to a secure parent or close caregiver. This is a very important point: being closely involved with a person who has a secure attachment is healing in itself.

2. For a few children whose controlling strategies may become so aggressive and punitive that they are seen to be socially unacceptable, the path is set for the development of a diagnosis of "adult personality disorders". In these cases, there may be occasional dissociative symptoms due to activation of the attachment system. These symptoms can quickly disappear if the individual resorts to his or her controlling defence by aggressive-punitive or compulsory caregiving behaviour (Liotti, 2011, pp. 239–240). This is a very good explanation of why so many children and adults, particularly men with a "disorganised attachment", resort to bullying and other abusive behaviours in order to cope with their feelings of insecurity or inadequacy. This certainly happens with couples prone to domestic violence.

3. An example of this is provided by a father who was severely beaten up by *his* father, as a child, because he did not behave as his father wanted. When this man became a father himself, he noticed that from the age of five, his son's disobedient behaviour enraged him, and he found himself beating him in the same way as he had been treated. Fortunately, through the loving understanding of his wife, he found the courage to have therapy and, by working through his early painful experiences, the need to re-enact his father's abuse disappeared.

4. Children brought up in traumatic and violent environments cannot escape the constant reactivation of their dysregulated attachment system so they develop dissociative attachment disorders as we saw with Figen after years of being sexually abused.

Right-hemisphere brain damage

If there is no attuned caregiver to restore the infant's psychobiological equilibrium, over-stimulation or under-stimulation of the neuronal circuits at critical periods of brain growth can lead to stress-induced unregulated cortisol and neurotransmitters secretions. For example, excess cortisol secretion is believed to be responsible for the atrophy of the hippocampus in women who have been sexually abused.

In addition, abnormalities in the brain's immune response brought about by microglia are currently being investigated. These very small glial cells are seen as protectors of the brain, keeping it clean and healthy. However, the most famous function of microglia is their role as the immune system of the brain. Like other immune cells in the rest of the body, microglia continually inspect the brain and, when they sense a threat, they become active and initiate the process of inflammation, which is the body's reaction against infection. Unfortunately, they can also cause damage or disease under the wrong conditions, and this is what is understood to be happening under conditions of toxic stress related to the disorganised attachment.

Excess activation of the stress response occurs when children are exposed to terrifying experiences of violence and neglect without the support of a caring adult. If no adult intervenes to protect the child, the stress response is further activated and can end up being set permanently on high alert. This results in damage to the areas of the brain involved in learning and reasoning to such an extent that the neurons are weaker and fewer, just when they should be multiplying.

We now know that severe early trauma also alters the development of the right brain, the hemisphere that is specialised for the processing socio-emotional information and bodily states. The early maturing right cerebral cortex is dominant for attachment functions (Henry, 1997; Schore, 2001; Siegel, 1999) and stores the IWMs of the attachment relationships. An enduring severe developmental impairment of this system would be expressed as a severe limitation of the essential activity of the right hemisphere involving particularly the prefrontal cortex and the limbic system, leading to emotional and cognitive deficits and a view of the world as a dangerous place. They result in an abnormal development which is often not apparent until adolescence (Sullivan, 2012).

Adolescence: the "second phase of socialisation"

Adolescence is often seen by parents and others as a time when their young ones lose their mind because of raging hormones, but Dan Siegel believes that these destructive myths are harmful because they prevent adults from understanding and supporting these young people during this very important period in their lives.

The adolescent is basically preparing to leave home and is driven by very strong emotions. Joining his or her peers provides the support that is needed to achieve this. The search for novelty provides new experiences and their creativity can lead teenagers to developing their own new ideas. They are, in the end, much better equipped to be independent and fulfil their aims in life.

However, during this phase, a lot is happening in the human adolescent's brain. The two most important areas of the right hemisphere involved in adolescence are the prefrontal cortex and the limbic system, which includes the amygdala and the hippocampus. The fact that the prefrontal cortex is affected has serious implications since it has many different and important roles:

1. It adjusts our emotional responses and integrates the body's internal state with our surrounding environment.

2. It regulates our levels of arousal via the reticular activating system as well as our ANS such as the *fight–flight–freeze* response.
3. It can inhibit impulses from the amygdala via the voluntary control of the mammalian vagus.
4. It enables us to attune and empathise with others.

Clearly, this vital part of our brain is essential for our survival and fulfilment in the community, enabling us to live in an attuned way and cope actively and passively with the stressors of daily life.

The limbic system's primary goals are emotional regulation and empathy:

1. The amygdala monitors nearly all sensory stimuli and is involved in regulating fear and aggression, in learning self-awareness, self-control, and interpersonal skills as well as preparing the organism for actions in the face of danger with input from the neocortex and activating the *fight–flight–freeze* response.
2. The hippocampus is very much involved in the making and integration of memories from different sensory modalities as well as influencing a person's mental state.

All these centres in the brain undergo significant changes during "normal" adolescence and it takes a long time for all parts of the brain to function well together. In some young people the amygdala may develop at a faster rate than the prefrontal cortex, and this is sometimes considered to be an explanation for risky behaviour. The temporary loss of integration at this period leads to impaired emotional regulation, mood swings, destructive behaviour, all of which can be enhanced by the changes and fluctuations of the sex and other hormones. But the result is a brain that has been enriched, pruned, and rewired to be more effective and integrated.

Parents often find their adolescent children very difficult and feel that they are no longer wanted but, the fact is that it is a very important time for parents to be involved as their child struggles between being a child and an adult at the same time. Reading Siegel's book *Brainstorm* may prove very helpful as it was written with the approval of adolescents and parents (2014).

There is some dispute as to how long adolescent issues can last but it is important for both parents and the community to take seriously its implications because it can span quite a few years. An article in *The Lancet* sums up the situation very well:

> Arguably, the transition period from childhood to adulthood now occupies a greater portion of the life course than ever before at a time when unprecedented social forces, including marketing and digital media, are affecting health and wellbeing across these years. An expanded and more inclusive definition of adolescence is essential for developmentally appropriate framing of laws, social policies, and service systems. Rather than age 10–19 years, a definition of 10-24 years corresponds more closely to adolescent growth and popular understandings of this life phase would facilitate extended investments across a broader range of settings. (Sawyer, Azzopardi, Wickremarathne, & Patton, 2018)

The *traumatic attachment* affects the same areas of the brain, but its effects are more pronounced and distressing as well as becoming permanent without social and/or therapeutic interventions, as will become apparent when we explore the main effects of the disorganised attachment.

It is important to realise that this is also a time when children who have suffered from attachment problems are at their most susceptible to change if the appropriate therapy can be made available to them and their families. It is also a time when an understanding supportive attuned adult can have a very positive effect on these young people.

Impaired emotional regulation and developmental trauma

The main problem for children with a disorganised attachment is the resulting loss of ability to regulate emotions. This is the most far-reaching effect of early trauma and neglect (Van der Kolk, 1989). It results in a failure to modulate sympathetic-dominant affects such as terror, rage, and, surprisingly, elation, or parasympathetic-dominant affects such as shame, disgust, and hopeless despair.

Shame is a particularly important emotional reaction in individuals with a vulnerable sense of Self and is particularly powerful in individuals whose sense of Self has been totally invalidated, such as victims of chronic neglect or abuse. As Gilligan made clear in his work with homicidal prisoners, the basic cause of violent behaviour is the wish to ward off or eliminate the feeling of shame or humiliation, a feeling that is painful and can be intolerable and even overwhelming and to replace it with its opposite, the feeling of power and pride. A "look" can be sufficient for man with a wounded Self to feel disrespected. As one of Gilligan's prisoners said: "Better be bad than not be at all" (Gilligan, 2001).

We are discovering that the developmental impact of early trauma, seen in the disorganised attachment, is particularly extensive and one of the main reasons for this extensive impact is the divided Self, born out of the need to develop the IWM of an idealised mother to survive. But, as Schore acknowledges, the other IWM of a "dysregulated self in relation to a miss-attuning other" (2001, p. 240), is also vulnerable to being hyperactivated or "triggered" and thereby induce violent behaviour. This will be vividly illustrated in our next chapter.

Traumatised brains and minds

As we saw earlier on, children brought up in traumatic and violent environments, at home or in their community, cannot escape the constant reactivation of their dysregulated "Self-in-relation-to-a-terrifying-dysregulating-mother".

The persistent activation of their *stress* response can also turn into a persisting fear state or "trait" under the control of the amygdala. Similarly, the volume of the orbitofrontal cortex is also reduced, which may account for more immediate *fight–flight–freeze* response, even when there is no real danger.

One could consider this to be an adaptive response to the terrifying and chaotic environment in which they live in poor neglected inner city areas. Children who are found to carry knives and commit knife crime in these environments often do so in order to survive in areas where drugs are sold and the streets are rife with rumours and fear. For these young people whose sense of Self is very vulnerable, a disrespectful look or an aggressive word can be threatening enough to trigger into action past IWMs of terrifying experiences at the hands of past abusers. The outcome can often be another wounded or dead child and a distraught family.

Some young men with a criminal history report that they get a "high" when stalking their "human prey" and male children faced with a neutral face often feel threatened or under attack. Girls, on the other hand, tend to dissociate and are often more anxious. It is said that their first response to threat is often to "tend and befriend". However, many are now involved in aggressive street gangs.

Vulnerability to complex trauma

Infants exposed to chronic abuse or neglect show a reduction in cortisol secretion during subsequent frightening episodes; this low cortisol response can lead to increased vulnerability to PTSD in later life as Yehuda found out when she was studying the victims of road traffic accidents. These victims had their blood taken for alcohol and cortisol levels and one would assume that having survived a frightening accident, the cortisol levels would be high. However, she found that the victims who developed PTSD had a lower-than-normal release of cortisol. Yehuda concluded that PTSD may in fact reflect a "biologic sensitisation disorder" rather than a post-traumatic stress disorder (Yehuda, 1997). Wang attributed this sensitisation to changes in their attachment system as she noted that many insecure children tended to show suppression of the cortisol levels over time (Wang, 1997).

We now know that childhood abuse and/or neglect are key factors in the development of complex trauma in veterans (Bernstein et al., 2022) and a secure attachment is the primary defence against trauma induced psychopathology. So, Yehuda was right, but that has not changed the way the American Psychiatric Association (APA), involved in creating the latest *Diagnostic and Statistical Manual of Mental Disorders* (*DSM-5*), view the importance of child abuse and neglect. They simply removed complex PTSD and refused to replace it with Van der Kolk's diagnosis for trauma in children which he called "developmental trauma".

British psychiatrists were able to show some independence of spirit in relation to their American colleagues by both improving and retaining the diagnosis of complex PTSD in the WHO's *International Classification of Diseases* (*ICD-11*) which is widely used internationally (World Health Organization, 2019/2021).

Epigenetic transmission of the traumatic attachment

Direct transmission

Figen's experience with her child shows one of the ways that the disorganised attachment and its accompanying traumatic attachment is transmitted directly to the next generation. During our work in the TSS at the Maudsley Hospital in London, several refugee women, who had been raped when in captivity abroad, subsequently reported that their babies' eyes reminded them of their abuser and had become the "trigger" that brought back the awful memories of being violated. They were suffering from complex trauma. These women had chosen to keep their babies and were very distressed to find that their baby had this terrible effect on them.

At such moments, the mother would be overwhelmed, both mentally and physically, by the terrible flashbacks of what she experienced at the hands of her assailant, and she would be unable to respond to her child's desperate need for comfort and reassurance. During flashbacks, traumatised individuals relive their past terrifying experiences as if they are happening all over again. Their infant faces a mother in a state of terror or dissociation; she is no longer there for her young one as her face and behaviour have become the cause of his terror. Her baby, in a state of extreme fear without any solution, will freeze and dissociate for self-protection.

It is interesting to note that these infants were all male, like their mother's abusers, so that it may be that this additional factor contributed to the triggering of their mother's traumatic experiences. The therapeutic team was well aware that mothers suffering from complex PTSD are unable to prevent themselves from traumatising their own infants *because* of the flashbacks that they experience. To spare them any further distress, their names were transferred to the top of our waiting list so as to receive treatment for their traumatic experience as soon as possible, and social services were recruited to help with the child care.

Epigenetic transmission via the womb

Following the terrorist attack the World Trade Center on 11 September 2001, Yehuda carried out a study on pregnant women in New York who developed PTSD as a result of this event. She subsequently studied their babies and found that these were born with lower levels of cortisol than normal, which made them more vulnerable to PTSD later on in life. This was the result of epigenetic transmission from the mother to the foetus carried out by methylation of certain genes which were prevented from producing the normal amount of cortisol (Yehuda et al., 2005). Similar low levels of cortisol were found in the children of Holocaust survivors.

Could such changes be an evolutionary adaptation to survival in a more destructive environment?

The implications of a dissociated Self in relation to therapy

Liotti (2011) maintains that the structural dissociation of the Self should be considered "primarily as an intersubjective reality hindering the process of consciousness rather than as a defence against mental pain", which is how many see it. This also concurs with what Siegel stated: "Our minds are created by the functioning of our brains and the ways in which information and energy flows within us and between us." He adds in relation to the mind: "The mind can be understood as patterns of flow and energy. As we will see, energy and flow within one brain, or between brains. In this manner, the ways in which energy and information flow within an individual and or between two individuals helps create the experience of mind" (Siegel, 2001).

One therefore assumes from this that, for Siegel, "stress" leads to a reduction in the complexity of the mind as it rigidifies and becomes less of a free-flowing open system. This is very important clinically as it explains why the flow of energy due to attunement and empathy declines with the severity of trauma; this is also important in relation to the treatment of these individuals.

Liotti is one of the very few psychoanalytic psychotherapists who really addressed the implications of the *traumatic attachment*: it certainly stresses the brain in early life by dividing the Self and actually altering the neurodevelopmental pathways of the affected infant. Faced with a divided Self, he reasons that the psychotherapy of pathological dissociation should be carried out in phases, the first of which should be that of achieving attachment security and only secondarily focusing on trauma work.

As will become apparent in the following chapters, to achieve a secure attachment, the Self must be integrated by removing the dissociation. This is borne out by the clinical cases we present in treatment using the TAIP to reverse the dissociative effects of the *traumatic attachment*. This leads us on to asking ourselves which disorders are affected by the presences of a divided Self and how do we identify them? The fact is that, according to the NSPCC in the UK, half a million children suffer from abuse and neglect every year. This means that there are thousands of adults who have developed a *traumatic attachment* in order to survive their childhood terror and, in so doing, they have developed split Selves.

What is the main manifestation of a split Self?

From the little work that we had done so far in the TSS, certain patients' failure to move on in therapy appeared to be linked to a past history of having suffered from childhood abuse. We felt stuck and this is what led me to develop the TAIP with the help of Johnson. I was lucky enough to have seen his work and learnt from it. However, one of the most challenging aspects of working as a therapist remains finding ways to deal with clients who, despite their stated wish to alter their behaviour, appear to find it very difficult to change and overcome destructive patterns.

Much has been written by psychoanalytic theorists about why clients behave in this counter-productive and apparently irrational way, starting with Freud for whom the discovery of what he refers to as the patient's "resistance" led to the concept of repression and the unconscious: this became the foundation for psychoanalysis. This "unconscious" resistance was identified by Fairbairn as the "moral defence" which he acknowledges gives the patient the powerful role of being to blame for whatever he has done to anger his parent and, in so doing, provides him with the hope of one day getting it right so as to finally get the love that he still yearns for (1952). As noted earlier, men and women suffering from the effects of the traumatic attachment find it very difficult to free themselves from its powerful embrace.

However, one man stands out for the huge impact of his work in this field; he is a physician, not a psychiatrist. Whilst Main and others were carrying out research into the disorganised attachment, an eminent and courageous doctor in San Diego, USA, called Vincent Felitti, was struggling to make sense of his patients' behaviour in a recently developed obesity clinic in Kaiser Permanente's Department of Preventive Medicine. Its programme was designed for people who were 100 to 600 pounds overweight. By 1985, he had observed that 50 per cent of the people who attended had dropped out whilst they were actually losing weight, not gaining it, and that they had proceeded to put it all on again.

This is a familiar experience for most therapists and psychiatrists who have had clients or patients who don't appear to be able to get better, however hard they try. Until we had discovered the TAIP, we did not really understand why quite a few of the people who had made the effort to have therapy would drop out for no known reason, or just remain "stuck"; however, we now know that individuals with a past history of disorganised attachment may well opt to cling to their unconscious moral defence in order to maintain their secret attachment to their idealised mother and remain in control of their lives.

Felitti was an unusual physician because, instead of giving up or speculating about possible causes for this behaviour, he decided to get to the bottom of this mystery by actually conducting face-to-face interviews with approximately two hundred "drop outs", using the same standard set of questions for everyone. He had nothing to report for weeks until, one day, he made a mistake and instead of asking, "How old were you when you were first sexually active?", he asked: "How much did you weigh when you were first sexually active?" The patient, who was a woman, replied "Forty pounds." Being unable to really take on board the implications of what he was hearing, he asked the same question again. She gave the same answer and then burst into tears and added, "It was when I was four years old, my father."

Felitti was shocked as he had only met one patient who had been sexually abused in his entire career. He soon found himself interviewing more and more patients who brought up the same history of child abuse. He thought, "This can't be true. Someone would have told me in medical school." Felitti then decided to ask five of his colleagues to interview one hundred patients in the weight programme only to find out that they turned up with similar disturbing stories: out of 286 patients they had interviewed, a clear majority had been sexually abused as children.

That was alarming enough, but Felitti was struck by other findings after interviewing a woman who had been raped when she was twenty-three years old. In the year after this attack, she put on 105 pounds. He then heard her mutter: "Overweight is overlooked, and that is what I need to be." This made Felitti realise that for these people who were 100 to 400 pounds overweight, they did not see their weight as a problem. For them it was a solution that made them feel better because it soothed their anxiety, their fears, or their depression. In other words, without food, these people became "dysregulated", as they must have done as infants when exposed to their abusive parent. Food for these people was what alcohol is for alcoholics, or drugs are for drug addicts: "a way of making the terrible pain feel better", as one of his patients said. Felitti felt that these explanations provided him with satisfactory motivations for his patients' behaviour and helped him feel sympathetic and supportive towards them.

He also wanted to share his findings with other professionals and, understandably, he chose as his first audience, the North American Association for the Study of Obesity, which included psychiatrists and psychologists. Their response was, I am sorry to say, predictable. He reports: "I was told that I was naive to believe my patients, that it was commonly understood by those more familiar with such matters that these patients' statements were fabrications to provide a cover explanation for their failed lives" (Stevens, 2012).

At around the same time, I had the same response during my psychotherapy training at the Maudsley Hospital when I was being supervised for my work with a woman who informed me that she had been sexually abused. My Kleinian supervisors told me, in no uncertain terms, that it was all in her mind and that I should not believe such stories.

In 1896, Freud was to come to the same conclusions as my psychoanalytic colleagues after giving his first paper on "hysteria" to the illustrious Psychiatric Society in Vienna where he revealed that:

> At the bottom of every case of hysteria there are one or more occurrences of premature sexual experiences, occurrences which belong to the earlier years of childhood but which can be reproduced through the work of psychoanalysis. (Freud, 1896c, p. 212)

> Sexual experiences in childhood consisting in stimulation of the genitals, coitus-like acts, and so on, must therefore be recognised, in the last analysis, as being the traumas, which lead to a hysterical reaction to events at puberty and to the development of hysterical symptoms. (ibid., pp. 206–207)

The abuser, he discovered was all too often a close relative and he could not have been more up-to-date in his conclusion when, referring to the vulnerability of the infant and the childhood brain, he stated:

> Injuries sustained by an organ which is yet immature, or by a function that is in the process of developing, often cause more severe and lasting effects than they could do in more mature years. (ibid.)

Freud therefore believed that the diagnosis of hysteria could be ascribed to what we would now refer to as complex trauma following an early history of sexual abuse and a resulting disorganised attachment.

However, his wonderful paper was met with an icy silence by his new psychiatric colleagues and the presiding professor said; "It sounds like a scientific fairy tale." Freud was very upset, and his reaction was understandable because he believed he had discovered, "through the process of thought that remained unconscious" that early trauma was one of the main causes of many types of mental illnesses. As a result of his colleagues' response to his most important discovery, "the solution to a more than a thousand-year-old problem", Freud was to turn his back on his patients and the reality of their traumatic experiences in order to be able to earn a living in Vienna (Zulueta, 2006a, pp. 161–163).

Returning to Felitti, he was luckier than Freud because an epidemiologist, who had attended the meeting where his results were dismissed, suggested to him that he carry out a study with thousands of patients from the general population. He then introduced him to Dr Robert Anda, a medical epidemiologist at the US Centers for Disease Control and Prevention who was very interested in studying the links between emotions and physical illnesses. Felitti agreed to carry out this research project and Anda then spent a year studying the research literature on childhood trauma before setting up the study in Kaiser Permanente. It involved 17,421 patients who agreed to help the team understand how childhood events might affect adult health.

Every patient filled out a detailed biopsychosocial medical questionnaire before undergoing a complete physical medical examination and extensive laboratory tests. Anda added to this a questionnaire that focused on what he named adverse childhood experiences (ACEs): these are defined as toxic stressful experiences occurring in childhood that directly harm a child, such as physical or sexual abuse, or that affect the environment in which they live, such as growing up in a house with domestic violence.

He selected ten major ACEs which included five types of abuse—sexual, verbal and physical, emotional and physical neglect—and five types of family dysfunction—a parent who is mentally ill or alcoholic, a mother who is a domestic violence victim, a family member who has been in prison, and the loss of a parent through divorce or abandonment (Bellis et al., 2016).

This was the first survey that looked at the effects of different types of traumas simultaneously. The surveys began in 1995 and continued through to 1997 with the participants being followed for over fifteen years. The results were astonishing, bearing in mind how little people knew what was going on in the lives of millions of children in the privacy of their homes. When the first results came in, Anda told his interviewer that he wept: "I saw how much people had suffered."

Some major facts emerged from this study which are highly relevant to our study of the disorganised attachment and its resulting *traumatic attachment*:

1. There was a direct link between childhood trauma and adult onset of chronic disease, as well as mental illness, doing time in prison, and work issues, such as absenteeism.
2. About two-thirds of the adults had experienced one or more types of ACEs. Of these, 87 per cent had experienced two or more types of ACEs. For instance, people who had

an alcoholic father were likely to have also experienced physical or emotional abuse. So, ACEs did not usually happen in isolation.

3. Most of these ACEs resulted in a higher risk of medical, psychological, or social problems as an adult. To explain this, Felitti and Anda developed a scoring system whereby each type of adverse childhood experience counted as one point.

4. The more ACE scores an individual had suffered, the more likely they were to suffer from a biomedical condition: for instance, with four or more ACE scores, the greater the likelihood of a cancer diagnosis compared to someone with zero ACE scores.

5. The more ACE scores an individual had endured, the greater the incidence of:
    i.   Smoking, severe obesity, alcohol, and drug abuse.
    ii.   Ischaemic heart disease, strokes, and chest diseases.
    iii. Diabetes, hepatitis, sexually transmitted diseases.
    iv.   Depression and attempted suicide.
    v.   They are also more likely to be violent, to have multiple marriages, and more auto-immune diseases.

6. One of the interesting findings relates to the risk of being a victim of domestic violence which is higher the more ACEs you have suffered as a woman and less so if you are a man. It also shows that the risk of perpetrating domestic violence is higher the more ACEs you have experienced as men or women. This confirms the existence of a template or IWM of abuse whereby victims tend re-enact their traumatic experience in terms of either being the abuser or the victim, another pathway for the transmission of the traumatic attachment.

7. Another surprising finding in this study is that over a third had attended college and 40 per cent had one college degree or more. They all had jobs as well. As Anda said: "It's not just 'them'. It's us."

New ACEs have had to be added to the original ten as they left out racism, peer violence, bullying, community violence, war, poverty, and environmental disasters.

Felitti made it his mission in life to share his and Anda's very important findings and publish more research (Anda et al., 2006). Without doubt, he has shown us how early damage to the infant mind, that is, body and brain, due to ACEs, is probably the most important determinant of the health and well-being of the US nation (Felitti, 2002). Similar results have been obtained in the UK (Bellis, 2016). The fact that these results challenge the effectiveness of the current medical model in dealing with the ill health of so many in our countries is because it is so closely linked to the pharmaceutical industry; this means that these findings are often ignored or rejected by professionals whose living depends on things as they are (Davies, 2022).

However, a large programme of trauma-informed care has taken off in the US and in certain parts of the UK. Based on the research on attachment that we looked at in the early part of this book and supported by the trauma work carried out by Bloom, Van der Kolk,

Herman, and many others, a different way of caring for those who suffer from the effects of ACEs is being developed called trauma-informed care (TIC). Unlike the current medical approach that focuses on asking "What is wrong with you?", individuals seeking help in a TIC setting are asked "What has happened to you?" We will be looking at this new approach when we examine new therapeutic ways that are now available for healing the fractured minds in the last part of this book.

However, one major aspect of Felitti and Anda's study remains unanswered: why couldn't the patients in his obesity clinic finish their weight-losing programme? Do the explanations given by Felitti's patients give a satisfactory reason for why they did not continue to lose weight? They clearly satisfied Felitti's curiosity, but many patients who suffer from the developmental effects of a disorganised attachment do not have explanations for their failure to complete their therapeutic programme, such as people suffering from addictions, unresolved grief, depression, or complex trauma to name but a few. The forthcoming chapters on the use of the TAIP will provide them and their therapist with the answers they seek.

Conclusion

What we have learnt so far, through the evidence presented by Main and her colleagues, is that when an infant is faced with a terrifying caregiver, who can be mother or another important attachment figure on whom the infant depends, they will behave in a disorganised way and end up "freezing". According to Schore, what is happening during the Strange Situation is that, after some initial movement towards the caregiver, driven by the attachment drive, the terrifying parent triggers the infant's ANS *fight–flight–freeze* defence response which results in dissociation, as observed in several infants in the Strange Situation.

And, as we know that abused and neglected infants, children, and later adults, demonstrate a paradoxical attachment to their abusing parent, Schore assumed that an internal process takes place when the infant freezes that ends up providing the infant with what he or she yearns for most—an "idealised" mother to protect him or her.

He describes how an IWM of this idealised attachment to mother develops to counter the terrifying lived experiences of being abused or abandoned by the infant's real mother: this requires a splitting of the Self into two IWMs of "me in relation to an idealised mother" to exist separately from the IWMs of "me-in-relation-to-a-terrifying-dysregulating-mother".

This is what is referred to as *structural dissociation* and the resulting paradoxical attachment is what is referred to as the *traumatic attachment*.

The dissociated infant Self remains traumatically attached to the idealised mother of his or her early life which means that the normal process of neurobiological development cannot take place due to the overriding effect of the dissociation that is splitting the developing Self into two. The effects of this pathological process become increasingly evident in adolescence and in adulthood, as was observed in other mammals (Sullivan, 2012).

What has happened to these infants is that the ANS' defence system has "hijacked" the infant's normal developmental pathway. Whilst this is visibly enacted in rats and monkeys by their infants clinging to their abusive mothers, the human child and, later, the adult, simply behave in accordance with the need of the split infant Self clinging to his or her imaginary mother in order to survive.

CHAPTER 4

Eliciting the traumatic attachment with the TAIP

Weaning in primates

The quality of primate life depends so much on the relationship between the parent and child that it is not surprising that human infants and children share common difficult experiences with their primate cousins before reaching the more independent state of adulthood. Let us see if anything like the effects of the *traumatic attachment* can be observed in the family life of chimpanzees with whom we share 96 per cent of our genes. Jane Goodall's account of her thirty years spent observing chimpanzee family life in the Gombe National Park in Tanzania provides us with vivid examples of their behaviour during the different phases of their lives. This is a species where the males play hardly any role in the early development of their infants and illustrates the difficulties that can occur when males are not involved in this phase of primate life.

Goodall was very interested in the links between chimpanzee infant behaviour and different types of mothering (Goodall, 1990, p. 27). One of the examples she gives is particularly distressing and resonates very much with what happens to human infants whose mothers are unable to provide them with the secure attachment that they require for a fulfilling social life.

Flo was a particularly successful female chimp. Her mothering skills were reflected in the success of her sons reaching the top of the social hierarchy and her daughter's competence as a mother in her own right. Mothering qualities in chimpanzee life become particularly obvious during weaning which normally occurs in the infant's fourth year. At this point in time, the mother is usually pregnant and is preparing herself for the arrival of her next infant: this requires her to prevent her current child from suckling at the breast and riding on her back—harsh measures which she has to adopt with increasing firmness and frequency.

> The birth of the next baby signals the beginning of a new era for the previous child. No longer can they claim the mother's full attention, no longer can they ride on her back or creep into the warm sanctuary of her nest at night. Infancy is left behind. However, although the mother can no longer lavish her full attention, she is still there to provide reassurance and protection. She will groom the older child far more than she grooms the younger and share food in response to begging. The new-fledged juvenile, therefore, even if upset initially, usually recovers quickly and becomes even more fascinated by the baby. (Goodall,1990, p. 162)

Unfortunately, Flo's last son, Flint, did not follow the normal route towards independence; his mother's pregnancy at such an old age deprived her of the strength and energy to wean Flint. When she tried to prevent him from suckling or riding on her back, his temper tantrums were so violent and aggressive that she gave in to him, again and again. As a result, he was still suckling when his sister Flame was born, and he would push his way into Flo's nest at night. "At the same time, he became increasingly depressed, playing seldom and spending long hours sitting close to Flo and grooming her." And then, Flo became ill and, one night, her infant Flame disappeared. When his mother had recovered from her illness, Flint resumed riding on her back and creeping into bed with her. Many months later, Flo died, and his life took a turn for the worse.

Goodall makes the point that even youngsters who are nutritionally independent may become so affected by the loss of their mother that they pine away and die. Flint was eight-and-a-half years old when Flo died and should have been able to look after himself, but it seemed that he did not have the will to survive without her.

> Never shall I forget watching as, three days after Flo's death, Flint climbed slowly into a tall tree near the stream. He walked along one of the branches, then stopped and stood motionless, staring down at an empty nest. After about two minutes, he turned away, and with the movements of an old man, climbed down, walked a few steps, then lay, with wide eyes staring ahead. The nest was one that he and Flo had shared a short while before Flo died. (ibid., p. 165)

His big brother and sister tried to help him and feed him, but he would always return to the place where his mother had died and then he, too, fell sick.

> The last short journey he made, pausing to rest every few feet, was the very place where Flo's body had lain. There he stayed for a few hours, sometimes staring and staring into the water. He struggled on a little further and then curled up, and never moved again. (ibid., p. 165)

This sad story makes me think of the infants in Main's Strange Situation, whose only recourse to survival is to invent an idealised mother in their minds. By spending the last moments of his life in the very place where his mother passed away, Flint appears to be enacting his desperate need to join her. Many of the people I have worked with, whose troubled early life left them with the same desperate yearning for the mother that never was, tried to do the same in desperate acts of suicide.

The work we are going to share in relation to the TAIP often feels as if we are dealing with a delayed separation process akin to "weaning" when it relates to the mother and, in some cases, when it is carried out in relation to the father or another caregiver who had a similar role for the child. It involves letting go of infancy and growing up to become fully adult. Several clients described in this book present with addiction and unresolved grief for their mother and as will become clear, these disorders can be resolved. Using the TAIP, they were able to let go of their "addiction" and finally grieve their unmourned parents and lost childhood, thereby resuming the normal cycle of life.

Discovering how to reverse the traumatic attachment

So, how did I find out about this innovative approach? I came across the work of the now Professor Bob Johnson by chance, when watching a programme on television describing the work of a psychiatrist in Parkhurst Prison. The prevention of violence is a subject of great interest to me, so when I saw what this colleague of mine was able to achieve with his patient and others who had committed homicide, I was amazed and naturally very curious. It opened my mind to the therapeutic possibility of being able to stop violent men and women from committing further destructive acts. As I thought through what took place in terms of Bowlby's attachment theory, which plays an enormous role in violent behaviour, I realised that what Bob Johnson was doing was reversing the *traumatic attachment*'s deadly grip on the adult minds of abused and neglected infants.

Making sense of Johnson's approach to curing mental pain and violence

As a psychiatrist in Parkhurst Prison, working on a ward for dangerous men, he appeared on the BBC, interviewing one of the prisoners called Lenny. This man, in his late forties, had committed homicide. By the time the film was made, he had shared with his psychiatrist his personal life history and his main traumatic experience, which was of having been regularly "battered" by his mother as a child. He admitted that he was frightened of her, and, with his therapist, he had begun to make links between his fear and his violent behaviour.

The interview that follows is conducted in the knowledge that Lenny battered his mate to death when the latter, who had been stealing with him on a wet evening, insisted that they spend the night in the comfort of his mother's house rather than under the leaking roof of a barn. When Lenny refused, terrified at the thought of turning up at his mother's house with their stolen goods, his friend responded by mocking him. Lenny picked up a log and battered him to death.

In a film clip of an early therapeutic session, Lenny appears quite rigid in the way he sits and responds to Dr Johnson, even though a trusting relationship has developed between them. His therapist, who has obtained informed consent to both film and to proceed with his therapeutic approach, says to him:

> (B is the therapist; L the patient)
> B: Say your mother was sitting over there (on the other side of the room), what would you say to her?
> L: I'd say "Mother, you can't hit me anymore, I am an adult."

The patient then slumps in his chair, looks down and then raises his hand over his mouth with an accompanying fearful expression—just like some of the disorganised infants in the Strange Situation conducted by colleagues of Main. His rigidity can be ascribed to the terror that he still feels as he imagines that his mother is in the room, as if her presence was no longer imaginary and he was still small and vulnerable.

> B: And you believe that?
> L: Yes, partly.
> B: Can you tell her you are an adult?
> L: I could try.
> B: You'd find it difficult?
> L: Yes, I would.
> B: Do you find that surprising, that you find it difficult to tell your mother you're an adult?
> L: Yes, very surprising.
> B: It is, isn't it? So, what will stop you? Say your mother was sitting over there, what would you say to her?
> L: I'd say "Mother, you can't hit me anymore. I'm an adult."
> B: And you believe that?
> L: Yes, partly. (Lenny replies as he did before, at which point Johnson laughs, a warm laugh.)
> B: You partly believe and partly don't! (This engages Lenny to laugh as well.)
> L: I don't know whether I could say that to her or not.
> B: What would stop you?
> L: (with conviction) Fear.
> B: Fear of what? What's she going to do?
> L: She might get up and clout me.
> B: Might she?
> L: Well she might.
> B: How old is she?
> L: Eighty-five.
> B: And she is going to do you an injury, is she? (Johnson challenges Lenny in a friendly voice.)
> L: (rather defensively) Oh she's still lively.
> B: Eighty-five. How big is she?
> L: Five feet, two inches.
> B: And how big are you?
> L: Six feet, three and a half inches.

B: It doesn't sound much of a match, does it?

L: No, but you can't hit a woman, can you?

This film illustrates how, by asking this dangerous man to face his mother in his imagination and tasking him to tell her that he is an adult whom she can no longer beat up, Johnson has elicited what looks and sounds like the IWM of a terrified child in relation to a very violent mother. This Child Self could have belonged to any one of the disorganised infants in Main's Strange Situation experiment.

To achieve this, Johnson has had to work on at least two fronts:

1. He has had to develop a relationship of trust with the adult Lenny who has allowed Johnson to put him through an experience that could so easily have been felt as humiliating and therefore dangerous for his psychiatrist. I believe that this level of trust can only be achieved when patients feel that their therapist is attuned to them and has a genuine desire to help them overcome their many difficulties, born out of their past experiences. Johnson does this by repeatedly supporting and encouraging the patient's Adult Self to help his Child Self face his childhood "demons" by declaring his grown-up independence from his mother and his resultant immunity from her attacks.

2. Johnson is also very much in touch with the depth of the terror that his patient experienced in his childhood and still experiences, as is made evident in the session. This is crucial because Lenny committed his crime when his mate challenged him to seek shelter at his mother's house. The very idea must have made him feel as terrified as he felt as a child.

The effect was to reactivate the internal representation of him, the "bad kid" victim, in relation to his terrifying punishing mother. This is encapsulated in his Child Self's IWM of a "dysregulated self in interaction with a mis-attuning and frightening other" as Schore put it rather technically. When his mate then mocked him for his refusal to face his mother, Lenny must have felt so humiliated that he re-enacted the IWM of the abuser–victim, only this time, he became the aggressor and his mate the victim whom he battered to death (Johnson, 1997).

As Gilligan wrote:

> Shame is the emotional reaction of a Self that has been totally invalidated and is extremely important in triggering violent reactions in victims of chronic abuse and neglect. The basic cause of violent behaviour is the wish to ward off or eliminate the feeling of shame and humiliation—a feeling that is painful and can even be intolerable and overwhelming—and replace it with its opposite, the feeling of power and pride. "Better be bad, than not be at all." (Gilligan, 2001, p. 29)

What we hear in the session is so interesting because Lenny, this big powerful man, cannot help voicing the terror of his Child Self when faced with his imagined mother who used to beat him up. By making Lenny imagine that he is in the room with his mother and by asking him to declare his adulthood, Johnson is asking the Adult Self to overcome the terror that his Child Self still feels. In so doing, Johnson is activating Lenny's speech area which is in the left hemisphere and thereby connecting his left hemisphere with his right hemisphere where the Child Self's implicit or unconscious memories are stored.

Could it be that by encouraging the Adult Self to express the reality of his adulthood in order to overcome his Child Self's terror of their mother, Johnson has brought the embodied Child Self and conscious Adult Self in contact with each other to overcome together their terrifying early experiences? In so doing, the dissociation that kept them apart across the hemispheres begins to melt and the healing of the fractured Self can begin to take place, as we have witnessed with many of our clients.

This explanation for what is taking place in Johnson's treatment which he calls Verbal Physiotherapy, is indirectly supported by an important positron emission tomography or PET study conducted by Rauch on traumatised patients suffering from PTSD (Rauch et al., 1996). They report that when these individuals were asked to describe their traumatic experience, the speech area known as Broca's area in the left hemisphere shuts down. (In my understanding, this reaction is related to the *freeze* response which we share with other mammals when in danger of being killed by a predator, which I describe in Chapter 3.)

By making his patient speak aloud to his terrifying mother, Johnson is activating his speech area and basically healing Lenny's traumatised mind by initiating the melt-down of the dissociation between the two Selves. It makes sense of the name he has given to his therapeutic modality, "Verbal Physiotherapy for Speechless Terror" (2018).

When discussing this video, Johnson points out that Lenny is not able to "think straight" because of his terror: to everyone else he appears to be an adult, but he cannot experience this because the presence of his imagined mother is enough to elicit his embodied split Child Self, the victim of his mother's abuse.

The last session of treatment

After eight weeks of gently coaxing Lenny to let his mother know that he is now an adult and that she can no longer hit him, Johnson records another session with Lenny. The latter now looks relaxed and confident: he has a strong voice, and he moves his arms and body freely when he leans forward to share something important with his psychiatrist. It made me realise how rigid he had been in the first interview when he was still frozen with terror.

His therapist asks him what he would do if his mother was coming across to hit him.

Lenny answers "Oh, in no way would she hit me now!"
"What would you say?" asks Johnson.
"I wouldn't have to say anything," he replies. "If she went to slap me, I'd just hold her arm!" He is smiling and laid-back.
Johnson laughs with delight and Lenny joins him, whilst repeating, "I would!"
"You did not have the confidence to do that before."

In response, his patient leans forward and says, "If this were to have happened years ago, had a doctor taken an interest—say when I was in my twenties, and said what you would say and *we conquered it* and I went to the house, and suppose I came home late, and she says blah blah blah and went to hit me, I'd say, 'Mother, you can't hit me luv, I'm grown up, you can't do it.'"

Moving forward in his chair, he addresses his imaginary mother: "You can kick me out of the house."

"'Cause it's your home," says Johnson, acknowledging that Lenny is right.

Lenny continues, having given his mum a face-saving way out of the conflict: "It's your house, but you can't hit me, don't try and hit me."

Johnson acknowledges the change: "You've never said that."

"I've never said that," responds his proud patient.

"You've never said that up to the last month or two, have you?"

"I've never had the confidence to say that, have I?" Lenny replies.

"That's right."

Lenny then adds, "You're brainwashed into fear. It's like a brainwash."

Johnson responds, "That's wonderful. That's very clear."

His patient became a model prisoner, but Johnson's revealing new approach was of no interest to his psychiatric forensic colleagues. Perhaps they feared it would challenge the penal system in which they work.

Johnson says that what he has found is that, by encouraging his patient to say, with his support, "Hello mother, I am an adult"—which happens to be the true, and Lenny recognises it to be true—he eventually gets used to saying it and can say it without difficulty. Johnson then informs us that what they are doing in these sessions is having a curious effect because it stops him getting angry and stops him getting violent in the prison unlike the previous Lenny who was always getting into trouble (Johnson, 2005).

Johnson strongly believes in the power of emotions since they are what make us engaged and active human beings. And, as we saw in his work with Lenny, he acknowledged the core emotion of infant and childhood trauma as being that of "speechless terror" and the power of "warm emotions to melt" this terror (Johnson, 2018).

Before leaving Johnson and Lenny, it is important to stress that this work is only possible if the therapist is both aware of the reality of the childhood terror and, at the same time, aware of the reality that Lenny is now an adult who no longer needs to fear his old mother. He is both understanding and supportive as he communicates nonverbally: "I am with you, and you can do it!"

Applying Johnson's approach in the Traumatic Stress Service

Many years later, in the TSS at the Maudsley Hospital, we realised that we had too many patients on our waiting list for therapy; at the same time, so many of the men and women who were in therapy seemed unable to work towards a successful conclusion with their therapist. They appeared stuck, and we felt that we were stuck with them: we recognised that we were facing the challenging issue of what is often referred to as "dependency in therapy" which occurs so often with individuals who suffer from the effects of complex trauma and dissociation; in other words, people who suffered from the effects of a disorganised attachment and the resulting *traumatic attachment*.

I did not see this as clearly as I do now, but I recognised that we often felt that our patients were behaving in a "childish" way by making impossible demands on us, especially in relation to their many difficulties in facing the end of their therapy. Public health services can ill afford the luxury of providing endless therapy and these patients' apparent "resistance" was a problem for us, as it had been for Freud and Felitti and continues to be for many other therapists treating the survivors of child abuse or neglect.

I then remembered the work of Bob Johnson who had spent some time on the same psychiatric ward as me in Charing Cross Hospital in London after his film was televised. He and I had planned to run a group for women who were suffering from the effects of childhood abuse. Unfortunately, we never did work together as I was appointed to develop the TSS at the Maudsley Hospital. However, I remembered how, when he interviewed his patients, he would always ask them whether they could say something like: "Mum, I am an adult or grown-up and I don't need you anymore."

What was so interesting for me was the fact that the patients took to this approach in considering their condition: it made a lot of sense for them. Could this be what we needed to do? I contacted Bob Johnson, and he kindly agreed to come to the TSS and share with the team the details of his work.

The essence of this approach is, in my view, to create a situation where the patient faces an imaginary parent who was the source of his (or her) terror as a child and who is still, inexplicably, as terrifying now, even in adulthood. Such an attachment can be understood as the mental representation or IWM of repeated experiences in which these children have felt both terrified and, paradoxically, desperately in need of their caregiver whose protection is felt as essential for their survival. This is the *traumatic attachment*. By telling the patient that he is now an adult, Johnson is simply telling the truth but in fact a lot more is happening.

For example, in the case of his work with the prisoner Lenny, Johnson had set up the equivalent of the Strange Situation by inviting this one-time disorganised infant Lenny to face his abusive terrifying parent. Then, by telling him to declare himself an adult in relation to his old mother, Johnson initiates the process of normal separation and growing up. With the support of his attuned and caring doctor, whom he could trust, Lenny repeatedly went through this ritual of overcoming the fear that belongs to the Child Self and replacing it with an increasingly confident Adult Self. Not surprisingly, as Johnson is in fact dealing with the dissociated Child Self, we are witnessing the healing, over time, of this dissociated Self until "We conquered It!" as Lenny declares at the end of his treatment. "It" is the terror-driven *traumatic attachment* and its associated dissociation that split the infant Self to ensure the infant's survival.

Johnson describes this process as the "melting of the *traumatic attachment*" resulting from the warm trusting relationship between the patient and his therapist in the face of a terrifying parental figure. As Lenny's fear gradually declines, the dissociation fades away and integration of the Self can take place. As Johnson noted, this "has a very curious effect because it stops him getting angry and it stops him getting violent", a noticeable and remarkable change as he no longer behaves as a dangerous prisoner. The Lenny we see in this session is, indeed, a much more lively and communicative human being. Johnson's approach made sense to us since most of our patients suffered from the long-standing effects of a disorganised attachment, as Lenny did. We realised that if we could reverse the dissociative effect of their *traumatic attachments,* both patients and therapists would benefit.

I decided to develop an equivalent procedure (Zulueta, 2006b, 2010b) to Johnson's which I initially named the Traumatic Attachment Induction Test, or TAIT, and subsequently modified to the TAIP.

The word "induction" acknowledges the fact that we hoped to "bring on" or elicit the *traumatic attachment* that we suspected had led to our patients' original dissociation and their resulting disturbed development and vulnerability. In other words, we wanted to develop a therapeutic tool that enabled therapists to access the hitherto unconscious IWMs of their patient's Child Self in relation to either their terrifying caregiver, as Johnson did, or the IWM of Child Self in relation to their idealised mother.

While Johnson asks his patient to challenge his mother by telling her that he is an adult and therefore she cannot hit him anymore, we were aware that such a sentence did not suit an interaction with an idealised mother, which is probably the most frequent situation we thought we would encounter with our patients. I therefore decided to try and elicit the characteristic embodied response of the Child Self in a separation test, like the Strange Situation, where the patient tells her mother, for example, that she no longer needs her as she did as a child. This appeared to induce a strong angry response from the mother in relation to both the "yearning Child Self" or the "terrified Child Self", which is illustrated in the next case example.

Introducing the TAIP in the therapeutic context

To have an idea of what the use of the TAIP involves, we can attend a typical assessment interview before we explore how it functions in more detail.

> A woman called Emma is being assessed for psychotherapy in the TSS. This is her second assessment session. She has shared her history of childhood abuse, both physical and emotional, and described her current painful issues. The therapist feels that she is very interested in the possibility of having therapy and that a good rapport had been established between them. At this point, the therapist offers Emma the possibility of conducting a brief, imaginary "separation test" which she says may help her to understand some of the reasons for her difficulties.

Having agreed to this, Emma is then asked to remind herself of the fact that she is now a forty-two-year-old woman and to share what she had achieved so far as an adult. This is partly to ensure that the Adult Self is in charge and agrees with what she is invited to do but it is also essential for the TAIP to involve the Adult Self as will be revealed the interview.

The therapist then invites Emma to imagine that her mother is sitting opposite her in the room and asks Emma to speak to her mother by repeating her previous adult statement and then to say the following words *whilst noticing what happens in her body*:

"Mum, I am now forty-two years old, I am an adult now and I don't need you anymore like I did when I was a child."

On attempting this exercise, Emma becomes quite pale and looks frightened as she tries to say "I don't need you anymore as I did when I was a child" to her imaginary mother. This interaction does not last for more than a couple of minutes before the therapist gently invites her to share what she is feeling in her body.

Emma tells her that she found it very difficult to say those words to her mother; she also noticed that her throat felt tight, that her stomach was churning, and that her heart was pounding. She admitted that she felt very frightened of her imagined mother because she was convinced, at that moment, that her mother was behind the door and would come into the room and beat her up!

This was strange, as Emma had reported earlier on that her mother had died twenty years before. This is important, as it informs us that she has not been able to mourn the loss of her parent. This issue of *unresolved* or *complex grief* came up in the therapy of all our clients who experienced difficulties in carrying out the TAIP. We deduce that is because of the fractured nature of the Self in the disorganised attachment. (I will be referring to this issue in more detail in Chapter 6).

In the discussion with the therapist that followed, Emma realised that a part of her was still as terrified of her mother as she had been as a little girl. She then realised that it was because of this overriding terror that she could not tell her mother that she did not need her anymore, even though she was now an adult working woman. Emma recognised these feelings of fear as belonging to her terrified Child Self and began to acknowledge how much they had affected her life by preventing her from standing up for what she wanted. She could see how this terror had bound her to her mother's iron will and she felt those same feelings may well have prevented her from grieving following her mother's death.

What is the TAIP and what it does, in brief

The "test" the therapist referred to is our new procedure, the TAIP, based on an imagined and simplified adult version of the Strange Situation. When asking our clients or patients whether they would like to do the TAIP we now refer to it as an "experience" rather than a "test" because of the latter's laboratory connotations.

When using the TAIP with a male client, the Adult Self is invited to imagine himself separating from his mother by telling his parent that he no longer needs her as he did when he was a child. Initially, this may seem an easy request to follow for an adult but, like the Strange Situation that uses a separation test as a stressful experience designed to expose the underlying degree of attachment insecurity, the TAIP aims to do the same.

What is surprising is that, when used with individuals who have developed a disorganised attachment, the TAIP exposes the embodied Child Self reacting in genuine fear to the idea of separating from a parent they actually believe to be present, as Lenny and Emma did. Lenny thought his mother would attack him in the room, and Emma was convinced that her mother was behind the office door and would come into the room and do the same! Clearly, for Emma, as for Lenny, this lived experience is based on very early somatic memories of terrifying experiences at the hands of their mothers in early life, transformed into mental representations or IWMs of these terrifying relationships which would continue to prevent them from growing up and becoming independent.

As we have already mentioned, Bowlby defined these relationships between the child and his or her caregivers as templates that form their IWMs, and his view of therapy is that:

> A therapist applying attachment theory sees his role as being one of providing the condition in which the patient can explore his representational models of himself and his attachment figures with a view to reappraising them and restructuring them in the light of the new understanding he acquires and the new experiences he has in the therapeutic relationships. (Bowlby, 1988, p. 138)

So, what is being elicited here is the underlying unconscious *traumatic attachment* involving the mental representation or IWM of the Child Self in relation to his or her mis-attuning and frightening mother. In other cases, it is the IWM of the Child Self in relation to the idealised mother that is being induced.

Adults who have developed a secure attachment with their caregiver have little or no difficulty in expressing their independence by letting their imaginary parent know that they do not need him or her like they did as a child. However, most of the patients attending the TSS were individuals whose early life experiences were marked by the effects of abuse and neglect, adult versions of the infants in Main and Solomon's study.

Just as these last two researchers were surprised to observe the unexpected behaviours of the infants after two short separations from their parent in the Strange Situation, so were the therapists in the TSS when they invited their patients to carry out the TAIP in relation to their imaginary parental figure, either within the context of a prolonged three-session assessment for therapy or during the therapy itself. The important thing to remember is that this procedure can only take place if the patient or client feels safe enough to carry this out with a therapist whose presence is felt to be supportive and "on their side", so to speak.

To obtain consent to conduct the TAIP, the therapist addresses the Adult Self in the room, and asks their age and enquires about their life's achievements. This is very important in terms of using the TAIP because it is the Adult Self who will become aware of the Child Self's existence when he or she addresses the imagined parent and simultaneously notices what is going on in his or her body.

The therapist initiates the TAIP by telling the patient to imagine that his mother, for example, is now sitting opposite him and then asks him to repeat the sentence giving his age and his adult achievements and then adding the following words, while noticing what is happening in his body: "Mum, I am an adult now and I don't need you anymore like I did when I was a child."

Patients often ask if they can call their parent by a different name or ask the therapist to repeat what they have to say. The therapist will encourage them to address their parent as they used to as a child and help them to repeat the words they need to use for the TAIP.

The words will refer to a separation experience from the attachment figure with whom the patient's Child Self is thought in some way to be traumatically attached to, either through terror, as with Lenny and Emma, or through the secret yearning for an idealised attachment which is often present in people who suffer from addiction, for example.

The sentence "Mum, I am an adult, and I don't need you anymore like I did when I was a child" conveys the fact that, though I am still like a child in my need for my mother, or another parental figure, I don't need to be that way and I am being given permission by my therapist to grow up and become an adult in my own right. The patient feels he can say this when he feels he can trust and rely on his therapist. Naturally, the words can be altered, so long as they convey the real possibility of separating from their caregiver in the safety of their attachment relationship to their therapist who plays a crucial role in facilitating this procedure.

These words act as a separation test to "activate the attachment system" but, unlike the terrified infants in Main's Strange Situation who are made to suffer, once again, the terror of a parents' absence, the adult patient is being offered the possibility of working through this separation with an attuned and encouraging therapist who understands how difficult and painful this task can be for the patient.

What follows, is unexpected for the clients who are introduced to the TAIP during their assessment interviews. They find it difficult to repeat the prescribed words as they struggle to overcome their embodied emotional reaction at the thought of separating from mother or another parental figure: this turns out to be very difficult or seemingly impossible because of the autonomic fear response that it elicits. The heart rate can go up, the stomach contract, the chest tightens, and speaking the prescribed words may feel really frightening or even almost impossible, either because they still feel a strong need for this parent or because they still live in fear of their parent's retaliation, as Emma did.

During an assessment interview, the separation experience is limited to a couple of minutes, following which the therapist gently intervenes by asking what their patient is feeling in their body and what thoughts they are having: this is the most important part of the TAIP. What many therapists using the TAIP have noticed is that their patients usually identify the sensations, emotions, and feelings that arise during this exercise as belonging to their Child Self, all of which had not been consciously available to them before they carried out the TAIP. With the help of the therapist, they start to make sense of this encounter with what appears to be their Child Self's IWM, still traumatically attached to the mother or father of their past; sometimes they can even begin to plan their future therapeutic journey as one in which letting go of this abusive or idealised attachment relationship becomes central to their progress in their therapy.

Identifying the traumatic attachment prior to starting therapy

For both clients and therapists, it can be helpful to know whether the therapeutic journey they are about to embark on together might involve overcoming the difficulties created by the *traumatic attachment*. The disorders identified by Felitti, such as addictions of various kinds, including obesity, domestic violence, unresolved or complex grief, and those encountered in the treatment of complex trauma and so-called borderline personality disorder, often lead to negative outcomes through no fault either of the clients or the staff involved in their care. However, as therapists are usually unaware of the underlying reasons for this apparent "resistance" to treatment, patients often end up carrying the blame and staff often act out their frustration in an unprofessional and even destructive manner, as we will see in a later chapter.

In our version of Johnson's treatment, using the TAIP, the process that is beginning to take place when it is first used during therapy can occasionally be enough to lead on to the healing of the divided Self; or can, as a final outcome, be facilitated in patients with higher levels of dissociation by following it up with a symbolic burial ritual of the Child Self. These various possibilities will be described in the next few chapters.

Indicators of a likely traumatic attachment

There are three main features in a patient's history that indicate that a *traumatic attachment* is likely to exist:

1. A strong "moral defence" expressed by feeling to blame or undeserving of any treatment.
2. Idealisation of a parental figure and evidence of splitting, such as one parent being seen as very "good" and idealised whilst the other is the "bad" one.
3. A history of resistance to change in psychotherapy or other treatments.

The TAIP can also be used during an assessment interview to explore in more detail how the *traumatic attachment* may manifest itself during the therapeutic journey by involving the patient in the process. Such an experience during the assessment can often shorten the length of therapy and make it less stressful for both therapist and patient.

> Sandra was a young woman with a history of severe neglect as well as symptoms of an eating disorder. When I offered her the possibility of doing the TAIP in our second assessment interview, she agreed to it but found herself unable to even think about telling her mother that she did not need her anymore.
>
> Even though she realised that she would have to give up this deep-seated yearning for her mother when undergoing therapy, she insisted that she still wanted to take up the offer of psychotherapy. This apparent "double think" is quite often encountered in individuals with a disorganised attachment. I assume that it is related to the fact that they have a divided or split Self: the Adult Self wants therapy to improve his or her life but the Child Self remains traumatically attached to the idealised mother and is terrified of losing her support.

> When I pointed out that a part of her, the Child Self, was terrified of the idea of "getting better" because this would make it less likely for her to get mother's attention and loving care, she smiled with a rather sheepish expression on her face.
>
> I then asked her: "How will this little one, who yearns for mother, express this need during therapy?"
>
> Sandra replied very simply: "By not eating."

Her truthful response enabled us both to plan for such an eventuality by involving the eating disorders unit during her therapeutic journey, which proved very helpful both for her and for her therapist.

This TAIP-led approach acknowledges the reality of the terrified or needy Child Self as a potential "saboteur" in the treatment of individuals who have suffered from abuse and neglect in their early life. This is manifest in many disorders arising from an early disorganised attachment. This is the core problem with many so-called "difficult to treat disorders" which we will be exploring in Chapter 6 and it can also be at the root of a common problem in child adoption, as we will find out here.

The use of the TAIP in therapy

Rationale

Bowlby had very clear ideas about how to understand the development of an individual's personality: "It is necessary to consider the environment in which each individual develops as well as the genetic potentials with which he is endowed" (1988, p. 64), to which we can also add the epigenetic potentials.

> The pathway along which the attachment behaviour comes to be organised and further that the pathway is determined to a high degree by the way his parent-figures treat him.
>
> A principal means by which such experiences influence personality development is held to be through their effects on how a person construes the world about him and how he expects people to whom he might become attached to behave, both of which are derivatives of the representational models of his parents that are built up during childhood.
>
> Evidence suggests that these models tend to persist relatively unmodified at an unconscious level and to be far more accurate reflections of how his parents really treated him than traditional opinion has supposed. (Bowlby, 1988, p. 65)

Bowlby is referring here to the IWMs. The concept of "working models" or "internal representations" has until now remained an abstract concept initially formulated by Bowlby and his followers to explain the different attachment behaviours of one-year-olds in the Strange Situation (Ainsworth, Blehar, Waters, & Wall, 1978; Hesse & Main, 2000). When referring to the existence of different representations of themselves in relation to their abusive or neglectful caregiver, Bowlby referred to these different IWMs as "segregated different states" acquired through life by "selective exclusion", which we would now refer to as *dissociation.*

According to Bowlby, when a child grows up, the adult consciously maintains a "wholly favourable image of the parent"; however, at a less conscious level, he nurses an image in which the parent is represented as neglectful, rejecting, or ill-treating him (Bowlby, 1988, p. 70). He goes on to say that people for whom this procedure plays an important part, "are handicapped in terms of their dealings with other human beings compared to people for whom it only plays a minor part" (ibid., p. 72).

For example:

> A set of responses a person is making may become disconnected cognitively from the inter-personal situation which is eliciting it, leaving him unaware of why he is responding as he is. He may mistakenly identify some other person (or situation) as the one which is eliciting his responses. He may divert his responses away from someone who is in some degree responsible for arousing them and toward some irrelevant figure, including himself.
>
> He may dwell so insistently on the details of his own reactions and suffering that he has no time to consider what the interpersonal situation responsible for his reaction might be. (ibid., p. 65)

We will see examples of these different types of reaction in the forthcoming chapters when addressing the difficulties encountered by patients, particularly the people who are given the diagnosis of "borderline personality disorder", in great part because of their high levels of dissociation.

The importance of the traumatic attachment in relation to adoption

There still seems to be a general belief that infants who have been adopted in early life do not need to mourn their lost mother, which means that adoptive parents are not informed that this may be an important issue to think about and work on when they adopt a child.

> Marion was one such a child. Unfortunately, she did not seek help until her late sixties. She was born abroad but adopted in the UK at the age of nine months. Her childhood was a very unhappy one as she felt that she had received far less love and attention from her adoptive mother than her siblings did. Once she left home to study and work, she struggled with an addiction to alcohol, was often bullied at work, and was unable to develop any good attachment relationships or have a family.
>
> Throughout her life, she had constantly blamed her adoptive mother for all her problems, and she now wanted help in dealing with these angry feelings because they prevented her from responding to her sister and brother, who often invited her to their homes in response to her loneliness. At some point in our second assessment interview, when she appeared to feel safe with me, I suggested that we try and carry out the TAIP in relation to her birth mother.

Marion strongly disagreed with this as she was convinced that all her problems were due to her adoptive mother. I reassured her by suggesting that we could do a second test in relation to her adoptive mother.

As she was carrying out the TAIP and imagining herself talking to her birth mother whom she had never met since she was adopted, Marion found out just how much she yearned for her and how angry she felt about having been put up for adoption. It was a painful shock for her, and she said that she wished she had known this when she was much younger, for it would have made such a difference to her life.

Marion could not get in touch with her birth mother as she had died, but her adoptive mother was still alive: I suggested that she might want to meet with her and share what she had now discovered. It might heal her relationship with her adoptive family and lead to happier moments in her later life. She left me, shaken but hopeful.

The role of the adoptive mother is often that of providing the necessary decoy to protect the idealised mother from the anger that the disorganised adopted child feels in relation to her loss. Marion's discovery was very important for me, too, as I knew how often things do go wrong between parents and their adopted children. There can be many reasons for these difficulties involving either the child's life experiences before the adoption or the way their adoptive parents relate to them. Early abuse or neglect at the hands of the biological mother often leads to a child being put up for adoption and therefore makes it likely that they may suffer from the long-term effects of a disorganised attachment, leading to an unconscious idealised attachment to their lost mother. This was the case with Marion. In such cases the yearning for the idealised mother prevents a good relationship developing with the adoptive mother on whom all the angry feelings related to being abandoned by the birth mother are projected.

I was attending a conference on adoption many years ago where a therapist, who was working with a mother and her adopted daughter, presented a video of them both: the mother was speaking to her daughter and her face and voice were so loving and gentle that she melted my heart. I also noticed the softening of the young girl's face as she listened to her mother. But then, suddenly, her features hardened, and she just cut her mother off. She disconnected.

I realised that the *traumatic attachment* had "stepped in" and wondered if the loving voice of her adoptive mother had triggered unconscious memories of her birth mother, whose voice and smell she had once "known" in her earliest days and whose loss she had survived by replacing her with an idealised mental representation to hang onto. At the same time, all her anger and distress over her adoption, was being projected onto the adoptive mother, as had happened with Marion.

This is a common unconscious defence in adoptees that needs to be recognised and worked with. Fortunately, more professionals are now aware of this phenomenon and work with adoptive families in helping them to recognise the impact of this often unrecognised loss, which is not easy for them but so helpful in the long run. In her book *Lost and Found*, Betty Jean Lifton, an adoptee herself, traces the adopted child's lifelong struggle to form an authentic sense of self in his or her search for wholeness (Lifton, 1979). Could this inner emptiness be due to the *traumatic attachment*'s divided Self?

A step-by-step summary of how to implement the TAIP

The use of the TAIP during assessments

The whole point of the TAIP is to find out if, underlying many of the adult patient's difficulties, is a hitherto unconscious younger Self-state that is still strongly attached to their childhood caregiver, either through their yearning for love or through terror, as was the case with Lenny and Emma. The use of the TAIP during an assessment differs from its use in therapy because it comes as a surprise to the patient (or client) who has no prior knowledge of this experience and what it entails. For this reason, I have nearly always used it in my second assessment interview. By that time, I can sense whether the patient trusts me enough and appears to want to understand why they think and act as they do.

Whether we use the TAIP during an assessment or in therapy, the same basic principles need to be maintained to make it work, but some variation is possible in therapy; this will become apparent as each author presents her work in the forthcoming chapters.

Basic steps and principles to keep in mind when carrying out the TAIP

The relationship between the therapist and the client

This needs to be an attuned and trusting one for the client to be able to share his or her feelings and thoughts without a sense of shame or humiliation.

Timing the use of the TAIP

The therapist will have mentioned the possibility of the TAIP, which is referred to as an "experience", earlier on in therapy when dealing with the relationship between her patient and his parent or parents. If the client is interested, she will have explained how useful it is to have it recorded on video and obtained the patient's signature on a consent form that stipulates that both client and the therapist will have access to it. It could also include an additional clause that allows the video to be shown to the therapist's supervision group.

It is usually carried out following a thoughtful dialogue focussing on the patient's attachment figure, but timing is a matter of experience, as is the choice of parent to focus on.

Checking the levels of dissociation

If the levels of dissociation using the dissociative experiences scale (DES) have not yet been measured, it is important that this should be done in order to be sure that the TAIP can be safely used with this client. The TAIP works optimally with patients whose levels of dissociation are between 20 and 40, which includes the diagnosis of BPD. It may not usually be appropriate for individuals suffering from higher levels of dissociation such as dissociative identity disorder without some earlier preparatory work.

The DES should be done again, after using the TAIP, when both therapist and client are aware that major changes have taken place, since this is a procedure that actually eliminates or reduces dissociation, and is the only one, as far as I'm aware, to do so.

Keeping the Adult Self in charge of the TAIP in the room

This is crucial in terms of using the TAIP because it is the Adult Self who will become aware of the embodied Child Self's existence when patients address their imagined parent and simultaneously notice what is going on in their body when repeating the therapist's words.

On the day in which the procedure is being carried out, the client will be asked if he or she feels ready to go ahead with the "experience". If the answer is "yes", the therapist will first focus on maintaining their Adult Self in the room by asking the client to give his or her age as well as an account of their achievements to date.

The therapist then tells their patient to repeat a sentence and to speak out loudly whilst noticing what is happening in his or her body during that experience.

It is wise for therapists to check with the client what they call their chosen parent before doing the TAIP, otherwise clients may inform the therapist that they call their parent by a different name after doing the TAIP. If that happens, the TAIP should be repeated, particularly if there was no response or a minimal one.

The separation test scenario

The therapist then asks their client to imagine their mother (or other parent) sitting opposite them and tells them to address her by repeating the following words. For example: "Mum I am thirty-five years old, I am now a qualified teacher, and I am married with two children. I don't need you anymore like I needed you when I was a child" to which the therapist adds: "Notice what happens in your body when you say those words." This last sentence addresses the possible existence of an embodied Child Self. It is very important that the client speaks out loud and not in their head.

How long should the actual TAIP experience last? In the assessments, I only gave it one to two minutes. However, in therapy, one could start with a short two-minute session, but it could last longer if used again later on in therapy and/or if both therapist and client feel that a longer experience would be a useful experience.

The client's reaction

Patients may find it relatively easy to speak the words out loud or they may find it very difficult and remain silent. The therapist responds in a gentle empathic manner, noting that the patient may be finding it difficult, but she will encourage him or her to try again whilst highlighting at the same time the importance of their body's response, focusing on which parts are affected and in what way, since the Child Self is an embodied response.

The client's physical experiences, emotions, and thoughts

This is the final outcome of this procedure and requires a respectful openness of mind and a genuine empathic curiosity in relation to what the client feels and thinks. This is the most important aspect of the TAIP as it is the time when the Adult Self of the patient can begin to connect the existence of his newly found Child Self with his past and current experiences and difficulties, as Emma did. He will then begin to see what is required for him to "grow up and take control of his life" with the empathic support of his therapist.

The therapist must bear in mind both the possible shock and embarrassment that the Adult Self may feel since patients can often find themselves in the grip of 'childish" emotions. She can empathise with these reactions and, by treating the client with compassion, she can at the same time enable the Adult Self to acknowledge that he is sharing the experiences of himself, his Child Self, at a very young age, on the receiving end of terrifying experiences at the hands of their common mother or having the now conscious experience of being inexplicably dependent on her.

By acknowledging with similar compassion the idealised attachment of the terrifying fear and possible anger of the Child Self, the therapist can enable the two half-Selves to exist together and, in a sense, begin to make contact and integrate across the dissociative divide of terror that was engineered by the *traumatic attachment* so early on in their life.

The video-recording of the TAIP

The video-recording of the TAIP is especially useful because it allows the patient and therapist to revisit the experience and acts as a powerful reminder of what took place in a session after the TAIP. I encourage therapists to use it quite often in their therapy as it enables the client and therapist to note the changes that are taking place over time. Video work is highly effective in the treatment of dissociation because it facilitates integration of the Self, as the clients see themselves in different states.

The video-recording also allows therapists to share and improve their approach either on their own or by sharing the video in supervision. It can also be particularly useful for research purposes.

Consequences of using the TAIP

The TAIP opens up a new way of understanding many of the negative experiences that both therapists and patients go through in therapy and gives them a new way of resolving them.

It is particularly interesting to discover, through the work of Felitti and Anda, how many of our social, medical, and psychological problems are probably the product of the *traumatic attachment* because they are so difficult to treat. It allows us to begin to imagine the possibility of changing the therapeutic outcome of these disorders for the better by using the TAIP.

Though Felitti is unaware of this therapeutic development, he plans to devote his professional life to unmasking the traumatic causes of many of the illnesses of the mind and body. Many doctors and psychiatrists still refuse to acknowledge his results because it threatens the status quo which ensures them a comfortable living.

Conclusion

The TAIP provides therapists with a lived experience that encourages and empowers their adult clients who suffered abuse and neglect as infants and children to become aware of either their childhood terror or their desperate yearning for love and safety embodied within the *traumatic attachment*. At the same time, as the therapist reminds his or her clients of the fact that they are now no longer dependent children, but capable adults, their Adult Self begins to feel safe enough, in the presence of such an attuned and encouraging therapist, to finally acknowledge the terrifying emotions they felt as children, as well as the fact that they need no longer be terrified or needy.

In so doing, the terror that divided the two split Selves begins to melt: the Adult Self and Child Self are being brought together by a therapist who is both aware of the reality of the childhood terror and, at the same time, aware of the reality that his or her patients no longer need to fear their parent's abuse nor do they need an idealised parent to survive. Like Johnson, the therapist is saying: "I am with you, and you can do it."

The TAIP, by engineering this get-together of the two dissociated half-Selves, enables attuned and respectful psychotherapists to finally reverse the destructive effects of the *traumatic attachment* by melting the terror that once set them apart for life. In so doing, the TAIP therapists can heal their clients' fractured Self.

Its powerful effects will be illustrated in the work conducted by Monique Notice, Jayshree Unadkat, and Leonor de Escoriaza (Chapters 7, 8, and 9). It is important to note that it can be used with different therapeutic modalities such as psychodynamic psychotherapy, Lifespan Integration (LI), eye movement desensitisation and reprocessing (EMDR), schema therapy, as well as group therapy, which will be described in the next chapter.

CHAPTER 5

Reversing the traumatic attachment via the TAIP to heal PTSD and BPD

L ittle did I realise that having written about the origins of violence, I would end up, a few years later (Zulueta, 2006a), as head of an outpatient service devoted to the treatment of victims of violence. It made sense to Professor Gunn, a forensic psychiatrist who had invited me, as he felt that the victims of the violent men he saw were also entitled to receive the care that they needed. Developing this service proved an exciting challenge for me, as all the patients suffered from the effects of trauma and were nearly all diagnosed as suffering from post-traumatic stress disorder (PTSD), a condition that I had not encountered often in my previous jobs. As the name of the service indicates, our role was to provide men and women suffering from the effects of trauma with the possibility of recovery. Most of these had complex problems that the local services could not deal with.

Over the years, inspired by the work of Judith Herman (1997) and Van der Kolk (2014), we developed a therapeutic service where we tried to adapt our approach to the different individual and cultural needs of the men and women who attended the service. As around half of them came from different countries in the Middle East, Africa, and a few from South America, this meant developing and using different therapeutic approaches and languages (Lab et al., 2008).

The staff provided a variety of different therapeutic skills to the people who attended, such as EMDR, LI, psychoanalytic psychotherapy, systemic family therapy and group therapy as well as trauma- focused cognitive behaviour therapy (TF-CBT), though this was later provided by Professor Ehlers in her treatment centre for patients suffering from simple PTSD (Ehlers & Clark, 2000). We also had the use of a local city farm, where the refugees and asylum seekers enjoyed the dance therapy introduced by Nina Papadopoulos, a dance movement therapist and research psychologist. They were also able to grow vegetables which they used to cook to a meal for each other once a week.

Surprisingly, EMDR proved to be the treatment of choice for many of the women who had been raped, irrespective of where they came from, because it is a therapy where the patient does not need to describe the trauma, which can be very humiliating for the victim.

In our attempt to address the cultural needs of these patients, I felt it was very important to offer them therapy in their first language: many of the therapists in the TSS spoke different languages and came from different cultural backgrounds, such as myself, but we also used interpreters when necessary, to engage with those who could not speak English (Zulueta, 1990, 1995).

Trauma from an attachment perspective

Having spent my previous years focusing on the role of attachment theory and research in my understanding of psychiatric conditions, it was with this frame of reference in mind that I began to look at PTSD. It is usually defined by its symptoms as outlined in *DSM-5*, the American psychiatric "bible", as if these reflect the reality: the fact is that the American definition of PTSD has changed with time and those who produce the manual show no apparent interest in recognising the physiological and neural circuits involved in this disorder (American Psychiatric Association, 2013; Pickersgill, 2014).

We now know that mammals such as elephants, dogs, camels, horses, and many others are known to develop similar symptoms when unable to act during terrifying life-threatening experiences: this shows that we share a common vulnerability which is due to our attachment system. If we go back to the young elephants who became violent after losing their mothers and their adult relatives, we saw how being able to interact with secure elder males provided the necessary remedy for their disturbed behaviour. We have also, in the early chapters of this book, learnt why this mammalian interaction is so important as we looked at the research carried out on the sharing of emotional pain between loving partners and the importance of social attachments which enable our behavioural and physiological systems to become attuned to one another, providing for each other a source of stimulation and emotional regulation (Field, 1985, p. 431).

When Erich Lindemann defined trauma as "the sudden disruption of our affiliative bonds" he was referring to our attachment bonds as they are defined in the field of animal behaviour (Lindemann, 1944). His definition makes the most sense to me after working in the field of trauma for fifteen years. All my patients noted varying degrees of difficulty in making and maintaining relationships and those who had been tortured by their fellow men, the most affected, had become living ghosts of their former selves, out of reach, locked in an invisible capsule of emotional silence, deprived of the "emotional oxygen" of life, the living web of attachments that define our sense of being.

Not surprisingly, with my interest in attachment, the first thing that I noticed on reading the literature on PTSD was that the most important risk factor for this disorder is in fact "the lack of social support" (NICE, 2005) at the time of the traumatic experience, during the experience, and afterwards. This factor is scarcely mentioned in Western "individualistic" cultures, but it is crucial because, by ignoring, it we leave out the possibility of an attuned-based approach to healing traumatised minds. For example, why did the young, traumatised elephants respond so rapidly to the presence of the two secure adult males who took over their care? It led to a reduction in testosterone levels and the normalisation of their behaviour with the suppression of their extended musth. By restoring a microcosm of the "living web of attachments" that makes male elephants what they are—peaceful sensitive social animals—these young adolescents were healed. Our need for one another is why children, who feel supported by a calm loving parental figure during a terrifying event, do not develop PTSD and it is much better for them not to be separated from their parents. When, during the war, my mother was sent to the safer countryside with her school mates, she said that she was constantly worrying about whether her parents were going to be killed in the bombing of London.

Many of the men I have treated, who fought in the same war, did not experience symptoms of PTSD until their partner died, years later, or, after they lost their role in the community through retirement. And, we have the example of the Kurdish refugee who did not develop any symptoms following his terrible traumatic experiences of war in his homeland and his long dangerous journey while he was safely ensconced with Kurdish people in London with whom he could attune and mentalize. Moving him to a hostile situation in Glasgow proved an expensive disaster as he ended up struggling with full-blown PTSD and requiring NHS care in the TSS where he was fortunate to have a Kurdish therapist who also spoke his language.

These examples confirm the importance of attachments as a protective factor in relation to PTSD, enabling people to retain the capacity to attune and empathise and to regulate their emotions. These findings also make sense of the fact that people who belong to tightly-knit communities usually withstand natural disasters and even violence without suffering from PTSD. This proved to be the case in Uganda in the 1970s, when a team of health workers went to help the victims of Idi Amin's civil war and found that there were vast numbers of victims of trauma but there were no cases of PTSD except, sadly, for the rape victims who had been ostracised because they were no longer deemed worthy of being a member of the family or the community (Zulueta, 2006a, pp. 203–205).

Our Western socio-economic system has dismantled many community structures, stressing the importance of the individual over the importance of the group, a culture where people are seen as independent and autonomous. This type of culture destroys the "living web of attachments" that once sustained the communities in which we evolved, leaving us now more vulnerable to the effects of trauma, be it man-made or due to natural disasters.

The official diagnosis of simple PTSD and complex PTSD

Although PTSD is now a well a well-known diagnosis, it is still controversial for two reasons: acknowledging human emotional vulnerability to the effects of violence, particularly in relation to war, does not go down well in societies which are based on the perpetration of violence by legal means. This was clear during the two World Wars. In the first, men afflicted by symptoms of PTSD were diagnosed as suffering from "shell shock" which was seen as a physical disorder. Hundreds of thousands of men left the First World War suffering from symptoms of what would now be called PTSD and, although some received a basic form of psychiatric treatment, they were largely vilified after the war. By the Second World War, psychiatrists concluded that these casualties were due to men who were prone to "neurotic tendencies" and so these were excluded from the American forces for the second war. However, large numbers of soldiers still showed symptoms of PTSD during the Second World War. Their condition was called "combat fatigue" (Pols & Oak, 2007).

However, PTSD as a diagnosis was not officially recognised until after the disastrous Vietnam War when thousands of traumatised American soldiers came home to be shunned by the public because of the unpopularity of the war and, as a result, they had nowhere to go for help. Doctors realised that they could no longer ignore these casualties. They were found to suffer from a *constellation* of symptoms which were assumed to be due to their terrifying and horrifying experiences during the war. This disorder was named post-traumatic stress disorder in *DSM-3* in 1980. It is now recognised in the WHO's *ICD-11* and in the American *DSM-5*.

However, despite this progress, resistance to the fact that traumatisation actually begins at home still persists. It was shortly after recognising the impact of trauma in Vietnam veterans that the women's rights movement started to make its presence felt in the United States and the issue of child sexual abuse and its terrible effects began to be recognised. Judith Herman, MD, described this condition in her book *Trauma and Recovery: The Aftermath of Violence— From Domestic Abuse to Political Terror* (1997), originally published in 1991 following her work with women who revealed that they had been sexually abused during their childhood (Herman & Hirschman, 2000, originally published in 1981). She described them as suffering from complex PTSD (C-PTSD) which was a more appropriate diagnosis for women whose traumas were associated with sexual abuse carried out by close relatives during their childhood. For her, the core experiences of this kind of trauma are "disempowerment" and "disconnection" from others. Therefore, recovery should be based on empowerment and the creation of new connections, which is why we used group therapy in the TSS for women who had been sexually abused in childhood.

Her model of trauma recovery was very much the model that we used in the TSS. It involved three stages: safety and stabilisation, remembrance and mourning, and reconnection and integration back into the community.

Simple PTSD

However, before looking at C-PTSD, it is important to recognise that PTSD may develop in adults who do not appear to have experienced a disorganised attachment: the terror and helplessness they experience as an adult when subjected to overwhelming traumatic experience may be powerful enough to set off the *fight–flight–freeze* response of the ANS, followed by dissociation. These individuals only present with symptoms of PTSD after one or two traumatic experiences in our experience. Those who attended the TSS tended to be "copers", men and women who prided themselves on being resilient and unemotional and who believed in the importance of a "stiff upper lip", or not complaining. For these people, their inability to cope with their traumatic experiences was a terrible humiliation: shame becomes an important issue in their treatment, as does the expression of emotions which betray weakness and lack of control. Tom was one such patient.

> He was a middle-aged ambulance driver from Hong Kong who was brought up by his strict mother not to make a fuss when he was upset. He presented with long-standing symptoms of PTSD as he believed in being stoical. Tom liked his work and had been involved in "picking up the pieces" after terrible accidents which he told me had meant having to retrieve the body parts of victims. These gruesome experiences did not bother him: he said, "it was part of my job". He could not understand why he could not get over his traumatic event.
>
> On this occasion however, he became a victim himself when he was severely burnt in his car as it suddenly exploded into flames and he was locked inside. He had to be cut out of the vehicle and driven to a specialist burns unit where he was immediately taken into theatre. A sheet was put over his head and part of his body as the doctors and nurses silently got on with the job of treating his burnt torso and limbs. Since nobody spoke to him and he could not see what was going on, he felt very anxious, but he never thought of simply asking for help. His stoic avoidant defence, adopted in his early life to prevent him from experiencing his mother's rejection when in need, "locked" him in this isolated state of suffering. It got worse when he was transferred to the intensive care unit where silence was required as various tubes were inserted into his body. He felt that he was not treated as a human being.

Tom was terrified and felt quite helpless since he could not bring himself to communicate his distress to the nursing and medical staff because of the shame instilled in him during his childhood. Instead, his *fight–flight–freeze* defence system took over, leading him to dissociate and he found himself reliving this terrifying experience through intrusive thoughts, visual flashbacks, nightmares, and recurrent memories. He consciously and unconsciously did everything he could to avoid anything that could trigger these dissociative experiences and ended up being unable to work. His symptoms of high arousal prevented him from sleeping and concentrating as well as making him hyper-vigilant and irritable. He was most of the time in the ANS Yellow Zone of the *fight–flight–freeze* response. As often occurs with PTSD, he also became depressed. Fortunately, following twenty-two sessions of TF-CBT his symptoms resolved.

Tom's story brought home to me the importance of social support in preventing PTSD during the traumatic event as well as afterwards. He missed out on all these opportunities because of his avoidant attachment.

Complex PTSD

We have already mentioned complex PTSD in relation to the mothers whose baby boys reminded them of the men who had raped them when in jail abroad and how their trauma was then transmitted to their infants through the terror that these infants experienced when their mothers relived the tormenting flashbacks of their own terrible experiences (Chapter 3).

Most of the patients taken on for treatment in the TSS suffered from symptoms of complex post-traumatic stress disorder (C-PTSD). It can be caused by exposure to a long-term event or a series of events that are of an extremely threatening nature, from which escape is impossible or very difficult, leading to a sense of helplessness.

Typically, it is the result of childhood abuse and neglect which, as we now know, implies the likelihood of an early disorganised attachment and its associated *traumatic attachment*. However, it is likely that certain interpersonal experiences such as torture, slavery, genocide, and prolonged physical abuse, where the individual has been made to suffer and feels helpless, may also lead to the development of complex PTSD without an early history of childhood abuse or neglect, particularly in people with other types of insecure attachments.

The APA in charge of *DSM-5* refused to acknowledge the existence of complex PTSD despite, or because of, the large numbers of research studies submitted by Van der Kolk and his team, validating its importance. They also refused to acknowledge the validity of Van der Kolk's new diagnosis for children, that of developmental trauma disorder, which was submitted with another mountain of evidence regarding the multifaceted grim reality of the developmental damage suffered by chronically abused children and adolescents (Van der Kolk, 2005).

In the United States, if a diagnosis is not included in the "bible" of the APA, it does not exist professionally, which means that its treatment is not paid for by the insurance companies that underpin the health service. The absence of a diagnosis also leads to absent funding for research which is a catch-22, as research is needed to provide the funding.

This is what Dr Insel, director of the American National Institute of Mental Health wrote after the publication of *DSM-5*:

> The weakness is its lack of validity. Unlike our definitions of ischaemic heart disease, lymphoma, or AIDs, the DSM diagnoses are based on a consensus about clusters of clinical symptoms, not any objective laboratory measure. In the rest of medicine, this would be the

equivalent to creating diagnostic systems based on the nature of chest pain or the quality of fever. (Pickersgill, 2014, p. 522)

Referencing the *DSM-5* panel members' financial associations with industry, one discovers that the majority of the members of three-quarters of the working groups have financial ties to the pharmaceutical industry, including ties to the pharmaceutical companies that manufacture the medications used to treat these disorders (Cosgrove & Krimsky, 2012).

> The latest revision of the manual expands the number and definition of treatable disorders including grief – which is classified along with major depression. The worst, most irresponsible DSM5 expansion targets children by introducing "Disruptive Mood Dysregulation Disorder" whose purpose is to further increase the "number of children "diagnosed" and prescribed a combination of psychiatric drugs without meeting bipolar disorder criteria. (Pickersgill, 2014, p. 522)

Since psychotherapy is the main treatment for complex PTSD, it probably was of little financial interest to the panel's members.

As C-PTSD does not exist in the United States, all patients with symptoms of PTSD are now diagnosed as suffering simply from PTSD. However, it was not long before the APA had to include a "dissociative subtype" of PTSD which was applicable to individuals who met the criteria for PTSD but who also experienced:

a. "Depersonalisation" or "out of body experiences", such as individuals observing their own body from above which can create the perception that "this is happening to me". Women who have suffered childhood sexual abuse often report this experience.
b. "Derealisation" symptoms in which "things don't appear real" that can create the perception that "this is not happening to me". (DSM-5, p. 74)

The research rationale for the dissociative subtype in *DSM-5* was that 15 to 30 per cent of the patients suffered from depersonalisation and derealisation and showed repeated traumatisation and early ACEs increased psychiatric co-morbidity, that is, phobias and BPD amongst women, increased functional impairment and increased intentions to commit suicide, all characteristic traits of complex PTSD.

The therapeutic rationale for this dissociative subtype of *DSM-5* was that these particular individuals tended to respond better to treatments that included cognitive restructuring and skills training in addition to exposure-based therapies (Lanius et al., 2010; Lanius, Brand, Vermetten, Frewen, & Spiegel, 2012; Cloitre, Petkova, Wang, & Lassell, 2012). In other words, these individuals, who were patients suffering from C-PTSD, responded well to therapies designed to treat this condition which involve a long period of stabilisation to develop the skills to regulate their emotions before working on their traumatic experiences. This approach acknowledges their inability to regulate emotions; if that is not done, working on the trauma on its own, as one does for simple PTSD, only leads to re-traumatisation, more dissociation, and a negative outcome. One is left wondering how many "negative outcomes" had to take place before the APA created this subtype which is in fact another acknowledgement of the fact that complex PTSD differs from simple PTSD.

Fortunately, the WHO's *ICD-11* has included complex PTSD (in the sections on "Disorders specifically associated with stress" and "Mental or neurobehavioural disorders"). The main symptoms are described here. These are in addition to the symptoms of PTSD (experienced by Tom) which are severe and persistent:

1. Difficulty controlling emotions which can manifest as explosive anger, persistent sadness, depression, and suicidal thoughts.
2. Negative self-view. These individuals often feel helpless or guilty and undeserving of anything good, as a result of unconsciously adopting the *moral defence* to deal with their abuse or neglect when they were children. Shame is very marked in both the women and men (Zimmerman & Becker, 2022a, 2022b).
3. Difficulty with relationships due to the inability to trust other people, and their negative view of themselves. As a result, these people may avoid making relationships or develop unhealthy relationships; they will also re-enact past traumatic experiences from the perspective of the abuser or the victim as happens with domestic violence.
4. Dissociation, such as depersonalisation and/or derealisation, as well as few or no memories of their childhood.
5. Loss of a system of meanings which can include losing one's core beliefs, values, religious faith, or hope in the world and in other people.

All of these symptoms lead to a significant impairment in these individuals' personal, family, and occupational lives but also in other important areas of life.

However, this *ICD-11* diagnosis fails to include important somatic complaints that Herman describes in her definition of complex PTSD such as fibromyalgia, irritable bowel syndrome, allergies, chronic fatigue, and pelvic pain as well as other gynaecological symptoms in female survivors of child sexual abuse. This is because trauma affects the brain *and* the body.

American research into the origins of PTSD

One of the most interesting aspects of PTSD is the fact that many people go through a traumatic experience during their lifetime but do not develop PTSD. In the United States, for instance, it is estimated that 60 per cent of men and 50 per cent of women experience at least one traumatic experience in their lifetime but only 7 to 8 per cent will develop this disorder in 2022. This selective vulnerability to PTSD has been known for some time but it was not until mental health experts in the US realised that there was an epidemic of PTSD among soldiers returning from the wars in Iraq and Afghanistan that research was carried out to uncover this mystery.

One of the reasons for this is financial: between 10 and 20 per cent of these men and women developed symptoms of this disorder and their treatment, and lost productivity cost billions of dollars. As a scientific journal reports "given such proportions, there is considerable urgency to discover the sequence of biological events that causes PTSD and to learn why some soldiers succumb and others don't" (Velasquez-Manoff, 2015, p. 58).

These research findings are very interesting in view of what we have learnt about the disorganised attachment. Researchers have identified that differences in brain structure and function and a heightened immune reactivity go hand in hand with an increased likelihood of developing PTSD as an adult. We know these two features happen also to be due to the effects of the disorganised attachment on the infant brain (Chapter 3, p. 47). There are also many studies showings that ACEs (which include traumatic experiences) increase the chance of developing PTSD in adulthood (Frewen, Zhu, & Lanius, 2019). This effect is also seen to be "dose dependent", that is, the more ACEs the person has suffered as a child the more likely he or she is to develop PTSD.

As far as I know, no one, apart from our clinical team, has been able to elicit and identify in adults suffering from complex PTSD the *traumatic attachment and its IWMs*. However, a factor that points in that direction also appears in this recent research since it has been found that American men who have experienced abuse and adversity in childhood are more likely than the general population to join the army to escape from their terrifying environments at home.

> This was certainly the case for twenty-three-year-old Jim, who presented with very severe PTSD after fighting in Iraq. He had joined the army because of the structured life that it promised for him which he thought would compensate for the terrifying chaos of his early life. Little did he realise that as soon as he experienced fear on the battlefield, he would be reliving, day and night, the same scenarios that he lived through at home in his childhood.

Faced with a terrifying experience that is a threat to their survival, infants and children find refuge in the freeze response which leads to the dissociative splitting of the Self. It appears that any terrifying experience that triggers that same traumatic unconscious memory can reactivate the *traumatic attachment* of their early life. People like Jim, who develop PTSD by reactivating an early traumatic memory leading to their disorganised attachment, are amongst those who develop C-PTSD.

The use of the TAIP in the treatment of trauma

The use of the TAIP in group therapy with women sexually abused as children

The reader may recall that a considerable number of patients in Felitti's ACEs study (Chapter 3) had been sexually abused and were presenting with many different medical and psychological conditions in addition to being unable to finish their therapy in his obesity clinic. This is a characteristic of many of the more severely dysregulated individuals who suffer from the emotional and somatic effects of their damaged attachment system.

At the TSS, we had many patients on our waiting list who had a history of sexual abuse. At that time, the only therapy that I knew of for these women and men was long-term individual psychotherapy which would usually last more than two years because of the dependency issues that would arise in the final stages of treatment. Herman believed that people suffering from the effects of complex trauma cannot recover in isolation. They need to discover some meaning in their experience, and this happens more often by joining others. Just as trauma involves isolation, recovery requires belonging to a community or group. With this in mind, we felt that the best therapy for the women on our waiting list who had been sexually abused as children should be group therapy.

In my search for such an appropriate group therapy for these women, I came across a book entitled *Ending the Cycle of Abuse: The Stories of Women Abused as Children and the Group Therapy Techniques That Helped Them Heal*, written by Philip Ney and Anna Peter (1995). It provides a detailed account of group therapy for these women using a structured approach over thirty weeks.

In its introductory pages it highlighted the need to teach the group members relaxation techniques for when they felt very anxious, as well as grounding techniques to keep them in the "here and now" rather than dissociate.

The use of a structure and the practical recommendations made a lot of sense to me, having run a group for men and women using "free association" to qualify as a group analyst. "Free association" is a psychoanalytic tool used by Freud that aims to deepen people's self-understanding by looking at whatever thoughts, words, or images come freely to their mind, which the group analyst then interprets according to the group analytic theories that we were being taught. This technique probably made sense and was helpful to less disturbed people being seen by most of my fellow trainees who worked mainly in private practice. However, I only had access to severely traumatised individuals who had been referred to the hospital where I worked at the time.

I soon found their levels of distress, anger, and potential for violence quite frightening, especially when the group lapsed into long periods of silence which they found very threatening. This is not surprising if one thinks of the disorganised infants and their reaction to Tronick's "still face" experiment, and the terror they so easily experience when their caregiver is not available to them. This was particularly relevant in the group as these patients were more than likely to have a history of child abuse and/or neglect.

It did not take long for me to introduce the group to what I referred to as the "sandwich model" of therapy: this meant that I began every group with a "check-in", asking each member to describe how they felt and what had happened to them during the past week, and we also ended with a "check-out" that assessed how each member felt before leaving the group.

This simple structural change markedly reduced the anxiety levels in the group, providing us with plenty to talk about as well as making each individual feel that they mattered and were not going to be left out, thereby increasing their sense of belonging and cohesion. My conclusion was that the more disturbed a person feels, the more they need a safe structure to provide them with a *secure base*, as Bowlby would call it, to achieve any real change. My examiners did not comment on my heretical "sandwich model" and I still qualified as a group analyst.

Reading Ney and Peter's book, I realised that the authors used the same "check-in and check-out" structure as well as combining different therapeutic modalities with experiential exercises during which the group members practised saying and doing things in the sessions. They also had homework to do which kept them focused on the tasks they were working on throughout the week.

These tasks addressed what we now know are such important issues for adults who have been severely traumatised in their early lives:

1. One of the first tasks was being able to give a name to their emotions because many did not recognise that their headaches or stomach aches, for example, were ways in which their bodies expressed fear, anger, or distress. The group was very helpful in assisting *each other* to overcome this inability to recognise or describe their own emotions, which is called alexithymia. It is one of the effects of severe abuse resulting from damage to the corpus callosum that connects the two hemispheres of the brain.

2. A lot of time was spent working on the symptoms and behaviours related to the *moral defence* which played a large role in their lives, such as the feeling that they were to blame for the way they were treated, their inability to confront their abuser, let alone blame their mothers for not protecting them, and their overriding sense of "badness" that made them feel they did not deserve anything good.

3. To compound the effects of the moral defence was the realisation that, at times, these women had contributed to their own victimisation: this would be understood and explained as a characteristic feature of traumatised individuals who find themselves re-enacting their abuse (Van der Kolk, 2014, pp. 179–181). In addition, the sensory pleasure that they sometimes experienced when they were being sexually abused made them feel that they had a part to play in their abuse. It helped them to learn that this was a normal biological response to being touched in certain parts of the body.

4. All these different experiences relating to their moral defence were naturally bound up with overwhelming feelings of shame, manifested in how they felt, spoke, and behaved.

I shared these findings with a colleague who wanted to run a group with me, and we agreed that this model could provide us with a helpful therapeutic modality for the sexually abused women in the TSS. The only difference would be that we would include the TAIP to monitor the extent of the *traumatic attachment* during the group therapy. It felt appropriate to do so since Ney and Peter focused on helping their patients become aware of their Child Self, who is often understood to be expressing her opposition to doing some of the healing work because of her need to maintain the *traumatic attachment* to her idealised mother. Members of the group often identified their Child Self through the headaches they often experienced during the group sessions which they interpreted as the Child Self's fury at having to do something she did not like because it felt threatening: the threat was due to the fear of losing the support of their idealised mother.

As Ney and Peter's aim was to prepare the women to let go of their Child Self, and thereby their attachment to their idealised mother in order to become independent adults, the TAIP functioned in parallel by preparing their Child Self to let go of the same protective mother and thereby integrate with the Adult Self as the dissociation, born out of terror, is dissolved.

Having never run this type of group before, we extended the duration to one year and we planned to address their *traumatic attachment* by including three sessions of the TAIP—one at the beginning of the group therapy, one in the middle, and one at the end of the therapy.

In 2002, myself and my co-therapist, finally met our new group of very anxious women. The first session was spent introducing ourselves to each other and sharing the ground rules for the group as well as an outline of what lay ahead. We encouraged the women to tell us why they wanted to be there and how they had managed to overcome so many obstacles to participate in this therapy. This was important, we said, because there would be times when they would feel like giving up on their treatment, so we emphasised "do hold onto the reasons why you are here".

In the second group meeting, my co-therapist and I introduced the group members to the TAIP, which they were encouraged to try out, one by one, as we went round the group. "Mother" was represented by a tissue box on its side, topped with a tissue in lieu of hair, sitting on a table at the centre of the group. The women were asked to recall their current age and achievements and then to repeat these same words to their mother, ending with the statement "I don't need you anymore as I did when I was a child." They were also told to notice what was going on in their bodies as they spoke.

Carrying out the TAIP only took a few minutes and was accompanied by a lot of groans and very anxious faces. We then asked each group member to feed back their embodied experience; all the women found it very hard to speak to their imaginary mother and one or two simply could not do it. They reported feeling a gagging or choking sensation in their throats, churning sensations in their stomachs, and fear, which was very severe for one of the women while she was trying to carry out the procedure. All of them were extremely surprised by these bodily reactions to their imaginary mother figure and they remarked on how this experience had made them realise how powerful their mothers still were in their minds; the mother they were referring to was the imaginary mother to which their Child Self was so closely attached.

During the first few weeks, the group focused on identifying and expressing their emotions to become more aware of the effects of the abuse they had been through, both in how they felt and the way they thought. This was naturally very painful and frightening and tested their commitment to the group.

This stage was followed by exercises where they could express their anger with their parents and the abuser in a non-destructive way and cope with their fears and the resulting feelings of guilt. This emotion, which is so closely connected to the moral defence, took a lot of time to "unpack" as it involved allocating responsibility where it belonged and dealing with their deep feeling that they did not deserve anything good.

What surprised me was to see that most of the women dealt with their abuser relatively quickly and were able to express their feelings in a direct way in the early stages of the group, but the need to protect their mother was very powerful and difficult to overcome because of the *traumatic attachment* of their Child Self to their idealised mother. In the end, they finally acknowledged that their mother was much to blame for not protecting them. Having dealt with their pain, anger, fear, and guilt, the women were encouraged to imagine saying goodbye to the life that they could have had if they had not been abused and neglected. This stage naturally connects with saying goodbye to their idealised mother, so we brought in the TAIP for the second time and asked the women to report on their somatic sensations and their feelings and thoughts as they told their imaginary mother that they did not need her anymore. All of them reported some reduction, both in relation to their fear and their physical sensations, but they said that the exercise still felt "scary".

Around this period, members of the group were encouraged to carry out a "ritual" in relation to the death of their Child Self as described by Ney and Peters. The authors' view was that this was necessary for integration of the Self to take place as the Child Self would otherwise get them into trouble and interfere with their parenting. If one sees the Child Self in relation to its idealised mother, one can see that the death of the Child Self is tantamount to letting go of the *traumatic attachment* to the idealised mother. Their ritual clearly provided back-up to the TAIP. Following the ritual enacted in the group, the women were told to carry out this burial symbolically, outside the group: "some type of burial, somewhere alone, quietly where they felt the child could be at rest" (Ney & Peters, 1995, p. 98).

We noticed that whenever the women focused on this issue, they all developed headaches which they attributed to their Child Self objecting to the project. I wrote in my notes that when I asked each member of the group to imagine the Child in the other, "the exercise brought them out of a quiet sort of depressed mood as they dared to describe each other's hidden Selves: they did this very warmly but with trepidation, in case they upset the other. It was very moving".

One woman, called Diana, was told by one member of the group that her Child Self was seen as "a very angry thumping tantrum-child with two bunches of hair". Others confirmed this view. The Child Self of another woman, Monica, was seen by the others as "a stubborn, no-I-won't-child" and Shirley's was "a very reasonable but not-to-be-budged child". These short examples illustrate how actively the women worked with each other on letting go of their Child Self, a task that a few of the women continued with until the end of the group therapy.

In the meantime, the group work centred around communicating in writing with those who had abused them or who did not protect them and, in preparation for the ending of the group, the participants focused on what they had learnt from their experience, what they would take forward to no longer "self-destruct", and how to love and care for themselves and others better. At the end of the group, an emotional time for all of us, both my co-therapist and I forgot to carry out the TAIP, but the group members did not, which indicated to us that they valued it, despite the difficult emotions that it elicited. The key part of the process of healing was being able to say with conviction and without fear: "Mum, I don't need you anymore as I did as a child."

All the women were followed up six months after the group. Our best outcomes were seen in about a third of the patients, those who overcame their *traumatic attachment* by having grieved the loss of their Child Self through carrying out the ritual at home. Each woman invented her own ritual: for example, one put a picture of herself in a boat on the Thames; another buried a picture of herself in the garden of her original home in Ireland.

One of the most important effects of the TAIP-based therapy is that once the women had mourned the loss of their childhood and idealised mother, they found that their relationship to their real mother changed for the better as they were able to view their parent from an adult perspective. It is useful to inform clients who are working on the TAIP of this outcome as they struggle to let go of their idealised attachment.

Having measured symptoms such as depression and their levels of dissociation before and after the therapy, we noted that for those who had succeeded in letting go of their Child Self, both results had returned to normal levels, which is remarkable. It indicates that the *traumatic attachment* is central to understanding dissociation and that its dismantlement through the combined use of the TAIP, and associated grief work, can be curative (Şar, 2014; Lyssenko et al., 2018; Zulueta, 2010a).

Those who had not yet succeeded in letting go of their Child Self but who knew how to do it, had improved to some degree. Those who simply found it too difficult to carry out the ritual were usually patients who had had no previous therapy. Members of these last two groups were offered the possibility of joining the same type of group for a second time.

This group therapy for women sexually abused as children was regularly repeated within the TSS and it was also offered to men who suffered from the effects of child sexual abuse. We also monitored changes in a less formal way at various stages within the group itself. Those who repeatedly self-harmed or abused alcohol reported a decrease. They also reported an increase in their levels of trust, decreased levels of isolation, and increased levels of social interaction, self-esteem, confidence, and self-care which were also observed by the therapists. They began to view their future in a more hopeful way, and some of the women began to reduce their medication and use their mental health services less frequently.

As a few of these women were attending local psychiatric services, one of the therapists would attend their community mental health team meetings to report on their progress or discuss any difficulties that they were having. By the time I retired from the TSS, this therapeutic model had been taken up by other psychotherapy units in the South London and Maudsley NHS Trust because of its effectiveness.

The triangle of abuse

One of the most important contributions to the group and to my learning experience was the introduction of the *triangle of abuse* which is described by Ney and Peters as involving the Victim, Perpetrator, and Colluder.

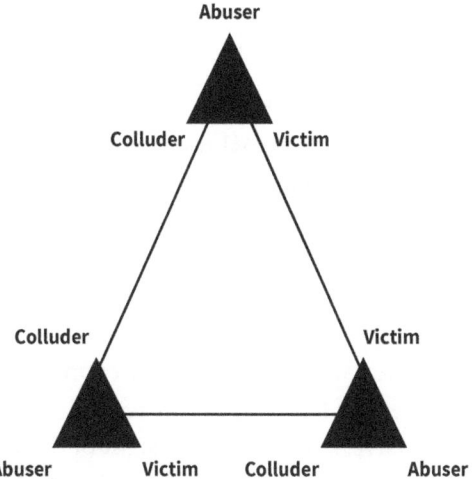

Figure 5.1 Triangle of abuse

It certainly changed my way of thinking about abuse and violence in general. The easiest way to understand it is to think of a fairly common example of abuse: an adult survivor of sexual abuse, like the members of our group, may find herself in a relationship with a man who ends up abusing her daughter because she fails to protect her; the once-survivor mother has now become the observer/colluder in this triangle of abuse, much as her mother probably was in relation to her own abuse.

One may well ask: Why did this adult survivor get involved with a potential abuser? Unfortunately, those who suffer from complex trauma tend to re-enact their abuse either as an abuser, as a victim, or, as we are learning, as an observer/colluder. As Van der Kolk states:

> These victimised people neutralise their emotional hyperarousal by a variety of addictive behaviours, including compulsive re-exposure to situations reminiscent of the trauma. (Van der Kolk, 1989, p. 401)

Trauma-induced compulsive re-exposure behaviour can be found in veterans who enlist as mercenaries, in sexually abused children who become prostitutes (Welldon, 1988), in physically abused children who recreate their violent abuse with their partners in adulthood through domestic violence and many other violent offences. These experiences can lead to the release of endogenous opiates which helps these women and men to regulate their emotional arousal.

In this way, the phenomenon of *repetition compulsion*, which results from the inability to integrate and process traumatic experiences due to the split Self, can also become addictive and thereby soothe the individual's pain (Gilligan, 1996; Zulueta, 2006a). Young people who cut themselves report finding peace and relief from their emotional pain, which as we know is every bit as real as physical pain.

The triangle of abuse is an important part of the mental representations of abused individuals and should play a part in their therapeutic journey despite the understandable reluctance of victims to be seen in any other role. It is also important for psychiatrists and psychotherapists to remember that patients who suffer from PTSD and C-PTSD can unfortunately traumatise their children, as Main discovered when she carried out her study of the disorganised attachment.

The reader may recall how the refugee women who had been raped and who subsequently had babies as a result of the rape, managed to traumatise their children simply through the way they behaved when experiencing flashbacks of their terrifying traumatic experience at the hands of their abuser. They were, in effect re-creating the triangle of abuse and had become the unsuspecting abusers of their infant boys, who were now both their victims as well as being their mothers' abusers, since it was the sight of their eyes, or possibly their male genitalia, that had triggered these women's flashbacks. The TAIP breaks the cycle of abuse by healing the vulnerable Self.

When one realises the level of disturbance suffered by most, if not all, of the women referred to us, it is not surprising that one year of this group work was not enough on its own for people who did not have any prior experience of therapy. It is a very short period of time for such vulnerable people like Aida, whose story I am sharing here:

> Aida, a fifty-three-year-old Moroccan woman was one of the people referred to the TSS for the treatment of her traumatic memories of child sexual abuse. Her referrer was a therapist who was seeing her in short-term psychotherapy for one of her many symptoms. She presented as a vivacious woman who was keen to make contact with me.
>
> Aida gave me a detailed account of her current difficulties relating to her poor sleep, disturbed by nightmares where she relived her sexual abuse. In addition, she was very frightened to go out on her own and depended on her very close relationship with her daughter as well as a tendency to drink too much.
>
> Aida was born in the UK, the eldest of three sisters. Her father was an abusive alcoholic who beat his wife and started sexually abusing her at a young age. Her mother was never able to

stop the abuse and even prevented her from informing the police or the medical staff, denying that the abuse had ever taken place.

To escape from her abusers, Aida married very young and had her daughter, Rana. Her husband left her, but she held a good job until she was forty years old, when she had a mental breakdown. She had struggled ever since.

She suffered from symptoms of C-PTSD. Aida not only relived her abuse at night but also in the day, when she often felt that it was literally happening all over again; these flashbacks and re-enactments usually ended up with a panic attack. In her attempts to reduce these horrific experiences, she avoided anything that could remind her of the traumas by dissociating. This left her feeling emotionally detached and numb, unable to have loving feelings and without any sense of a future, although she wanted one.

Controlling her emotions was a problem for her, as it is for all who suffer from the effects of the disorganised attachment; she was hyper-vigilant and aroused, which added to her sleep problems, and she could be physically violent with her daughter. She had also tried to take her own life in adolescence. Her concentration and memory were poor and as she could not go out alone; she depended on Rana who was now an adult.

Aida's mother, who had died a few years before, finally admitted to her daughter that she had been abused. Despite this awful acknowledgement, Aida just wanted to feel that her mother loved her, and she protected her by seeing her as "a victim of circumstance". It was clear to me that she was still very distressed by her loss and that she had not been able to mourn her mother's death because of her *traumatic attachment* to her. In our second assessment session, having obtained more information about her history, I checked out her levels of depression and dissociation, which were high for someone with C-PTSD but made sense in relation to her history of emotional neglect and sexual abuse in early life. Since I felt that she was very motivated to engage in therapy and that she trusted me, I decided to carry out the TAIP.

I told her that we often used a test that might prove helpful in understanding what was going on for her. She agreed to using it and I started by telling her to notice any changes in her body when I asked her to repeat certain words for me. I then asked her to imagine her mother sitting before her and to say to her: "I am an adult. I am fifty-three years old and am the mother of a daughter. I don't need you anymore like I did as a child."

It was clear that she was overwhelmed by her attachment to her mother even before the TAIP and this became more obvious when carrying out the procedure. She sobbed, telling me how much she needed her and depended on her.

Once she had calmed down, she told me that when I referred to her as a fifty-three-year-old and the mother of a child, she was saying to herself "that's all wrong" and she ended up telling me that she never could believe that she had actually been her daughter's mother: this was her Child Self speaking. This last interaction between Aida and me shows how important it is to get clients to define their adulthood by describing their grown-up achievements *before* doing the TAIP. I had failed to do so in this case by defining her Adult Self for her and asking her to repeat those words that came from me and not from her.

She could see that she behaved with her daughter very much as her mother had behaved with her, especially as Rana looked so much like her grandmother. She told me that she had accused Rana of "not helping her to become independent and holding her back". This is yet another reference to the Child Self speaking.

I suggested that she and Rana alternately re-enact their relation to their mother, either as mother or as daughter, thereby repeating the rejection they had both lived through which made them both very upset and led them to fight verbally, and even physically, when Aida hit her daughter.

This role reversal between mother and child is frequently found in patients with a diagnosis of "borderline personality disorder" whose levels of dissociation are high.

Both complex PTSD and BPD result from the effects of the disorganised attachment and its *traumatic attachment*, so why is one diagnosed as a traumatic disorder and the other as a personality disorder? This example shows how unreliable the diagnostic boundaries are between these two disorders (Zulueta, 2009).

Aida's attitude to therapy and her degree of insight following the TAIP was a very good reason not to label her with a BPD diagnosis which can often be seen in a very negative way.

"Borderline personality disorder"

Our next experience of using the TAIP is in relation to women whose diagnosis of BPD is a source of criticism and anger. While I worked in the TSS, we used the diagnosis of complex PTSD, which was appropriate since it recognised these patients' histories of childhood trauma.

Many of the people who suffer from BPD tend to become intensely dependent and very angry with those with whom they are involved. They often suffer from extreme mood swings and impulsive behaviours, which makes their management and treatment very difficult.

As they tend to switch from idealising one person and denigrating another, the resulting "splitting" that occurs between members of staff can be very destructive. The latter will often describe these patients as "manipulative" and "attention seeking" and their demands are then met with anger and rejection, often recreating the very same conflicts these women experienced in their early life.

Without some way of making sense of these individuals' behaviour, both their therapy and management can easily become reactive, disciplinarian, and even abusive. As a result, individuals diagnosed as suffering from a BPD in general psychiatry often feel stigmatised, misunderstood, and rejected and their psychiatrists often consider them incurable.

It is interesting to note that the "splitting" in relation to the patient's treatability even takes place at a diagnostic and therapeutic level because, outside the wards, psychotherapists have developed many different therapeutic approaches which often greatly improve their clients' mental state and behaviour such as Jeffrey Young's schema therapy model (Young, Klosko, & Weishaar, 2003; Arntz & Jacob, 2013) or Anthony Ryle's cognitive analytical therapy (CAT) (Ryle,1990).

Origin of the symptoms of so-called "borderline personality disorder"

This disorder is very much the result of childhood trauma and neglect, more so than any other personality disorder. The rates of physical, sexual, and verbal abuse combined are in the range of 60 to 80 per cent. The severity of this condition is very much related to the degree of abuse, as is the amount of self-harming (Bressin & Gordon, 2013). It is also the personality disorder that is more likely to report a history of adoption, paternal alcoholism, divorce, and parental desertion as well as parental failings such as a neglectful mother and an abusive father. The affected women often do not recollect their sexual abuse (Mosquera, Gonzalez, & Hart, 2011).

As a result of these experiences, the women who suffer from this disorder feel extremely insecure.

Many authors on the subject identify the disorganised *traumatic attachment* in infancy as the origin of BPD and point out that therefore these individuals have a fragile sense of Self with very high levels of dissociation akin, at times, to a dissociated identity disorder or DID (ibid.). This is yet another traumatic disorder resulting from extreme abuse and neglect, which Dr Valerie Sinason, one of the few psychiatrists trained in psychotherapy, has studied and bravely exposed one of its horrific origins, satanic sexual abuse rings in the UK. This has been at a personal risk to herself (Sinason, 1998).

An alternative diagnosis for BPD, the disorganised attachment disorder

For many suffering from the symptoms of BPD, this diagnosis is now not only seen as detrimental to the treatment of many who are diagnosed with it, but the fact that it has now been classified as one of several personality disorders both in *ICD-11* and *DSM-5* poses another problem for those who suffer from its effects: they think that this diagnosis does not acknowledge the traumatic origins that I have outlined above.

In view of these valid criticisms of the diagnosis of BPD, I suggest an alternative diagnosis that recognises its traumatic origins: disorganised attachment disorder (DAD) and will refer to it in future. I also note that the same symptoms are referred to online as those of a disorganised attachment in adults, a much more appropriate way of describing the condition.

The current diagnostic symptoms of DAD or BPD are outlined below in italic accompanied by my explanation for their development in relation to the damage done by the *traumatic attachment* to their early development:

1. *Frantic efforts to avoid real or imagined abandonment.* It is as if an adult has turned into an infant or child who cannot bear to be left alone when separated from her mother

or father because she has not reached the stage of development that enables the child to hold in her mind their absent parent as a source of comfort. This reminds us of earlier scenes in the Strange Situation where infants show a "disorganised type" of behaviour following the return of their abusive parent and end up "stilling" or "freezing" (Chapter 3, p. 47).

These adults' development remains "stuck" at that point because it is then that the ANS defence system hijacks the normal development of their attachment system.

When triggered by subsequent similar traumatic experiences in adulthood, these individuals find themselves re-enacting their infantile response. It is important to remember that although we see it as too extreme for their age, it is literally how they feel, never having had a parent to help them regulate their emotions.

Though the *DSM-5* makes the point that one should not include suicidal behaviour here, the fact is that I have personal experience of attempted suicides which were due to a Child Self's attempts to join a dead mother.

2. *A pattern of unstable and intense interpersonal relationships characterised by alternating extremes of idealisation and devaluation.* This makes us think of the Child Self of the *traumatic attachment*, a dissociated Self where one part of the Self is hanging onto the idealised mother while the other part of the Self is terrified of the rejecting or abusing parent. If we recall that IWMs represent relationship templates that can be re-enacted by survivors of abuse as the victim or the perpetrator, this strange behaviour begins to make sense to us but not to the woman who is experiencing them. She is taken over by those emotions.

I suspect that the recurrent suicidal behaviour, gestures, and threats are part of the same phenomenon.

3. *Identity disturbance.* We need to constantly remind ourselves that, while these individuals can often function very well as professional adults in one Self-state, most of the other Self-states result from a vast array of abusive and neglectful experiences which they experienced very early on in their development. The multiplicity of their abusive experiences results in a highly dissociated Self, which is what distinguishes these women and men from those suffering from other personality disorders or C-PTSD.

4. "When I came to see you, I was all over the place. I didn't know who I was," said Chloe, one of the women I worked with, whose experiences are described below.

5. *Self-mutilating behaviour* is often carried out to obtain relief from pain and anguish since cutting or burning releases endogenous opiates.

6. *Impulsivity in at least two areas that are potentially self-damaging, such as substance abuse, spending, sex, or binge eating.* I think this explanation does not consider the motivation for these behaviours which, like addiction, provide these women with temporary relief from the terrible emotional pain they feel and reduce their chronic feelings of inner emptiness which is their frequent complaint.

7. *Chronic feelings of emptiness.* This experience of an empty hole at the core of their sense of Self, is very well described by two of Monique Notice's clients in Chapter 7 who we know suffered from the effects of the *traumatic attachment*. It is an extremely distressing lived experience for these women.

8. *Inappropriate intense anger or difficulty controlling anger and frequent displays of temper, constant anger, recurrent physical fights* arise as a result of early terrifying experiences of abuse which are being triggered or reactivated by any similar minor slights or abuse; their anger only appears "inappropriate" out of context because we fail to take into account their traumatic history combined with a reduced capacity to regulate emotions resulting from the damage to the orbitofrontal area of the brain (Silbersweig et al., 2007).

9. *Affective instability due to marked reactivity of mood such as intense episodic irritability, anxiety, or dysphoria lasting a few hours, and only rarely more than a few days* are due to a failure to regulate emotions.

The psychotherapeutic treatment of BPD or DAD

When training to be a psychotherapist at the Maudsley Hospital, one of my first patients exposed me to most of these destructive behaviours. Whilst our sessions did not leave me feeling completely overwhelmed, they were very distressing and, at times, I did wonder if there was a better way of helping my patient. This was before the more cognitively based approaches, such as Anthony Ryle's CAT (1990) and Young's schema therapy (2003) had been developed, offering a structured and collaborative approach to working with such patients. My supervisor was a very experienced psychoanalyst inspired by Kernberg's transference-based psychoanalytic approach.

> Mina was a twenty-five-year-old woman when we first met: she was half-Indian and half-English, from an affluent family living in London. She had suffered from emotional abuse and physical neglect during her childhood as her mother was often ill and in hospital. Her father, who was emotionally abusive to his wife, was often away on business.
>
> Mina was only six years old when her mother died, and she was left in the care of her father. He employed Indian nannies to look after her and began to abuse her sexually. He was a very intimidating man who threatened her in all sorts of ways so that she never dared to tell anyone about her abuse while she attended school. When she was seventeen, her father suddenly died of a heart attack abroad.
>
> At this point her English grandmother took over her care and helped her to get into university. She managed to get a good degree, being very bright, and obtained a well-paid job. During this time, she had many relationships with men, but they all ended badly which made her cut herself and take drugs to cope with the loss. At the age of twenty-four, after losing yet another boyfriend, she took an overdose and was admitted to hospital. This is when she was referred to my supervisor who suggested that I take her on for psychoanalytic psychotherapy, which lasted years.

During the first few years of therapy, Mina did manage to develop a long-term relationship with a man whom she married, and she also formed an attachment to me; most of the time I was idealised but at other times I was denigrated. Any mention of separation, due to work or a holiday on my part, led to explosive anger and threats, as well as a lot of distress. These temporary losses clearly triggered unconscious memories of her lost parents and especially her mother's death. When away from me, she needed to feel that I was "there for her", otherwise she felt I was abandoning her, like her mother had done by going into hospital and then dying.

She initiated our first therapeutic ending by telling me that she and her husband planned to live in France for his business. However, after a few months, I learnt that she had not moved and had been admitted to a private hospital following an overdose. She also wanted to resume her therapy with me, which my supervisor and I agreed to.

In our first sessions following the break, Mina told me that she now realised that she would always need me, even if I saw her for fifteen years! This made her angry and I felt that she wanted to keep me as an idealised mother and thereby avoid working on her losses as she began to realise how many negative feelings she had towards her parents. "When that happens," she told me, there were "no good feelings". Connections with the past were dangerous. The moral defence linked to the *traumatic attachment* had to be maintained because for the Child Self it meant survival.

Sometime later, following twice-a-week therapy, I felt we had gone back to the beginning when Mina declared "I need you all the time". "What you offer me is no good because it just is not enough!" "I can only stand a therapy with no breaks." "You should have made me better." Each time I had to be away, she would become enraged.

Finally, after four years, during which she enacted many of the disturbing behaviours I outlined earlier, Mina decided to end therapy with me. We agreed on making a date some time away, so that she could work towards separating from me, which would help her to mourn the loss of her parents.

Following this decision, we did enter a phase when Mina worked harder with me as she struggled in her attempts to make sense of her feelings and her behaviour and, as the end date approached, she began to experience memories and emotions relating to the loss of her mother. This seemed positive at one level, but they were very painful. We were in the shadow of her mother's death and Mina's anger was always close to the surface.

A few sessions before the official date when we were going to part, Mina decided that we must stop doing this work. She was feeling very low and was furious as she did not think that she could go through the loss of her mother. It was too painful. She wanted to try to live without therapy.

Again, I was very much aware of her need to hold onto her strong moral defence, which is the way traumatised children maintain their idealised parent and blame themselves for what they endured. She confirmed my fear when she admitted she was afraid of being a "good patient", meaning doing the therapeutic work that she felt was expected of her. She also said that being angry with her parents was one way of keeping them alive. She felt that having to face their loss might make her "fall apart" and she did not want to go through that, both for her sake and that of her husband's. She wanted to live a normal life.

At our last session, she left me in a rather matter-of-fact way. I feared that we were recreating the abandonment she had experienced as a child. However, the roles were reversed: by being the one who left, she enacted her mother, and I was the abandoned child; but would that role reversal be enough to protect her? She did have my phone number, so I was potentially still there for her.

Sometime later, I was informed that she did try and take an overdose, but she survived, and she let me know that she was under the care of another consultant in her area and was being given regular support rather than psychoanalytic psychotherapy.

Naturally, I felt tremendous relief to know that she was alive and in good hands. I did not have the knowledge I now have which would have made me realise a lot earlier that this lengthy psychoanalytic therapy, albeit under expert supervision, was not recommended for individuals like Mina. This was because, as a person whose Self was so profoundly split by the *traumatic attachment*, she rightly felt that she did not have the resources to mourn the loss of her mother with such an approach, let alone deal with the sexual abuse and loss of her father. She wanted to live, and she knew better than me what she did not need. I learnt from her many things and the most important was what Dr Clare taught me on my first day in psychiatry: "listen to your patients".

I have shared this piece of work in some detail because it does illustrate how difficult it is to help people with a severe DAD (or with BPD) if one does not understand the role of dissociation resulting from the *traumatic attachment*. The psychoanalysts in the Department of Psychotherapy at the Maudsley Hospital who trained me never mentioned dissociation: for them only repression existed.

I often dreaded our sessions, as Mina managed to make me feel very upset, worried, angry, anxious, and inadequate. When on the receiving end of her anger, at times it was a bit like being flayed alive! However, I never lost the sense that she did not want to be as verbally aggressive as she was with me but, since I was making her suffer, she was going to fight back as best she could.

The inability to mourn the loss of important attachment figures is one of the main obstacles, if not *the* main obstacle, to making a full recovery for those who suffer from the effects of the *traumatic attachment* and its dissociated Self.

Using the TAIP to heal DAD or BPD

Chloe was referred to me when I was a consultant psychiatrist in psychotherapy at Charing Cross Hospital, where I developed and ran an NHS out patient psychotherapy service. She presented as a feisty young woman of twenty-five who was clearly suffering a lot with a history of self-harm and serious overdoses as well as a terrifying *traumatic attachment* to her mother.

I felt warmly towards her because of her defiant spirit and the precise way in which she expressed herself. We seemed to be getting on, and although she fulfilled the criteria for complex PTSD and so-called BPD, which I knew would be a serious challenge, I offered to see her for psychotherapy on a weekly basis.

Chloe is the person mentioned in the introduction to this book, who told me to take on the task of sharing our findings relating her experience of the TAIP. Having finally decided to do this, I recently met with her on a few occasions to discuss this book and her role in it.

We had kept in touch since our last session, many years before, and I was aware of what she had been through since then. She discovered that she was gay, got married and had a child before she divorced. Chloe obtained a law degree and now works in schools helping children with difficulties. She recently lost her father. As Chloe put it simply, "I now live my life in the real world."

On one occasion, when we were meeting to prepare for this chapter, we looked at some of my old notes relating to her diagnosis and I noticed that she looked a bit upset. She then wrote to me the following email which she has given me permission to share here.

Chloe's notes and my response

> It was hard to read the notes about me, it felt very clinical. My life experiences reduced to a few lines of clinical diagnosis. It was sad to read.
>
> Remembering the past brings up feelings of frustration, annoyance, and some anger that it got to that stage in the first place.
>
> However, now my anger doesn't turn against me, my energy is aimed at a broken system that doesn't help children enough.

Her reaction to seeing my clinical notes left me feeling sad that I had upset her by reminding her of the times when I was the Doc Z who could listen to her bravely sharing her pain and distress only to appear to reduce her life experiences to a few lines of clinical diagnosis. Of course, these were not my psychotherapy notes where I recorded from memory in my own words what took place every time we met for a session.

However, her reaction does highlight the gap that exists between the awful reality of her past abusive experiences which psychiatrists simply label as "mental health conditions" or worse without showing any interest in what Chloe and others like her have been through. Somehow, by giving a "scientific diagnosis" to peoples' behaviour without any reference to what is really causing this behaviour, the psychiatrist appears to be refusing to acknowledge the fact that these people have survived levels of violence that, if carried out on adults, would be considered criminal. At times, the childhood stories that I hear, like the one that Chloe shares here, are tantamount to torture, especially as the violence is being carried out on children who cannot defend themselves and which, we now know, disrupts their entire development with far-reaching, damaging consequences in adulthood.

So, by turning these individuals' life experiences into so-called medical "symptoms and disorders" we are not attending to the reality of their lives nor are we acknowledging their suffering. Is it because we cannot cope with the fact that so many children are going through this, and so little is being done to prevent it? Or does it stir up our own unacknowledged suffering? After all, most of us are in this field because we have experienced ACEs, not to the extent that Mina and Chloe have, but enough to feel the need to avoid reminders of our helplessness at the hands of an abusive parent.

Chloe's notes continued

Perhaps to make me realise what my use of symptoms and diagnoses ignore, Chloe has described her childhood in notes which I am replicating here. (Her mother's voice is in bold type, as is mine.)

> By the time I was six years old I hated her.
> I wished she was dead.
> I knew I wasn't normal. I knew things in our house weren't normal.
> I cried once to a lady and told her how unhappy I was.
> She hugged me. She wiped my tears. She sent me home.
> I hated her too.
> We moved house several times before I was eight. Finally settled in a huge smelly and busy place where people talked funny and didn't like me or the way I talked either.
> I became a master of disguise.
> I looked out at the world.
> But … the world could not GET me.
> Me. I was safe.
> She could rage, holler, beat and chastise.
> Nothing could penetrate the safe cocoon I'd so cleverly built for myself. all by myself. I was so proud of myself. I'd done something right.
> Best of all it was quiet.
> I have a younger sibling who remembers very little of our life—I'm glad she doesn't.
> I, me. Remember everything.
> Left home alone in charge of my sibling. She comes home, sees we are still awake—puts two chairs either side of the living room—
> **run you little **** - RUN.**
> Each time I pass the chair I receive a hefty blow to my head—
> a whack to my face—
> **RUN! RUN! RUN! RUN!**
> **—you have energy to be awake— ***** RUN!**
> When I finally collapse – she leaves me there.
> I was seven.

Play for me!

—uuuummmm

Oh pleeeeease …

I don't want to.

PLAY!

It really wasn't worth saying anything as it always ended up worse for me.

One morning—

I don't feel well.

If you are sick, go to the doctors, I have work.

Front door bangs shut.

I went by myself. I had tonsillitis.

I was eight.

At nine I was still wetting the bed.

One night after not succeeding to convince her I was fast asleep, I got dragged out of bed. Found out I'd wet the bed and the soiled sheet got wrapped so tightly around my face I passed out.

By ten it was either the beatings or the bereft—which one would it be?

Footsteps up to the front door would leave my heart pounding.

SHIT—keys dropped.

BANG—BANG—LET ME IN!

On the upstairs landing I saw my sibling. Go back to bed and pretend to be asleep.

The front door opened. Her figure wobbled straight to the kitchen.

are you hungry I am what do you want I want something make me something what have we got come here do you love me I'm such a mess I'm sorry I'm hungry make me something not that why are you so stupid leave I'll do it sit down—no not upstairs sit there and wait you useless ***

mmmm I'm safe now—I laughed at how silly it was. Me—downstairs—in the kitchen at 11.30pm in my nighty, freezing cold feet watching her trying to cook …

*** BAMMMMM

Something hard and cold hit my face—**I'M TALKING TO YOU DO YOU HEAR ME—BAMMMMM** another blow to my head.

BAMM

BAM

BAMMM

I don't remember anything else.

I was ten.

I spend my life peering out. I come out to check if my sibling was okay.

She knows how to GET me.

If I don't respond—she goes for my sibling. I can't.

I really can't let that happen.

I don't let that happen.

I'm here. Come and get me.

I hate her.

She cries.

By eleven, I am so cut off from myself and everybody. I've forgotten what it's like to BE any other way.

I go to school, come home, eat, sleep, I go to school, bunk off school, try to escape—smoke dope—I don't really like it.

By seventeen, I'm a shell. I go to college. An older girl there takes one look at me and gives me the number of a counsellor.

My journey begins.

I don't remember how old I was when I was first admitted to a psych ward. Probably about twenty. I'd taken an overdose. I don't remember if I really wanted to die or not.

This was the start of a roller coaster of psychiatric-based events.

I clearly remember that first time I met DR. Z. in a stuffy therapy room in a large NHS inner-city hospital.

How are you feeling?

Long silence ... that there are pieces of me ... scattered everywhere.

Perhaps we could work at putting them back together?

So, we tried.

With patience, understanding, and the help of Dr Z, we worked together to find ways of bringing the shattered pieces of myself together. And we did.

We started with the more formal psychiatric route of delving into one's past (to see what went wrong)—however this just didn't work as every time we tried to do this, it sent my brain and me whirlwind crazy.

After a few attempts of this I remember marching into her office and saying to Dr Z "I can't do this anymore we have to find another way to make it different ..."

For most of the sessions I would look at Dr Z's feet. And they took on a safe personality of their own.

I have sporadic memories of the actual sessions. What I do remember the most is the physical that feelings would come up:

- Hearing my heartbeat in my ears
- Every muscle being tense
- The light around me being (too) bright
- Not being able to feel the ground underneath my feet
- Stabbing hot poker pain in my stomach
- Scrambled egg brain/trying to think through treacle
  My heart being crushed in a vice.

I do remember these moments too. We were by then in the Maudsley Hospital as Chloe had successfully obtained funding to follow me there for the rest of her therapy.

She was right, we had to find a way to work that did not trigger her past traumatic experiences. I knew only too well how useless that was from my earlier experience. So, I decided to work "in the here and now". We would sometimes end up sitting on the floor when a Child-Self was around. And I became very self-conscious of my feet as Chloe would interpret my emotions through the movements of my feet; she was usually correct, which was a little embarrassing.

However, this was collaborative work, and I felt much more at ease, focusing on an approach that encouraged mentalization and the integration of self-states. I would pick up something she said or the way she said it and we would try and understand what lay behind it; we ended up discovering emotions that she had learnt to hide and understand how she operated when frightened to avoid re-enactments. I also shared with her ways of managing her emotions.

One of the most visible changes that she finally achieved was being able to look at my face rather than at my feet, such had been the levels of terror in relation to the mother whom I could sometimes represent in the transference.

She finally ended therapy, a very different and confident person, who was studying to obtain a job. She had made good friends and was in an intimate relationship. She also felt that she could now "handle" her mother. What was very interesting is that, just as she was about to open the door to leave, Chloe turned round and asked me: "If I have a baby can I come and see you to meet my baby?"

I instinctively responded "Yes, of course", feeling that it was important for her to leave with a sense that we were still connected.

Two years later, Chloe rang me up asking me for an appointment. I met with her in a private room. She looked very well, and I learnt that everything was going well in her life: she was about to start a new career, having got a job and passed her exams. What was really distressing her however was that—having achieved all this—she now felt the same destructive and suicidal urges she had had all those years ago, before coming into therapy. I felt my heart sink: her Child Self was clearly terrified of losing her *traumatic attachment* to her idealised mother.

When I asked her about her relationship to her mother, she sounded irritated. I asked her why and she told me that her mother had not congratulated her on her success in her exams.

Picking up her anger, I thought of the TAIP and asked her if she would mind carrying out this test that we had developed.

She agreed to it so I told her that I would ask her to repeat some words after me and I asked her to notice what happened in her body as she spoke. I also added that I would look away so as not to make her feel embarrassed (which we no longer do as it has not seemed necessary).

Then I said to her: "Your mother is now sitting opposite you, and I would like you to say to her "Mum, I am now a grown-up woman with a job and a career before me, I don't need your approval as I did when I was little." There was a silence and then she swore out loud. She was very angry to find out how frightened she felt at the thought of doing without her mother. She noticed that her stomach was churning, and her heart was beating fast. She also realised that this meant that a part of her was still terrified of her mother and still desperate to get her love and approval. However, strengthened by her newly found confidence and aspirations, she was determined to "let go" of this part of herself, her Child Self.

I gave her the ritual we had used in the group for women who had been sexually abused in childhood (Ney & Peters, 1995, pp. 88–107) which meant choosing a day to devote to burying her Child Self, symbolised by a picture or object representing this little Self, and then letting it go in some way, for example, either burying it or sending down a river. She would then be likely to feel strong emotions welling up inside. As I remembered that during our therapy she had always been terrified of crying as she believed she would simply melt into a puddle, I added: "Go to your room and let the tears come. Imagine that you are on a beach with big waves washing over you and there is also a rock for you to hang onto when the waves break over you."

She left me with renewed energy, and we met for a second appointment two weeks later when she told me that she had not been able to fix a day to do it but that she would. Our third appointment took place after Christmas.

Chloe's notes continued

As for the TAIP

I remember that we used an empty chair with a blue fabric seat.

Five words changed my life.

"I don't need you anymore"

Afterwards:

I remember lying in bed and the gut-wrenching pain of crying so forcefully I thought I'd drown.

It consumed my whole body.

Waves of feelings would jolt out of me.

Probably for my self-preservation—I don't remember what I did after that at all.

Had a similar pain starting in exactly the same place in my body—my solar plexus—when (years later) I left my baby son for the first time (with a friend).

A sense of emptiness

A tight and urgent pull (to go back).

I had to fight very hard to overcome this sense or urge to go back (to him).

Unsteady on my feet. Not quite sure of my steps

Not quite able to be in the moment.

Although this time I didn't feel like I would drown—I had other people around me—supporting me.

Had a similar one when found out my dad was going to die/only had a few months to live.

The overwhelming gut feeling took over

But I didn't drown—I had someone to call and cry with and other people around me to talk to. It's no surprise that people take drugs, drink, are violent or anything else rather than feel "that" pain.

I never thought of myself as being a brave person.

However, thinking about all this—I was very brave to put myself through/face that kind of pain.

After Christmas, Chloe appeared looking wonderfully happy and proud of herself. She had undertaken the "ritual" and had also found herself crying for hours, mourning the loss of the childhood she never had and realising that her mother could never give her the love that she had yearned for (Bloom, 2000).

In this way, after three sessions over six weeks, she ended her last phase of psychotherapy, free from any self-destructive feelings. She then asked me playfully to guess what she had done at Christmas and proceeded to report that she and her sister had had a pleasant family occasion with their mother.

As we were about to end the session, Chloe stood up to face me and said: "It is now my turn to tell you something that you need to do: you must write about the way in which you enabled me to live as a normal person." She also advised me to use the TAIP in the assessment of other patients with similar histories of abuse, since this experience was so valuable for her in achieving a full recovery.

It is interesting that she ended by warning me that my psychiatric colleagues would laugh at me for suggesting such a possibility.

Sometime later, I was in a seminar with psychiatric colleagues discussing the treatment of people who suffered from so-called BPD. I told the professor in charge that we had developed a way of curing this disorder, which was met with derision, just as Chloe had warned me.

I challenged him to meet with the person who had experienced this new approach and to let me know what he thought after interviewing her. I had already asked Chloe if she would agree to such a meeting.

On the day of the appointment, this professor in forensic psychiatry met with her for more than half an hour. When the interview was over, she left, and he came smiling towards me and exclaimed: "Don't tell me she ever had a diagnosis of borderline personality disorder!" He was adamant that there was nothing wrong with her and walked away as I tried to describe the volumes of hospital notes on her case. Such is the closed mindset of some of my colleagues. Meanwhile, twenty-five years later, Chloe continues to live her life in the real world.

Chloe has the last word

> As for the clinical diagnosis of "borderline personality disorder",
>   When I came to see you, I was all over the place. I didn't know who I was. So, I guess "my-person" was disordered in some way as I didn't really know who I was at all.
>   However, to say that that it can't be cured or that a person can't find themselves, and with the right support in place in their life, to actually get to know who they are, is just not true.
>   I am the living testament to this.
>   Chloe

I only wish I had known about the TAIP when I was working with Mina and when a colleague and I developed and supervised the running of a group combined with individual therapy for individuals suffering from BPD or DAD (Zulueta & Mark, 2000). This approach was designed to contain the splitting which can be so easily disruptive during their therapeutic progress.

The role of the disorganised attachment in trauma-induced disorders

In my view, having worked with many of the different manifestations of terror's effects on the human mind, PTSD, complex PTSD (C-PTSD) and DAD, and the misnamed "borderline personality disorder" can all be seen as a way of describing and classifying people's responses to increasingly severe levels of traumatisation. Since we are now looking at trauma from an attachment perspective, we can begin to think about the possible role that the disorganised attachment and its accompanying *traumatic attachment*, may have in how humans respond to subsequent terrifying experiences as adults.

We know that the disorganised attachment in early childhood leads to the creation of the *traumatic attachment* and leaves its victims with a divided Self in addition to a fundamental reorganisation of the way the person experiences and reacts to the world compared to securely attached children.

What we don't yet know is when or if children stop responding to their parents' abuse and neglect by developing a *traumatic attachment*. We may recall that baby rats only reacted to their mother's inadequate care by developing the equivalent of a *traumatic attachment* to her for the first ten days of life, after which they would avoid her. Does this occur in human children? We have no evidence of it so far.

I suggest that simple PTSD acquired in adulthood, due to one or two traumatic events, does not result from the *traumatic attachment* if recovery takes place fairly promptly, with or without any psychological intervention. This may be more likely to happen if the affected person has developed an insecure avoidant attachment, like Tom. Simple PTSD can be seen as the response of an individual to an event that has triggered the *fight–flight–freeze* response and engendered a dissociative response without the involvement of the traumatic attachment and the splitting of the Self. Such people would not react negatively to doing the TAIP and they should respond to appropriate therapy without resistance to ending. However, this is hypothetical and needs to be confirmed through the use of the TAIP in such cases.

Those adults who respond to a single event with symptoms of PTSD and find it very difficult to recover and end their therapy, are probably individuals who experienced parental abuse and/or neglect in their childhood and developed a *traumatic attachment* which lay dormant until triggered by a specific event that evoked the earlier traumatic experience. These individuals would have a positive response to the TAIP and could develop complex PTSD or even BPD (or DAD) as illustrated by the war veteran Jim and many others.

The more severe type of trauma diagnosed as a personality disorder or BPD is inappropriately classified as these individuals, usually women, but not necessarily so, have in fact experienced more terrifying experiences in their infancy and childhood than any other person with a diagnosis of

PTSD. As I explained above, their condition should be called "disorganised attachment disorder" (DAD) as it is, in essence, the adult version of the disorganised attachment.

If we bear in mind the role of the disorganised attachment during human development and after, we can make much more sense of these trauma-induced conditions and we can understand why the TAIP can have such a powerful reparative effect on the divided Self that underlies C-PTSD and DAD.

So far, we have been able to discover its effect by using the TAIP with women who suffered from sexual abuse in childhood during group therapy. All responded with fear to the use of the TAIP as it elicited their Child Self in interaction with their parent who either terrified them by abusing them or by neglecting them emotionally: to say "I don't need you any more like I did as a child" invited either their parent's fury or the terror of losing the person on whom they depended most in their early life.

Conclusion

It is not surprising that the current psychiatric concept of trauma as defined by *DSM-5* does not suit the international work that is being carried out with the millions of people who have had to emigrate from war zones or climate disaster areas.

We have seen how the diagnosis of PTSD in the United States is given the importance of a scientific medical condition when, in fact, it is only based on clusters of physical symptoms without few, if any, objective scientific measures to confirm its validity and without reference to protective factors such as personal or community resilience or ACEs such as racism which can exacerbate the symptoms of trauma or can itself be traumatic experience which results in PTSD (Cénat, 2023).

Professor Renos Papadopoulos, director of the Centre for Trauma, Asylum and Refugees at the University of Essex, has recently published a book called *Involuntary Dislocation: Home, Trauma, Resilience, and Adversity-activated Development* (2021) on the treatment of migrants. It provides a powerful in-depth critique of the American psychiatric way of looking at PTSD, pointing out that the first casualty of trauma is complexity. By developing the Adversity Grid for those who work with migrants, he also provides them with a tool that can address the different ingredients that are likely to contribute to their responses to their involuntary new experiences away from home.

There is no doubt that we would benefit from such an approach, having discovered that the combination of experiences or symptoms and behaviours, labelled as a "dissociated subtype" of PTSD in the United States and complex PTSD in *ICD-11* as well as BPD or DAD, only manifest themselves following:

1. A traumatic experience that elicits terror and associated helplessness in interaction with
2. A vulnerability factor, such as a disorganised attachment associated with a *traumatic attachment* and/or transgenerational or epigenetic predisposing factors and

3. In the absence of a supportive social context or, more specifically, an attachment matrix such as used to exist in Ugandan communities prior to colonisations and which we described with our traumatised young elephants.

I am sure that other factors will become apparent and with therapeutic tools like the TAIP, a more sophisticated grid in relation to these traumatic conditions could be developed.

In the meantime, we are learning about the crucial role of the *traumatic attachment* in the aetiology of traumatic disorders. Our next chapter reveals that it has also been found to be fundamental to the development of different disorders which all share one common factor: they are often described as "difficult-to-treat disorders". This discovery surprised us all.

CHAPTER 6

The role of the TAIP in understanding and healing "difficult-to-treat" disorders

The use of the TAIP in understanding and treating homicidal and other violent individuals

As the TSS was part of Professor Gunn's forensic psychiatric unit, I often had the benefit of assessing patients with a forensic history. The following encounters illustrate how helpful the TAIP could be when it came to giving these men an understanding as to why they had committed their crimes. They could usually connect the emotional state they were in at the time of the crime with experiences of abuse during their childhood. This often opened up for them new ways of thinking about themselves and the work they needed to do with the forensic mental health staff.

The brief story of a young man who wanted to kill his father

Peter was a thirty-three-year-old man who had been referred by his therapist for an assessment because he had a history of repeatedly self-harming, attempting suicide, and trying to kill his father. He would only attend therapy when he felt low and then miss several sessions, which prevented him from making any progress.

Peter joined me with his therapist. He looked young for his age and, although anxious, he was keen to give me any information I needed. His early life had been a very violent one during which he witnessed his father kill his mother when he was six years old. After his mother's death, his father ended up in prison with the result that his paternal grandparents adopted him together with his older sister and younger brother who was disabled as a result of his father throwing him down the stairs.

Their adoption "was the worst thing that could have happened", he told me since the grand-parents used to beat the children and were constantly drunk. He was bullied at school and left, aged sixteen, without any qualifications, to join the army. He thought the army "was brilliant" as it enabled him to get away from his grandparents. Unfortunately, he developed peritonitis which led to a medical discharge. It was then that he met his first partner and found out that his father had come out of prison.

Peter threatened to kill him by throwing him off a cliff and later carried out an "armed" robbery with an imitation firearm in order to buy a gun to shoot his father. He received two consecutive community orders for these offences.

Meanwhile, he was in a relationship with Jane, who is mother to their son and daughter. It was when she started to work that he felt that he had lost control and he began to take the children out with him to drink, just as his grandfather had done with him and his siblings. He also began to abuse Jane physically for which he was charged with assault and bodily harm. They have separated, but he misses the children. He told me he lives with another woman.

Throughout his adult life, Peter had been in and out of psychiatric hospitals for episodes of depression, during which he would often cut himself or take overdoses.

He had also started to have flashbacks of his mother's death and other symptoms of PTSD, such as being unable to sleep and becoming threatening and aggressive.

His therapist added that his suicide threats and his insistence on murdering his father only occurred when he was feeling "down" and, at such moments, he would think of his father and then he would want to kill him for messing up his life.

He was being treated for PTSD and depression in relation to witnessing his mother's murder and he was also on antipsychotic medication.

Peter seemed to be developing a good relationship with me and he clearly trusted his psychotherapist who knew him well, so I decided to carry out the TAIP in our first and only session.

I usually measure people's levels of dissociation using the DES (Bernstein & Putnam, 1986) before carrying out the TAIP. His was 50 when I saw him, which was high, but I was told that it is lower when he is not depressed. He also told me, as we were going through the DES question-naire, that when he felt "low" he had experienced thinking that he had actually killed his father and that he had handed himself to the police because of this belief.

This was interesting, as it confirmed what I was already thinking, which was that he felt in some way impelled to carry out this murder when depressed. It also indicated that he had different states which concurred with his high level of dissociation, compatible with a diagnosis of a dissociative identity disorder.

I explained to him that we had developed a test that we had found to be helpful for people struggling with similar issues to his and I asked if he would like to try it. He was very interested, so I told him that it would involve reminding himself that he is now an adult, father of two children, and then to repeat some words after me and to notice what happens in his body when he tried to say these words.

I proceeded by asking him to imagine that his mother was in the room and to say out loud that he was now a thirty-three-year-old adult with two children and to tell her that he no longer needed her as he did as a child.

His reaction was immediate as he exclaimed: "I am six years old," thereby acknowledging the Child Self in relation to his idealised mother. This reaction is understandable because Peter did not actually acknowledge his adulthood before facing his imaginary mother and being asked to say, "I don't need you any more". This response shows that it is very important to make sure that the Adult Self is in the room before moving into the separation reaction that elicits the Child Self if we want to move on to integrating the split Self.

It was clear that the vivid picture of his mother was still very much in his mind. He could not imagine in any way separating himself from her or doing without her. He said that just thinking about the possibility filled him with tension and pain in his chest and abdomen, the embodied reaction of his Child Self to the TAIP.

He recognised very quickly that this meant that she was very much in his mind, and that he was very attached to her. He acknowledged that he yearns for her whenever he feels abandoned or "down".

Peter then told me that after his mother was stabbed by his father, she was carried away on a stretcher and, as she left the house, she said to him, "I will see you again", which she never did. He then admitted that she had also asked him to kill his father because of what he had done.

In Bowlby's terms, he had an embodied experience of the IWM of his Child Self bound to his idealised mother in reaction to the possibility of being separated from her. This led him to share another experience that he had when he was fourteen years old and spoke to his mother through a medium. She asked him why he hadn't killed his father, which made him feel guilty.

We were able to see that the main trigger for his low moods and his depression was reliving the experience of "abandonment". "When my mother left, I lost everything," he said: his mother and his father as well as his home.

We were thus able to make the very important connection between his Child Self's yearning for his mother, which takes over or is "triggered" when he feels "abandoned", and his need to kill his father to please his mother, a mother he has not been able to mourn because of his fractured Self.

Peter then told me that when Jane left him, he felt he had "lost everything" all over again, just like when he was a six-year-old boy. This was a terrible shock for him. "Now," he said, "I would do anything for Katy", his new girlfriend. If she goes out to buy something in the shops, he has this awful experience that he will never see her again and he must phone her.

I asked Peter what happened in his mind when he felt "low".

At such times, he said, he felt that "everything was gone", which suggests that he feels numb and cut off from all emotions. He "freezes" and dissociates. It is at such times that he wants to feel pain, which leads him to cut himself. It gives him relief to see the blood appear. His overriding thought, at such moments, is that "I am going to see my mum and have a cuddle with my mum."

The only thing that stops him from taking the next step in such moments is the guilt of what he will put his children through from the loss of their father. This is what leads him to dial 999 or to tell somebody rather than to be found following an overdose.

I returned to his mother's wish for him to kill his father and what he felt when she asked him why he had not killed him. He said that he had told her that he had tried twice to do so, and then Peter became quite upset and said, his eyes welling with tears: "But, I don't want to kill anyone. I don't understand why I suddenly become so different and feel I can do it!"

We were able to link these important statements with his vivid experience of panic in relation to the minute or two when he tried to tell his mother that he no longer needed her during the TAIP. He recognised how certain triggers, such as loss or fear, could precipitate him to experience himself as a six-year-old in relation to his mother whom he yearns for. He then saw how his attachment to his mother, already traumatic enough, is perverted by the need to placate her and please her by avenging her through killing his father.

He could see the link between the two and how this was brought on by moving into a Self-state where he becomes the child in need of his mother, his idealised mother.

We have here the IWM of his Child Self yearning for his idealised mother. In this way he escapes the clutches of the Child Self in relation to the traumatic experiences of his past.

Eliciting the *traumatic attachment* is clearly of fundamental importance in both understanding and enabling change to take place for this young man.

I stress the importance of "understanding" as it is a real embodied understanding where "just thinking about the possibility filled him with tension and pain in his chest and abdomen"; as that embodied experience takes place it is as if a movement towards integration appears to follow. (This phenomenon is clearly illustrated in the sessions presented by Monique Notice, Jayshree Unadkat, and Leonor de Escoriaza in the following chapters.)

Following our assessment, Peter began to attend all his sessions with his therapist. She informed me that he acknowledged that our meeting was something of a turning point for him. He found the presence of both me and his therapist very "containing" and, after this meeting, he felt able to make more sense of his difficulties.

With the help of a forensic psychiatrist who was also involved in his care, he was referred and admitted to a therapeutic community called the Henderson Hospital that offered in-patient psychotherapy. He appeared to make good use of his time there, having worked on his different states whilst being supported by the community to manage his strong emotions when he felt depressed.

For those who wish to learn how to use the TAIP, my experience with Peter is very revealing because I could have inadvertently triggered a flashback of his mother's traumatic death when I asked him to imagine his mother before repeating my words, especially as he suffered from PTSD with flashbacks of his mother's death. This did not happen and, in my experience of working with people suffering from complex PTSD, the use of the TAIP has never triggered a flashback or reliving of a past traumatic experience. Those who do work with clients suffering from PTSD know how easily it can happen and how prolonged such effects can be. The fact that using the TAIP never elicits flashbacks suggests that a different neural circuit of the brain is involved.

The short story of Robert, a one-time long-standing patient in Broadmoor Hospital

Robert had been referred to the TSS because he had moved out of Broadmoor hospital where he had been for several years, having received many convictions for robbery, criminal damage, and assault, causing bodily harm as well as threatening an individual with a fake weapon to obtain money. At that time, he was diagnosed as suffering from "paranoid schizophrenia", now referred to as schizophrenia of a paranoid type.

The UK mental health charity, MIND, gives useful information and support to people diagnosed with a mental health disorder, acknowledging for instance that Black people in the UK are more likely to experience discrimination, racism, social deprivation, and migration than most white people (https://www.mind.org.uk/information-support/types-of-mental-health-schizophrenia/). Many have a past family history of slavery or abuse in their home countries, when under colonial rule, which makes them more vulnerable to the traumatic experiences of institutional racism that they suffer in the UK. These kinds of highly stressful life experiences may lead to developing a psychotic illness that has been labelled as "schizophrenia". Similarly, these negative experiences may deter people from seeking help earlier on, or they were not able to obtain professional support until they become severely disturbed. My more open-minded psychiatric teachers soon made me aware of how often this happened, even in the Maudsley Hospital.

The forensic outreach team in charge of Robert's community rehabilitation wanted him to be assessed in relation to his traumatic experiences in Broadmoor Hospital, where he complained of having been abused several times. He was also trying to live in a supported hostel in the community and was studying to be a car mechanic in college, where he felt rather lonely. This meant that his main social contact was going to be with his father.

I learnt from his notes that his parents were of West Indian origin and that he had experienced a violent childhood as his father used to beat both his wife and his son. She often left the home to shelter at her mother's and finally separated from her husband when Robert was only three. At this point, his father took over his son's care. Robert found it hard at school and got into trouble for bad behaviour, so much so that he ended up being either in care or with his father for most of his childhood. His mother suddenly died when he was six and he was still struggling to come to terms with this loss.

When Robert came for his assessment interview, he presented as a friendly thirty-four-year-old fashionably dressed black man with a good sense of humour; however, not surprisingly, he also appeared a little anxious.

We explored his early life and particularly his relationship to his dad. Like many adults who have experienced violent abuse and loss in childhood, he would alternate between presenting a rather idealised picture of his father interspersed with fleeting references to being frightened of him and feeling let down by him. The resulting discourse was at times rather incoherent, bearing the hallmark of the "dysregulated Self in interaction with a mis-attuning and frightening other" (Schore, 2001, p. 240).

The presence of disorganised attachment's *traumatic attachment* became more evident when I interviewed him for the second time and hoped to carry out the TAIP in relation to his father, who was now one of the main people involved with him, which I imagined could be difficult for Robert.

When I began explaining what this test involved, he pointed out that he came from a culture where it would be disrespectful to tell a father that he was not needed anymore. I knew this was true since I had African friends who expected their grown-up children to continue talking to them with far more respect than Western families do.

So, Robert and I had to work out whether he was prepared to modify the TAIP so that he could use it to access an experience that might help him become more independent.

Robert still found this difficult, and I felt that his resistance was also about moving into the community after so many years in Broadmoor Hospital. We spent quite a lot of time in relation to his fear of getting back into the real world as he had tried to do this before but ended up having to return to Broadmoor Hospital. The staff there had, in a way, become his alternative family and he was not equipped to deal with their loss because of his *traumatic attachment*. This problem may apply to many young men who keep reoffending after being discharged from prison.

Our next hurdle was getting his permission to record our interview for the benefit of the forensic outreach team who were supporting him in his rehabilitation. He was worried that his father would get to see it and that it would hurt his feelings. I stressed that the video would be in Robert's safe keeping, to help him as he settled into the community.

Finally, I simply said: "Just see what it feels like to say I don't need my dad anymore."

Robert, who had been extremely talkative, suddenly went quiet, and remained so for nearly two minutes, silent and almost immobile, except for the occasional sigh and flip of his hands in a gesture of despair.

I remarked that he looked very sad, and asked him what had happened, what was it like?

"I don't really know," he replied, tears running down his cheeks.

"Things as a youngster, the past. Body calm … Thinking as a youngster … scars … I've never known where they came from."

He shows me "a scar here" pointing at his right leg "and a scar on my side" showing me his left side.

He then said: "Something came up in my mind … went blank. I couldn't think of my childhood, only … It was as … cold … sometimes I would sleep rough, I used to run away, and when I came back the police would pick me up, I'd be hit again … He's hurt me several times … If I was to say to anybody … It was my dad sometimes … sometimes I could not believe it was my dad. Some things he hasn't told me and the rest of the family has not told me so when I ran away it was to be looked after, to be free from my family shouting at me, giving me the blame. So, in one sense what he'd done to me but then there again …"

In the face of so much suffering, it is hard to know what to say other than to reflect back, in a compassionate way, the enormity of the pain he endured during his childhood.

To introduce some hope, since he was with me for an assessment for psychotherapy, I spoke about the therapeutic work he could be doing with the psychologist who had attended our session. Robert soon made it clear that he was keen to start and finally left me with a smile.

My colleague, an excellent psychologist who worked in the TSS, took him on for brief psychotherapy, teaching him how to regulate his emotions and to improve his ability to recognise the shifts between his idealising Self-states and the reality of his abuse. This would involve using the video we had recorded in my interview with him. Robert initially left it in our care, so that nobody could look at it, but, when he succeeded in moving into his own accommodation, he took it home and used to look at it quite often to help him with his rehabilitation. He subsequently acquired new skills and a more realistic and adult relationship with his father.

The potential role of the TAIP in a risk assessment for homicide

Our earlier interview with Peter using the TAIP revealed that he was being driven to kill his father by his Child-Self's desperate yearning for his idealised mother's love. That is why he was in the care of a forensic psychiatrist. There was the risk that when he was depressed and felt "down", he might attempt to carry out his mother's wish by attacking his father. At some level he could also be driven to do this because of his own hatred of his father.

I will share here two other interviews using the TAIP with men who had committed homicide: both expressed a strong wish to kill their violent fathers.

For confidential reasons, I cannot give many details of their lives, but I can share enough of their background to make sense of the way each one responded to the TAIP in relation to their father.

Edward was an Indian man in his early forties, who lived in the UK. He was being treated for severe complex PTSD with "borderline traits" and depression in his local psychiatric service. He was referred because he was not responding to the therapy and was having to take a lot of medication to calm himself down.

His parents were both from Mumbai and came to the UK as a young married couple to earn their living as shopkeepers. Both were extremely abusive, in their different ways, towards their son. His mother had two daughters to bring up and could scarcely attend to her son's needs. When he cried or protested she would hit him so hard he was made unconscious. His father had a terrible temper and believed that boys should be brought up through fear. He invented cruel punishments, including locking him up in the dark cellar without food for days and beating him up to the point that he had bruises all over his body.

Social services finally intervened, and Edward was moved to a residential school for difficult children where the staff were reasonably kind and able to contain him by encouraging him to take up sports and competitive games. They suggested that he join the Army Cadet Force in his teens; he enjoyed this so much that he subsequently joined the British Army which was a good way of getting away from home. However, he liked taking risks and was often given dangerous assignments to do on his own. It was during these expeditions that he found that he had a strong urge to kill, beyond what was required of him. This worried him a lot, especially as he was thinking of starting a family.

When I met him, accompanied by his male social worker, he was no longer in the army. He presented as a well-built Indian man who was cooperative but also very anxious about the interview. What came over very strongly was the guilt he felt for what he had done, which, combined with his inability to move forward in therapy and his childhood history of abuse and neglect, all made me think of the role of the *traumatic attachment*.

I was able to carry out the TAIP in relation to his father during the second of the two assessment interviews we had, after he had given me permission to do this. Having learnt how violent he could be when triggered, I did not want him to feel I was provoking him in any way so I asked him to remind himself of all the things he had achieved as an adult before letting him know that his father was in the room and then I said "I would like you to notice what happens in your body as you try and say to him: 'Dad, I am an adult now, I don't need to hate you anymore.'"

(I used this word rather than "fear" as I felt fear could make him react violently. By giving him the choice of hating or not, he is more in control of the situation.)

Edward immediately responded by saying, "I want to hate him" and both the social worker and I noticed him making a slight movement forward of his shoulders as if he was about to attack his imaginary father.

I asked, "Did you feel anything in your body?"

"Yeah, here," he replied, indicating his shoulder area.

I asked, "What was it?"

"An energy surge … I'll be honest with you; I wanted to leap forward and kick him hard!"

I responded: "Was that a feeling that you recognise from your past experiences in the Army?"

"Yeah, you get that, I don't know, you get that surge in your body and that almost excitement that you want to hurt and …" "The only reason I don't feel like that towards my mum is because she is a woman …"

I asked him, "Are you surprised you had that feeling and the connection with the Army?"

"Yeah, without a doubt, 'cos I used to get that urge," and he gave another example: "And it's just, I don't know. I can't explain, it goes through your body you know."

Edward did not take up the offer of therapy in the TSS and I think that there may have been more than one reason for this refusal. Not only did he feel terribly guilty about what he had done in the army, but that same guilt fed into the "moral defence" that abused children adopt by being the bad one in order not to blame their parents for the abuse they have experienced at their hands.

In Bowlby's terms, both Peter and Edward's Child Self had to split into two IWMs to survive by hanging on to an idealised parent in one half of the Self and, at the same time, to be the culprit in relation to all those terrifying interactions when he was abused by his parents, represented within the other-half Self.

When I suggested to Edward that he still had a desperate hidden yearning for love and care from his parents and an invisible umbilical cord that still holds on to that hope, he looked at me and said: "Come to think of it, I sometimes contact my dad just to make sure that his life is shit and I get comfort from it", and he told me that he did the same with his mum.

Healing the fractured homicidal mind through equine therapy and the TAIP

A colleague of mine who worked in the field of criminology and who was carrying out research on young people in prison asked me one day if I would consider assessing one of the young men he had listened to who was in jail for a murder he had committed in the company of his criminal family when he was aged fifteen. My colleague had a good relationship with him and Dan, as the young man was called, had asked him to help him find a psychotherapist for when he was released from prison in a few months' time after a period of ten years. He did not want to turn out to be a criminal like his father.

I made it clear that I was no longer taking on clients for psychotherapy, but I offered to carry out an assessment interview.

A few months later, Dan and my colleague turned up to see me in a private room. He had been forewarned that I used the TAIP which he could access in my TED lecture on the internet (Zulueta, 2015b).

Dan was a friendly and intelligent young man of mixed ethnic background who was clearly eager to avoid the criminal life of many of his family members. Like all the men I have met who have committed violent offences, Dan suffered from the effects of a very violent and chaotic childhood.

He had made the most of his prison life by learning various skills and he was now living in the Essex community where he would regularly meet with his probation officer and attend a psychiatrist for his symptoms of complex PTSD and depression. My role was to find him a therapist and to share my findings with these professionals.

When I carried out the TAIP in relation to his violent father his response was interesting because, like Edward, he experienced a strong urge to attack him, and he said that he wanted to kill him.

This meant to me that Dan was at risk of committing a violent offence and it was important that I find some form of treatment that would help him regulate his emotions, the first stage of any therapy for complex PTSD. It occurred to me that I knew an equine therapist who had in fact treated army veterans suffering from PTSD with some success. The effects of this therapeutic approach are summed up here:

> This Equine Assisted Therapy (EAT) is being increasingly used for a wide range of physical and mental health conditions, including PTSD. EAT asserts that horse-human interaction experiences during therapy can potentially foster insight and behavioural changes in patients, as these interactions offer a platform for eliciting thoughts, feelings, and behaviours

related to patients' lives outside treatment. Furthermore, horses are especially conducive to this process as they are naturally hypervigilant and sensitive to verbal and nonverbal cues, providing patients instantaneous feedback during the horse-human interactions, which, in turn, afford patients and therapists opportunities to foster emotional awareness, reflection, and attunement to thoughts, behaviours and forms of communication. (Equine Assisted Therapy, 2022)

Fortunately, she agreed to offer Dan equine therapy at no cost, which was extremely generous. As a result, once a month, I would meet Dan, on the train to her equine centre, and I would record on video the sessions involving him with his two "therapists". It was very moving to watch this young person communicate and respond so quickly to the animal whom he trusted so much more than any human. His human therapist was also very encouraging and sensitive to his needs which led him to develop a good relationship with her that continued beyond his therapy. We carried on with these monthly sessions for about a year.

I was able to record on my iPad the magic of attunement taking place between these three individuals. Later, in a quiet corner of the carriage, on the train journey back to our respective homes, Dan and I would watch these recordings together. He would study what took place and we would discuss his findings from an attachment perspective which he subsequently found very useful in caring for his very young children at home.

Both my colleague and I have remained in contact with Dan. When he asked for some help with his adopted adolescent son, they both benefitted from "video interaction guidance" therapy (https://www.videointeractionguidance.net/), an attunement-based therapy, which we have discovered can be an extremely effective form of interpersonal therapy for traumatised individuals, and which I will describe in the next section.

Two years after I first met Dan, I carried out another the TAIP session with him in relation to his father who had died a few months before. It was a moving moment when he told me that he no longer feared or hated his father; he only wished that he had also been able to benefit from the therapy that he has had to change his life. He was also able to mourn his loss.

These remarkable changes indicate that the fractured Self had healed, and I no longer considered him at risk of committing homicide. The probation officer made his own decision in relation to Dan and continued to meet him for as long as was necessary. We now hear from him that he is teaching boxing to young people who have suffered and reacted as he did when they were young. He is also working with horses and is an involved and supportive father.

The use of alternative attunement-based therapies in the prevention of violence

The role of video interaction guidance in the prevention of domestic violence

There are several attunement-based therapies that are very effective in the treatment of disrupted attachments, as I was to discover in my last few years at work. Equine therapy is one, as we witnessed with Dan. Video interaction guidance (VIG) is another, as mentioned above in relation to Dan and his teenage son and which I will describe in detail in Chapter 10. However, since we are dealing with the treatment of violence, I would like to share my experience of its use with a newly trained therapist or guide called Lupita working with street children in an NGO called Foundation Junto Con Los Niños (JUCONI) in the town of Puebla in Mexico. My role at the time was to observe and note if their clients were benefitting from the staff's recent training in VIG.

She presented her work on video with a father in his late thirties who had been in prison for domestic violence. It takes severe levels of violence to end up in prison in Mexico. He was now released and wanted to have access to his four-year-old son. His wife, understandably, refused to give him permission. He insisted so much that JUCONI took him on as their client which made it possible for him to meet with his son to see if he could benefit from VIG. In the UK, this man would probably have been given a diagnosis of antisocial personality disorder, which is known to be very difficult to treat and he would not have been offered psychoanalytic psychotherapy because he did not appear to be "psychologically minded", which refers to a tendency to understand or explain behaviour in psychological terms.

In addition to the VIG sessions, he was also following the attachment-based therapeutic programme that JUCONI had developed to help parents reunite with their children.

VIG video sessions of father and son in Mexico carried out in Spanish

Strengthening families affected by trauma using VIG

First recording of a father and his son.

The father, Juan, and his son, Pablo, are on the floor of a room with toys all around them; the father, who clearly does not know what to do, is seen turning over cards whilst his son examines the toys. Pablo takes the first initiative by showing Juan a blue toy which the father receives in his hand. The son glances at the camera and continues moving toys on and off a nearby shelf whilst the father watches; he appears tense and is probably very anxious.

A clip selected for the first shared review appears on the screen and is a photo of the son handing him the blue toy and the father receiving it whilst they look at each other.

First shared review

Juan, a Latino-looking man with a substantial moustache, is sitting facing the screen. He seems very tense. Lupita is in a chair next to him and turns towards him; she looks relaxed and friendly and tells him that her motive in sharing this video is to show him interacting with Pablo. She then says, with her warm smile, "There are some very good moments that I liked, very positive moments between you and Pablo that I would like to share with you."

He continues to look tense with his eyes fixed on her laptop screen.

"Do you want to see it?" she asks.

"Yes", he replies, his eyes still fixed on the screen, but his expression is a tiny bit softer, less anxious. She says: "We are going to look at the last photo" and smiles. His eyes are still fixed on the screen.

"What do you see there?" she asks him.

He says something I cannot understand that ends with "… what I did". She looks at him and then at the screen and makes sounds of appreciation.

Emerging change in another session

Juan and son are seated at a round table covered with sheets of paper and pens. Pablo points to something on a shelf opposite him and then looks at his father who follows the direction of his finger to the item on the shelf as his son asks if he can get it. The father nods in approval and says something. His son gets to his feet and takes a small basket from the table and walks with it to the shelf. The father appears to be encouraging him and says, "Choose what you want." His son says something to his father as he looks at him and the father and son end up looking at each other as the father agrees; this is clearly a moment when the two of them are connecting.

Next video where the two are standing by a shelf

Pablo asks, "What do you want?" Father replies, "Do you have apples?" in a gentle kind voice. He is learning to play with his son and is moving into the Green Zone.

Seventh shared review

An amazing change has taken place: "Don Juan", as Lupita calls him, is sitting in a relaxed manner with his right arm leaning on the arm of the sofa which he is sharing with Lupita. He seems calm and involved as he looks at the screen of Lupita's iPad. She turns towards him and asks him with a smile on her face: "What did you see Don Juan?"

"I put words to his activity," he replies with a warm smile and laughs as he says: "And now I don't know if I am hearing properly but …" He comments on the fact that his speech is louder. He remarks that at times (in the past) he has spoken very softly and couldn't be heard. He is now smiling most of the time and clearly pleased with what he has achieved. He continues to look at the screen.

Lupita turns towards him and then at the screen, smiling and expressing her pleasure at what he is saying. She then asks more about him noticing that his voice is louder.

"I gave it more volume," he replies and she replies, "Exactly", confirming what he said.

Their relationship is improving, and he clearly trusts her, feeling that she is attuned to him.

After a few more sessions of VIG

Juan and his son Pablo are in a Wendy house: the father is seated and looks at his son who is standing on his right side, facing the screen and playing with a jug and what looks like a plastic ice-cream. He pours some imaginary liquid over the ice-cream which he then gives to his father. Juan takes it and smiles with pleasure as he removes the ice-cream from the blue cup and laughs as he pretends to drink out of the cup. He then says something and his son turning towards him emits high pitched sound of excitement: "Tiiii!"

Pablo is now facing us, playing with a plastic mobile phone while his father looks on over his shoulder. Pablo smiles to himself as he puts the phone to his ear and begins an imaginary conversation with Mummy, which I do not understand. He then turns round and gives the phone to his father who asks: "Who are you speaking to?" Pablo replies: "To Mummy" and hands him the phone which his father puts to his ear and speaks.

His voice is gentle and reassuring as he asks his imaginary wife: "What are you doing? working? … with Pablo … Pablo is playing."

And as he speaks, his son is standing in front of him with such a joyful face, laughing as he looks at his father talking to his imaginary mother. He turns towards the camera, and possibly towards Lupita, to share his delight in getting his parents back together through play. Isn't it every child's dream when they have separated?

There is no doubt that by this stage both son and father are bathing in oxytocin and are in the Green Zone.

The healing of the father's traumatic attachment through the son and Lupita

A subsequent clip shows Pablo doing carpentry with his father and they are talking to each other as the father supervises Pablo and at one point teases him.

Sometime later, Juan obtained permission for a supervised visit to his son and family at their home and, after several months, he moved in with his family; no further violence occurred following this stage which indicates that VIG did heal his past wounds. This took months instead of years of more traditional psychoanalytic psychotherapy.

When JUCONI presented its work using VIG to the wealthy men and women who funded the project, one of the wives lent over to tell me that she wished such an approach could be provided for their families. I think that is an important message for us all; everyone, rich and poor would like to have a happier family life.

Returning to the work carried out by Lupita and Juan, there is no doubt that the wish to parent his son had a very important role in motivating this man to get involved in therapy. I think that the VIG therapeutic approach has a huge role to play in offering men the opportunity to get in touch with emotions that they normally wouldn't allow themselves to feel because they are not considered "manly enough" or make them feel ashamed. Through caring for their children, men learn to experience and communicate emotions that enable them to develop a new creative and fulfilling role in society, a role that men often feel deprived of.

The hunter gatherers in the forests of Borneo in the 1950s, called the Punans, were directly involved in the care of their children with their wives, but they were probably the only men in the world to deliver their partner's babies!

Anna Machin, in her book *The Life of Dad: The Making of the Modern Father*, describes how men undergo significant biological changes in fatherhood and how their contribution complements mum's to the benefit of their children (Machin, 2018).

The use of the TAIP in the successful treatment of addictions and unresolved grief

Addiction to alcohol and drugs

Funding for UK services for addictions was cut in 2012 by 30 per cent following controversial NHS reforms which reflected a political ideology that considers substance use disorders to be only self-inflicted life-style choices rather than being linked to health conditions. The results are distressing because they are avoidable: for instance, we are now seeing increasing deaths due to opioid addiction or dependence on other drugs for chronic pain because the NHS treatments are being reduced, leaving poorer people with no alternative but to self-medicate their suffering.

In 2017, Colin Drummond, a professor of addictions psychiatry wrote in an article in the *British Medical Journal* (Drummond, 2017) that '"savings" in specialist services are increasing pressure elsewhere in the NHS":

> Shocking images of drug users sprawled unconscious or standing statue-like in an intoxicated state have begun to surface in the media recently.
>
> Meanwhile deaths involving heroin and/or morphine have more than doubled since addiction services were transferred from NHS control to local authorities in 2012 and are now at the highest level on record. Last year there were more than 15,000 drug related, and over 1 million alcohol-related, hospital admissions. (Drummond, 2017)

Since then, the government has promised increased funding over three years to rebuild drug services in most deprived areas (https://www.bbc.co.uk/news/uk-59533858). However, the number of deaths due to drug overdoses continues to rise with over 4,000 deaths in 2021. Many countries, including Scotland, are introducing "drug consumption rooms", staffed by professionals or trained volunteers who can provide emergency care when needed and which can also facilitate access to other health and social services. The UK government remains opposed to these "overdose prevention sites", despite the good results achieved in other countries (Ng et al., 2017).

In Vancouver, for example, the site was associated with a 26 per cent net reduction in fatal overdose rates in the vicinity and is especially useful for highly marginalised people with no fixed abode (Transform, 2019). In the United States there are very few such sites and opposition to them is currently threatening their existence.

There is no doubt that drug users are stigmatised despite the fact that Felitti showed that drug abuse was related to ACEs (Felitti, 2003).

In the United States, however, one doctor stands out for his approach to the treatment of addiction: Dr Daniel Sumrok believes that addiction should be called "ritualised compulsive comfort seeking" and his service is based on addressing the person's ACEs through psychotherapy, medication assistance, and by helping them find a "ritualised compulsive comfort seeking behaviour that won't kill them or put them in jail" (Sumrok, 2017; Stevens, 2022).

I never thought that the use of the TAIP could possibly contribute to the care of people who suffer from alcohol or other addiction as I know only too well how difficult it can be to recover from these conditions. Many well-known psychiatrists like Van der Kolk and Gabor Maté have been emphasising that all addictions result from the experience of trauma in the womb or in early life. Felitti's ACEs study and subsequent related studies make it quite clear that there is a profound correlation between these experiences and addiction (Felitti, 2003).

This implies, yet again, that the disorganised attachment and its resulting *traumatic attachment* could be actively involved in these conditions; both Monica Notice and Jayshree Unadkat will be presenting examples of how the use of the TAIP, followed by a period of mourning relating to the loss of the idealised mother, appears to heal alcohol addiction as the craving disappears and so does the behaviour that goes with it.

Types of addiction

Large studies will need to be carried out to confirm these findings and to elucidate which of the many addictions respond to this approach. There are so far three types of addiction:

1. Physical addictions to addictive substances such as nicotine, alcohol, opioids, etc. These are usually treated by counselling and detox like Monique's client Beryl who tried many times to give up her drinking until she used the TAIP.
2. Impulse-control disorders like gambling which can be so destructive for individuals and their families and yet so difficult to treat.
3. Behavioural addictions which are defined as a compulsive need to engage in certain behaviours such as food addiction, pornography watching, exercise, work, shopping, playing video games. But perhaps the most important in our current times is "greed", defined as an insatiable desire for material gain (be it food, money, land, or animate/inanimate possessions) or social value, such as status or power.

We are living in a culture that rewards individual greed for money and power and we can see its destructive effects all around us. Unfortunately, if these addicted individuals can continue to amass their fortunes and resulting power with impunity, there is little we can do to stop their destructiveness. Rabindranath Tagore, in his book *Sadhana*, in the essay on the Realisation of Life (1916), sums up its effects:

> The greed of gain has no time or limit to its capaciousness. It's one object is to produce and consume. It has pity neither for beautiful nature nor for living human beings. It is ruthlessly ready without a moment's hesitation to crush beauty and life.

I think we can recognise these traits in many of our leaders today. As Gabor Maté so correctly said in one of his presentations, "addiction to power is always about the emptiness you try and fill from the outside" (Maté, 2012). We now know that empty hole comes from the fractured Self of the *traumatic attachment*. Greed is one of the many manifestations of the disorganised attachment. At its core lies terror, making it a treatable condition.

Whether these different disorders are related to an early disorganised attachment has yet to be explored by using the TAIP, but they are all seen as "difficult-to-treat", which we are discovering is often associated with the presence of the *traumatic attachment*.

Complicated or unresolved grief

In the summer of 2008, research published by Mary-Frances O'Connor, a professor at Columbia University and her colleagues made a few headlines in the science journals because of the paradoxical nature of their study's results. It was entitled "Craving love? Enduring grief activates brain's 'reward centre'" (O'Connor et al., 2008).

Grief is a painful life experience but successful adaptation to the loss usually takes place for most people (Bonnano et al., 2002). However, in a substantial minority of people, it can develop into complicated grief, previously known as chronic, traumatic grief (Ott, Lueger, Kelber, & Prigerso, 2007) or unresolved grief. It is characterised by "debilitating pangs of painful emotions, with intense yearning, longing and searching for the deceased, and preoccupied thoughts of the loved one". Those who are affected feel "stuck" and are often unable to resume a normal life.

The most interesting aspect, as far as we are concerned, is that people have noted that it's as if "the normal grieving process is unable to take its course". This unrelenting unfinished mourning can affect 10 to 20 per cent of people who have lost someone close to them.

O'Connor and her colleagues carried out functional magnetic resonance imaging (or FMRI) on eleven women who experienced complicated grief (CG) and compared them with those of twelve women who experienced non-complicated grief (NCG). They had all experienced the death of a mother or sister to breast cancer in the previous five years and were matched in relation to demographic characteristics.

The scans showed which parts of the brain are active during a given moment. Each woman was asked to look either at a picture they had chosen of their dead relative with their recorded words superimposed to remind them of the death or at similar pictures of strangers.

The parts of the brain involved in physical and emotional pain were activated in all the women when they saw the picture of their dead mother or sister. The pain system, as we know, is implicated in both physical and emotional pain (Chapter 2).

However, the scans of the women who suffered from complicated grief also lit up at the same time in another area of brain, the *nucleus accumbens* (NA) which plays a role in family attachments, such as sibling or maternal attachments, and involves dopamine and oxytocin. Dopamine is an important brain chemical that influences our mood and feelings of reward and motivation. Oxytocin is a hormone and chemical messenger produced in the brain best known for its key role in childbirth and breastfeeding. However, it is also called the "love hormone" for its role in parent–child bonding and couple bonding (Chapter 2).

Knutson et al. focus on "the association between the NA" and "yearning" as a neural response found in addiction (Knutson, Adams, Fong, & Hommer, 2001) because this disorder is like an addiction. To try to make sense of this they write:

> Many who suffer from addiction-like disorders experience them as afflictions, similarly, we are not suggesting that reveries about the deceased are emotionally satisfying, but rather may serve as craving responses that may make adapting to the reality of the loss more difficult.(ibid.)

Knowing, as we do, how addiction to alcohol involves the Child Self's strong attachment to the idealised mother, it is perhaps not so surprising to find that the same brain area of the NA is involved in complicated or unresolved grief.

Both Monique and Jayshree's clients (in Chapters 7 and 8, respectively), who overcame their alcohol addiction by integrating their divided Self, thereby letting go of their attachment to their idealised mother through the TAIP, found themselves finally able mourn the loss of their mothers as well. It seems to us that the lighting up of the NA may well be linked to the activation of the women's attachment to their idealised mother. This should disappear if and when the Self is no longer divided, and mourning can take place.

It makes us wonder if the activation of the NA may occur in all conditions where we discover a *traumatic attachment* which would make it a very useful research tool or a biological marker.

Clearly, what is missing in this important study are the personal histories of these women since we know nothing about their childhood experience and the nature of their attachments to either their mothers and sisters.

O'Connor's findings could represent the experience of the divided Self of the individual in a state of intense attachment to the person's idealised mother when faced with the painful loss of the real attachment figures, be it mother or sister. Grieving requires integration, which is not possible with a split Self, so the women cannot move on. They might benefit from the TAIP as will be illustrated in the next chapters.

The role of the TAIP in dissociation

In his famous paper of 1933, "The confusion of tongues between Adults and the Child", the psychoanalyst Sándor Ferenczi wrote:

> We talk a good deal in analysis of regressions into the infantile, but we do not really believe to what great extent we are right; we talk a lot about the splitting of the personality, but do not seem sufficiently to appreciate the depths of these splits. (1988, p. 200)

Referring to mental patients with hysteria who sometimes dissociated by adopting strange postures similar to those found in organic conditions, he continued: "If we keep our cool, educational attitude even *vis-à-vis*" patients in such states,

> we tear to shreds the last thread that connects him to us. The patient gone off into his trance is *a child indeed* who no longer reacts to intellectual explanations, only perhaps to maternal friendliness; without it he feels lonely and abandoned in his greatest need i.e. in the same unbearable situation which at one time led to a splitting of his mind and eventually to his illness; thus it is no wonder that the patient cannot but repeat now the symptom-formation exactly as he did at the time when his illness started. (ibid., p. 200)

He then reminds his psychoanalytic readers that "patients do not react to theatrical phrases, but only to real sincere sympathy". Ferenczi is clearly advocating an attuned approach to our clients who suffer from conditions such as DAD or BPD and other disorders born out of dissociation of which there are many, as we are still to find out. In addition, he also noted, all those years ago, the fact that when a child has been sexually abused "*the weak and underdeveloped personality reacts … by anxiety-ridden identification and by introjection of the menacing person*" (ibid., p. 203, original italics), which is what Fairbairn referred to when he developed the concept of the moral defence (Fairbairn, 1952).

He also writes:

> Detailed examination of the phenomena during an analytic trance [dissociated state], teaches us that there is neither shock nor fright without some trace of splitting of the personality … [as] part of the person regresses into a state of happiness that existed prior to the trauma—a trauma which it endeavours to annul. (ibid., p. 204)

Isn't he referring to the idealised attachment to mother which developed to protect the child from the dissociated horrors of the abuse?

Nearly a century later, in 2014, the Turkish Professor Vedat Şar comments on the recent revival of "interest in the science of psycho-traumatology and dissociative disorders, but he adds that studies in this field still remain marginal in number despite their highly creative and promising nature" (2014).

Şar notes that, unlike several other psychiatric disorders, there is not yet any specific drug treatment for PTSD and dissociative disorders, and "in addition, dissociation may accompany almost every psychiatric disorder and may influence their phenomenology as well as their response to treatment", as we are finding out.

He notes that dissociation can disrupt one or more mental functions, affecting consciousness, memory and/or identity, but also thinking, emotions, sensorimotor functioning, and/or behaviour. The orbitofrontal region of the brain is considered to be affected by trauma in early life (Schore, 2009).

Clinical appearances of dissociation

When describing the different clinical appearances of dissociation, Şar mentions substance abuse and points out how important it is to recognise the "role of dissociation for the prevention and the successful treatment of substance dependency among adolescents and young adults" (Şar, 2014, p. 175). Two other disorders where dissociation often plays a part are dissociative depression, often linked to sexual abuse and neglect, and BPD (or DAD). It is of interest that he is also critical of this condition being labelled as a personality disorder because it often includes features of a dissociative identity disorder.

The other clinical dissociative disorders that Şar mentions are repeated suicide attempts, conversion symptoms, acute dissociative disorder, dissociative amnesia or fugue, and schizoaffective disorder.

In adolescence in particular, which we know is the period when the effects of the split Self begin to manifest themselves more obviously, young people can suffer from motor uneasiness and affect dysregulation due to a dissociative disorder which resembles attention deficit hyperactivity disorder (ADHD). Child and adult forms of ADHD may also resemble a dissociative disorder: for example, when its symptoms can be confused with PTSD, comorbidity is possible (Ruiz, 2014).

This diagnosis is a controversial one: the Citizens Commission for Human Rights (CCHR) sees it as an example of how the psychiatric industry has redefined, rebranded and marketed normal behaviour as mental illness. It is based on a list of symptoms which, as Van der Kolk points out in an interview, can have a different aetiology and was voted into existence by a show of hands by the APA, which also promotes the use of drugs as treatment. It horrifies Van der Kolk that children should be labelled with a mental disorder: "You can think of yourself as a disordered person for the rest of your life!"

Gabor Maté doesn't see ADHD as a disease but recognises its links to early childhood trauma; he was diagnosed with it himself and was given medication, but he does not recommend this approach. His book *Scattered Minds* (2000) explains the origin of the symptoms people experience and provides a healing programme for adults and children which, in my view, actually describes what it is like to have a divided Self, because of the *traumatic attachment*.

We now know that it takes a certain amount of time for the clinical manifestations of the disorganised attachment to be identified as different clinical diagnoses so perhaps ADHD, with its variable symptomatology, is the manifestation of an interim state. The use of the TAIP in adult clients with ADHD would help us determine if this is a possibility.

Other dissociative disorders

A paper written by Lyssenko et al. in 2018, shows that dissociative features are also present in many other mental disorders such as schizophrenia, eating disorders, panic disorders, affective disorders, and obsessive–compulsive disorder (OCD). They point out that these dissociative symptoms are very important clinically because they are linked to maladaptive functioning and symptom severity in some disorders, for example "executive functioning and self-regulation skills in so-called BPD, alexithymia in panic disorders, anxiety and depression in Obsessive Compulsive Disorder (OCD)" (Lyssenko et al., 2018).

In addition, they state that dissociative symptoms can predict a non-response in the psychotherapeutic treatment of PTSD and panic disorders.

To measure the degree of dissociation, they recommend using the Dissociative Experiences Scale or DES (Bernstein & Putnam, 1986) which was described earlier, or a version that is easier to score, the DES-II (Carlson & Putnam, 1993), both of which have high validity and reliability. Having noted the results of the first and comprehensive meta-analysis on the DES by Van IJzendoorn and Schüngel (1996) twenty years earlier, the authors present their own meta-analysis to provide an evidence base of the prevalence and distribution of dissociation in adults suffering from mental disorders:

> The largest dissociation scores of over 30 or more were found for dissociative disorders, PTSD, BPD (or Disorganised Attachment Disorder as we name it), and conversion disorders; the lower range of scores, below 30, were found in substance related and addictive disorders, eating disorders, schizophrenia, anxiety disorder, OCD and affective disorders. (Lyssenko et al., 2018)

Regarding BPD, it showed dissociation scores like PTSD in twenty-seven studies, and the authors also point out that, although it is diagnosed as a personality disorder, it is closely associated with traumatic stress and has rates of ACEs higher than 50 per cent.

Lyssenko and her co-authors conclude that dissociative symptoms prevail in nearly all mental disorders and therefore an evaluation of dissociation should be part of every psychopathological assessment.

Their final statement pertains to the work we are sharing in this book: "Future studies should engage in a transdiagnostic perspective to enhance the development of treatment modules to deal with dissociative symptoms." Johnson grasped the nettle of dissociation when he focused on melting the terror induced dissociation in his patients. His approach is different from mine, but he was the first to show that it could be done; I owe my current work to him (Johnson, 1997, 2005).

However, excited as I was to have discovered the TAIP because of its unexpected and positive results, I was also worried: how could this apparently simple TAIP-driven approach appear to achieve such extraordinary results by healing people suffering from long-term addiction, violence, complex grief, BPD and complex PTSD?

Once again, Şar came to the rescue when he wrote (2014): "Dissociation and dissociative disorders can be treated successfully because they originate from a mechanism which is not pathological of itself." I do not know if he thought of the *traumatic attachment* at this point, but it certainly fulfils that function. He concludes: "Hence, dissociation and dissociative disorders are reversible subject to appropriate treatment." But, he adds that: "Dissociative patients who are not treated appropriately become highly complicated, manifesting one of the most difficult-to-treat conditions."

He also points out that dissociative disorders render the subject vulnerable to abuse, which I have sadly witnessed in my work.

Nature's different ways of healing the traumatic attachment

It seems that whilst evolution led to the development of the traumatic attachment to increase the survival of recently born mammals, the same evolutionary forces provided them with a natural remedy through their subsequent interactions with other members of their own species, as we saw with the delinquent young elephants.

In contemporary Western society, Schore states, our intimate attachment bonds can provide both an attunement experience and the potential to repair the damage brought on by past traumatic experiences, but this is less likely to happen with strangers in the current role of healers, a role once held by shamans or community healers in small primitive societies where everyone knew each other.

However, some traces of the magic of attunement are still around: I recall overhearing my experienced psychoanalytic supervisors remarking, with some surprise, on how several young trainees, with little or no experience, were able to achieve remarkable results without any knowledge of psychoanalysis. Could it be, I wondered, that many of the theories that we were being taught on how to respond to our suffering patients could get in the way of our natural attuned empathic responses? They certainly did in relation to clients or patients who gave us a history of childhood abuse which we were told not to believe.

The role of dissociation in the re-enactment of sexual abuse in psychotherapy

> The fact is that the therapeutic relationship is an attachment relationship to which both the client and the therapist bring their attachment history. And here lies the problem: the client who needs therapy is usually someone with an insecure attachment. When this attachment is of the disorganised type this will be the result of a history of childhood abuse and neglect with all that that implies. (Zulueta, 2015a)

We now know, through our study of trauma and ACEs, that the higher the ACE score the greater the incidence of being sexually assaulted as an adult and the greater the likelihood of being a victim or a perpetrator of domestic violence. These individuals have an unconscious propensity to re-create their abuse within the therapeutic setting; whether this happens or not will depend on the therapist's degree of attachment security. This is because their early abusive attachment experiences can be re-enacted later on either in the role of victim or in the role of abuser, depending on the context.

Most therapists are required to have therapy as part of their training but few work on their past traumatic experiences or use the ACEs questionnaire to get some idea as to their potential vulnerability. Felitti told me that when he gives lectures, he usually asks his audience to complete the ACE questionnaire anonymously; to his surprise our profession has the highest level of ACEs compared to other professions.

Many doctors go into medicine to give patients the care that they did not receive in their childhood (Vaillant, Sobowale, & McArthur, 1972). Bowlby was aware of this too and spoke of "compulsive carers" who want to give their patients the care they themselves never had.

This can result in the therapist or doctor becoming over-dependent on their clients' improvement which can lead to anger and rejection if this does not happen. All too often, male therapists find ways of rationalising their perverse re-enactment of their patient's sexual abuse with catastrophic results for their patients who then lose all trust in therapists, often needing readmission to hospital or attempting suicide (Zulueta, 2015a). These clients rarely have the self-confidence or the means to take their therapist to court and their abusing male therapists are often allowed to continue seeing patients, as I found out in my attempt to support a young woman who had been abused by her therapist in a private psychotherapy service. Therefore, a genuine compassionate understanding of our own traumatic past and that of our more disturbed clients is so important in the field of psychotherapy.

However, I must add that, despite such knowledge, we will inevitably find ourselves re-enacting in minor ways certain traumatic experiences of our patients. If this happens, Alan Schore's advice is very helpful as he tells us to acknowledge the pain we have inflicted and to apologise for this. Sometimes, we realise retrospectively that what we did or failed to do must have felt very much like the kind of action our client's abuser did; in such cases I refer to this experience as "being in the shadow of the abuser" and I explain to my patient how people who have been abused often find themselves reliving abusive situations, either as the victim or as the abuser. I may end up inviting my client to let me know when she feels this is happening in our sessions. As a result, these negative therapeutic experiences can actually become a turning point in therapy as a more cooperative way of working together is established, as happened with my patient Chloe following her last suicide attempt.

The role of dissociation in the re-enactment of past abuse in domestic violence

The re-enactment of past abuse, so often observed in domestic violence and in traumatised patients during treatment, does not make sense until one looks at it from the perspective of the *traumatic attachment* which, by splitting the Self, has made it impossible to process past traumatic experiences. As a result, any whiff of a past traumatic experience can trigger the reliving or re-enactment of that original experience, leading to a repetition of that trauma, either from the perspective of the abuser, victim, or colluder. This makes the phenomenon of re-enactment one of the most destructive aspects of trauma, as we saw with the homicidal men referred to earlier. It also explains the behaviour of hostages who paradoxically support or even claim to love their captors such as Patty Hearst, the American daughter of the publisher William Randolph Hearst in 1974.

Unfortunately, many professionals involved in dealing with domestic violence do not take this into account when they are dealing with domestic violence relating either to child abuse or female victims of male abuse. In the case of Figen, the Turkish mother who was aware that to have a male baby spelt trouble for her (Chapter 3), those involved in her care refused to listen to her when she asked for an abortion, and again, when she asked for her child to be removed from her care.

Police and social workers involved with severe cases of domestic violence are often unable to make sense of their client's behaviour when she returns to her abuser at the risk of her own life, unless they have learnt about the effects of dissociation. Domestic abuse can be such a destructive and deadly experience for so many families that I hazard here a simplified explanation involving an imaginary man and a woman.

> Often both partners suffer from the effects of a disorganised attachment so, they both have a vulnerable sense of Self because it is a fractured Self. The violence has been going on for quite a long time. When triggered by a threat to his vulnerable split male Self, which may appear quite minor, but which has symbolic significance, such as meal not served on time, the man is enraged and feels he must punish his female partner. He is in the Yellow Zone of *fight*, leading to the Red Zone of dissociation.
>
> Both partners are re-enacting an earlier childhood experience of terrifying abuse from the perspective of the abuser and victim. We know, from earlier studies, that the IWMs of these attachment experiences encode a template of an abuser attacking a victim, which can be re-enacted from the perspective of either the abuser or the victim, even though both were victims as children (Troy & Sroufe, 1987).
>
> In a male-dominated society, the male naturally opts unconsciously for the more powerful role as abuser and, in his fury, attacks his partner. This experience triggers her past IWM, and she has little option but to be the victim. The dissociative destructive re-enactment takes place and, when it ends, if the woman is still alive, they are both in another mental state with their terrifying destructive experiences now safely behind the wall of dissociation of their split Selves.
>
> Sometimes, the man, who is no longer emotionally connected to his rage, will apologise and promise not to do "it" again and the woman, who is no longer emotionally connected to her pain and terror, often forgives or forgets for the time being.
>
> The *traumatic attachment* has done its job: as infants, their shared idealisation of their abusive or neglectful mother and/or father enabled them both to reconnect with her whilst those terrifying memories were kept safely out of the way behind the wall of dissociation.

There are increasing numbers of domestic abuse where women are the abusers and men the victims, but the damage caused by the women is far less, so we do not hear about these cases.

Unfortunately, witnessing this terrible domestic atrocity is absolutely terrifying for children who often fear losing not only one parent but both. It is one of the worst of the ACES and carries within its IWMs the potential for violent re-enactment down the generations. In particularly severe cases, the man can involve his children in the act of domestic violence and attack them or both partners can re-enact their past terrifying experiences of abuse on their children which can end up in murder (Zulueta, 2006a, pp. 11–17). Domestic violence should be taken far more seriously by the government, the police, and the legal system than it is.

The implications of dissociation in psychotherapy

Returning to our therapeutic work with the TAIP, Liotti recommended, when working therapeutically with traumatised people, that it is best to attend to the dissociation before trying to process the traumatic experience (Liotti, 2011). We now have the tool to do this with the TAIP.

When treating people suffering from complex PTSD, psychotherapists usually start with a "stabilisation" phase during which they help their clients learn to regulate their emotions by using different techniques or approaches. This empowers the survivors of abuse and usually has the effect of strengthening their therapeutic relationship with their psychotherapist. I suggest that this would probably be a propitious time to suggest carrying out the TAIP; the outcome of this procedure is likely to help both therapist and client map out the course of their future therapy which may in fact be much shorter than expected as a result. However, the patient may reject this suggestion or simply fail to carry it out. This is likely if his or her levels of dissociation are very high, and it is an appropriate response. The TAIP can be offered later on during the therapy.

Potential research possibilities with the TAIP

Our journey of discovery using the TAIP has enabled us to expose the underlying *traumatic attachment* that appears to be at the root of so many very different psychiatric disorders.

The people we have described suffering from the effects of addiction of different kinds, violent behaviour, unresolved grief, complex PTSD and its more severe manifestation, wrongly named "borderline personality disorder", all respond in the same way to the use of the TAIP: their Adult Self gives way to their Child Self.

In addition, most of them complain of an embodied experience of a hole or vacuum that many spend their time trying to fill, often to no avail, which we interpret as the manifestation of their dissociated Self.

As a result, we can conclude that, as long as the Child Self remains stuck to its idealised mother to safeguard itself from the terrifying dangers across the dissociative divide, normal development from childhood to adulthood cannot take place.

The degree to which human emotional development is hampered by the *traumatic attachment* appears related to the individual's levels of dissociation which in turn reflect the degree of terror the Child Self experienced at the hands of his or her caregivers. Or to put it more simply: terror in infancy and childhood leads to a failure to regulate emotions and to a variety of different emotional conditions that we have been working on.

Clearly a lot more of research is needed to both consolidate our clinical findings and to explore whether the connection between the *traumatic attachment,* as elicited by the TAIP and dissociation, is repeatedly present in different disorders that are difficult to treat. If this proves to be the case, its reach is enormous, and the implications could be very important and positive in terms of the therapeutic treatment and outcome of these disorders.

What are the areas that could benefit from further research using the TAIP?

In relation to dissociation

There is little doubt that large studies are needed to confirm the validity of both types of results achieved by using the TAIP with "difficult-to-treat disorders": eliciting the traumatic attachment and reversing its dissociative action (Nemeroff, 2012).

Şar mentioned the treatment of dissociative identity disorder or DID as multiple personality disorder is now called (2014, p. 172): this is very likely to respond to the TAIP but we have not developed a therapeutic procedure to safely attend to its multiple levels of dissociation.

The other dissociative disorders described by Lyssenko et al. (2018), such as eating disorders, panic disorders, OCD, affective disorders, and schizophrenia remain unexplored in relation to the TAIP.

It would also be important to check if the TAIP elicits any response with disorders that do not have any dissociative features or disorders that do not show the same resistance to therapy.

Many measurements can be used to establish the value of using the TAIP in healing dissociative conditions but the most important for establishing the effectiveness of the TAIP is currently a reduction in dissociation to normal values which indicates that the Self is integrated.

Every therapist using the TAIP should assess their client for dissociation by using the DES-I (Bernstein & Putnam, 1986) or the shorter DES-II (Carlson & Putnam, 1999) before and after the therapy has ended, having also established the client's diagnosis according to the *DSM-5* (APA, 2013) and/or *ICD-11* (World Health Organization, 2019/2021).

In relation to brain scans

Inspired by the work of the neuroscientist Professor Mary Frances O'Connor and her team on unresolved or complicated grief, I think that it would be very useful to study the role of the NA in addictions in general since the authors suggest that it is active in these conditions as well as in complicated grief. As we now know that the *traumatic attachment* is involved in other conditions as well, could the lighting up of the NA become a research tool or marker to indicate the presence of the IWM of idealised *traumatic attachment*?

It would also be very useful to carry out brain scans during a TAIP to see what changes are taking place while the client's brain responds by revealing the *traumatic attachment* and later by integrating the dissociated Self; the latter would be a recording of how a brain changes when moving from being in a state of disorganised attachment to a secure attachment.

This may be technically difficult to achieve as the client needs to feel safe and supported in a therapeutic context. However, Rauch et al. (1996) managed to carry out a study using positron emission tomography (PET) scans with clients suffering from PTSD which showed the changes in their brain as the clients read their traumatic script; for example the shutting down of the speech area in the left hemisphere and the activation of the limbic area, particularly the amygdala which warn us of danger by activating the stress response in the right hemisphere (Rauch et al., 1996).

Changes in brain activity could probably be observed during both the "revealing" of the *traumatic attachment* and the "mending" of the split Self.

In relation to all psychiatric disorders and possible ACE-driven medical treatment

One of the interesting aspects of our work is witnessing how the TAIP has enabled us to expose the underlying *traumatic attachment* that appears to be at the root of so many different psychological disorders. So far, we have recorded the presence of the TAIP in clients who suffered from addictions of different kinds, anxiety disorders, violent behaviour, unresolved grief, complex PTSD, and its more severe manifestation, wrongly named BPD.

Lyssenko and her co-authors report that dissociative symptoms occur in nearly all mental disorders such as eating disorders, panic disorders, affective disorders, and schizophrenia.

If these different disorders were to respond to the use of the TAIP in the same manner as the ones we have presented here, this could alter significantly how these disorders should be treated and it could lead to much more positive outcomes for these individuals.

As our therapeutic work has focused on psychological disorders, we have not taken into account any of the medical conditions that may accompany these different mental disorders. I mention this as Felitti's research led to the discovery that the more ACEs an individual had endured, the greater the incidence of ischaemic heart disease, strokes, chest diseases, diabetes, hepatitis, and auto-immune diseases. This is not surprising, as we are now discovering how closely mind and body are linked. A recently published study in *Nature* and summarised in a more accessible form in *Science Daily* reveals that:

> A connection between the body and mind is built into the structure of the brain. The study shows that parts of the brain area that controls movement are plugged into networks involved in thinking and planning, and in control of involuntary bodily functions such as blood pressure and heart rate. (Gordon et al., 2023)

The authors called this circuit the somato-cognitive-active-network (SCAN). Whether it is implicated in the studies that we are doing, we don't know, but it is important to have more evidence as to the existence of this crucial connection.

The therapist's training in relation to the use of the TAIP in research

Whilst many more psychotherapists will need to train in this approach for it to be generally available and for research to take place, this should not take long as it requires a weekend online course followed up by a series of monthly online group supervisions. Trainees will present their work and accompanying videos during these sessions and thereby acquire the skills in applying the TAIP and using the different instruments to measure change mentioned earlier.

The use of the video with the permission of the client or patient is very important as it can be used to identify interesting reactions and new developments and is also a way of checking that the TAIP is being correctly applied as described in Chapter 4.

We recommend that, once trained in this procedure, psychotherapists will continue to share and supervise their work with others to both improve their skills and record their findings. We hope that many therapists will want to be involved in future studies, as outlined above, so that we can establish if the *traumatic attachment* is to be found in all "difficult-to-treat disorders" and to establish when the TAIP does or does not work in both identifying the *traumatic attachment* and in healing the split Self. With time, a more formal training system will be developed, along with a form of accreditation.

As we have indicated, the TAIP can be used with a variety of individual psychotherapeutic modalities such as psychoanalytic psychotherapy, LI, EMDR, group therapy, and probably with other approaches such as the various schema therapies, where the TAIP has not yet been tried.

Conclusion

My use of the TAIP with forensic patients has finally brought to light the missing link that I was looking for when I wrote my book *From Pain to Violence: The Traumatic Roots of Destructiveness*. I concluded that "violence is not an innate biological instinct: it is the manifestation of both our disrupted attachment bonds and our shattered self" (Zulueta, 2006a, p. 344). I never imagined that, by developing the TAIP and using it to explore the minds of homicidal patients, I would be able to locate the cause of their disrupted attachments and their shattered or divided Self, both due to the development of the *traumatic attachment* in their childhoods.

However, could discovering that violent behaviour is mainly due to the effects of childhood abuse and neglect have any effect on the way forensic patients are understood and treated?

My forensic colleagues work with individuals who are in prison because they have committed serious crimes, and they need to be punished; can punishment and an empathic understanding of what led them commit their crime co-exist? Having recently read Dr Gwen Adshead's remarkable book *The Devil You Know: Encounters in Forensic Psychiatry*, I am hopeful because her approach to these men and women is compassionate and non-judgemental, whilst keeping within the boundaries of her profession (Adshead & Horne, 2021). They respond to her by revealing some of their thoughts and feelings; for many, it is probably one of the few times that they have been treated with so much respect. Many of my forensic psychotherapy colleagues work in this way but they may fear that by successfully implementing the TAIP, the wounded Self of the homicidal man might heal, and then how would he react to being kept in prison? In my view, his newfound capacity to show remorse may help him use his time in prison to come to terms with his crime and prepare for a better life when he is released.

Whilst my work with homicidal men could be seen by some to be contentious, the good results achieved by Monique Notice and Jayshree Unadkat with addicted clients is good news in every sense of the word. We hope that therapists working in addiction services will take up the offer of training in the use of the TAIP and apply it with their clients. They are not at risk of doing themselves out of a job, as there are thousands of potential clients seeking help in this area!

The next three chapters describe some of the therapeutic work carried out by Monique Notice, Jayshree Unadkat, and Leonor de Escoriaza: all three are dedicated to helping their clients heal their past childhood wounds and lead a normal life with a sense of well-being.

Monique and Jayshree began working with the TAIP long before we were aware of the importance of using the DES and of many other findings that I have shared in this book. It is through their work that we have gradually developed our understanding of both the effects of the *traumatic attachment* and its reversal by using the TAIP, mostly in the context of private practice, except for the work on addiction.

CHAPTER 7

"It feels like a big empty hole inside"

Monique Notice

My journey with TAIP began on 4 February 2012 when I attended the annual Herts and Essex symposium to hear a talk by Dr Felicity de Zulueta. Her talk was titled, "Trauma and Attachment Today". I attended alongside my colleague and my then supervisor at the drug and alcohol agency where we worked at the time. I was a final year student on the MA degree that I was doing at the time.

At the end of her talk the three of us looked at each other and knew we had just listened to something very special. Her talk was describing PTSD from an attachment perspective. My supervisor, who was so dedicated and always looking out for ways of helping our clients at the agency, immediately started to think that this might somehow benefit them.

My initial motivation for joining the clinical research group that Felicity offered was to get a better understanding of the *traumatic attachment* as I was desperate for any ideas at all that might help me to help my clients who were struggling so painfully with their addictions.

I did not end up working in an alcohol and drug agency by choice, but this proved to be one of the richest experiences in my early psychotherapy career. As a trainee therapist and with only my nursing experience of working with people who had addictions to inform me at the time, I had very bleak expectations of being able to help someone with these issues. At the time, my nursing colleagues thought that patients with drug and alcohol addictions would never give up and get better: an unspoken, but at times spoken, belief.

As therapists, how do we think about addiction? Maté (2018) writes that brain development in the uterus and during childhood is the single most important biological factor in determining whether a person will be predisposed to substance dependence and addictive behaviours of any sort. Dr Felitti conducted a study on over 17,000 Americans and his conclusion was that "the basic cause of addiction is predominantly experience-dependent during childhood, and not substance dependent". Of course, many are of the opinion that genetics do play a role but not as big a role as medicine often maintains.

Initially, I was hesitant to use TAIP as part of my therapy. My training, as a psychodynamic psychotherapist made me feel rather nervous about introducing this intervention, and a recording device, into the therapy room. I was soon put at ease when Felicity explained how effective this can be as part of therapy.

Addiction and unresolved grief: "the big empty hole inside my stomach"

My work with Beryl started when I was a trainee at a drug and alcohol agency. She had been going there on and off for thirteen years, seeking help with her alcohol misuse. So, imagine my shock when the manager of the agency called me to her office and said, "I have a very tricky client for you. She has been in and out of the services for thirteen years and I want you to sort her out quickly. Don't let her mess you about. She has a habit of doing that."

At that moment I felt a huge range of emotions: first, anger, as I was only a trainee. How exactly was she expecting me to "sort her out" in twelve weeks? At the time the standard length of therapy was twelve weeks, which could be extended for varying reasons. I also felt scared, scared that I would fail and, at the time, this fear was based on my preconceived ideas that it was next to impossible for an alcoholic to give up the habit. Luckily, we ended up working together for nearly three years.

> Beryl was a fifty-seven-year-old woman who had three adult children and had been married twice and was now single. She had four grandchildren. She did not see two grandchildren who belonged to her eldest child, Martin, who no longer spoke to her and had not done so for many years. Her second son had eight-month-old twins whom she was only allowed to see when she was not drinking. This limitation on seeing the twins was very painful for her, as seeing them was one of the few delights that Beryl experienced at that time of her life.
>
> During our first sessions it was important for her to express how unsupportive both her ex-husbands had been. She struggled in her first marriage with her husband being unfaithful and unhelpful. She had two young children in quick succession and was soon left to be a single mother to them when her first husband left.
>
> Beryl said she felt judged at the AA meetings. This was to be a pervasive theme in her therapy: feeling unsupported by people. She highlighted how difficult it had been for her to have been bedridden for five years, hooked up to a continuous supply of oxygen to keep her alive whilst waiting for a lung transplant, which she had six years prior to seeing me.
>
> She was desperate to be in a relationship. She presented with psychological as well as physical issues. She was the fourth of five children. She described her childhood as "ok", with her mother doing, "everything" for her and her father hardly ever being present in the family home and, when he was there, he ignored her. For the most part she did not get on with her younger sister as she always felt that her sister was given preferential treatment.

She recalled that when she was about four years old her mother "went away for about ten days". On her return her mother said to her, "I have a present for you." Beryl recalled that her mother placed a "live breathing baby into my toy cot". She remembers feeling devastated that her mother went away and returned with a baby girl, and she thought, "Why does she want another girl, was I not good enough?" This was to be the start of a very fraught relationship between Beryl and her youngest sister.

Beryl also has very limited use of her right arm because of a car accident in which she was involved at age nineteen. In previous years she had undergone a lung transplant due to a genetic condition that had grossly impacted on the function of her lungs; this had left her bedridden and suffering with severe shortness of breath for some years and led to her youngest daughter, Sarah, becoming her main carer at the age of twelve.

Sarah, was eighteen when she came to see me and Beryl still found her a huge challenge and described her as selfish and uncaring, especially towards her.

Her main presenting symptoms were her depression and her addiction to alcohol, which I initially thought was limited to one bottle of wine per night, but I later found out that she would drink two or three bottles per night. This was highly contraindicated by her doctor, because of her physical condition.

As this was her third counselling experience in relation to her drinking, I asked her, "How do you think counselling will be different for you this time?" She said that she had only been half living, due to her daily consumption of wine. She hoped to be able to give up drinking and to be able to be more present and live her life more fully. She hated the fact that she was often "too drunk" to even remember watching her favourite television programmes.

Beryl spent a lot of the time during her sessions describing how let down she has felt by people, including her children, and how disappointed she felt with different individuals in her life. She was very caring and concerned about others and could not understand why people could not behave in a similar way towards her.

Very early on in our sessions, she often expressed her disappointment with her closest friend, Janet, whom she had met at AA. She said she envious of her as she was seeing a man whom she had met at AA.

Beryl spoke about feeling lonely and did not enjoy living alone but she also deeply mistrusted people: this interested me, as did the way she idealised me, which I was to discover after she missed her fourth session because of a fall down her stairs which left her with heavy bruising to her face. During the fifth week of our therapy, she rang to say that she could not attend as she needed an operation on her face for the injuries she had sustained. I was asked by the agency's manager to ring her and remind her that if she missed any more sessions, she would be put back on the waiting list. At this point she promised that she would be there the following week even if she had to get a taxi there (this was a huge expense for her as she was on a limited budget). During this call she said to me, "I cannot go back on the waiting list. I would hate to lose you. You have helped me so much. You are amazing."

Her idealisation of me continued throughout our work. I was mindful of this and often explored what it meant for her.

I was also very aware of the feelings that she elicited in me. I remember when I first met her, I thought that she looked like, "a typical alcoholic". This might have been a prejudice or a fear of mine: a prejudice because, in those early days I had a very unhelpful picture in my mind of how our work would progress; and I was fearful because I felt very hopeless in relation to how much I would be able to help her overcome such a severe problem.

On the other hand, I was very struck by how eloquent she was. I really enjoy sitting with people who use words in a creative way. I also admired her courage and often wondered how I might have fared in her position with so many disabilities due to her severe illness. I realised that I became very fond of her and maybe this was the main reason for being so fearful of being disappointed by her.

Our sessions went by so quickly, and I often found myself savouring every minute of the time I spent with this very courageous woman.

When she returned on her sixth week, I was aware of just how pleased I was to see her. The session seemed so brief, and at the end of that session, I thought, "I could easily have carried on listening to you for another hour."

She spoke about her operation and how for the first time in her life she felt that she had friends. She was overwhelmed with gratitude for the number of well wishes, cards, and text messages she had received. She said that she had felt empowered by our last session and was feeling confident that she would be able to cope if her friends let her down. We discussed her fear of being left alone. She said that all her life she had struggled with being left alone. She recalled being about six years old when she and her brother, who was four, got home from school to find that their mother was out. She was terrified and ran out of the house trying frantically to find her mother who was nowhere to be seen. When she returned home, she accidentally got locked in the pantry and desperately screamed and knocked on the window for help.

Her mum returned home eventually, and her response was: "Oh well, I have a right to pop out sometimes." This felt very unsupportive to Beryl. She said that this felt like the same kind of disappointment she felt when her mother brought her baby sister home without preparing her for the imminent arrival.

The relationship with her second son was not the kind of relationship that she wanted. She was very proud of his achievements but was unhappy that he could not accept her with her drinking.

During her second marriage, she had attempted suicide by overdosing on antidepressant tablets after an argument with her husband that left her feeling humiliated after he walked out on her. She was discovered unconscious by her older son Martin and her brother. She later said that she felt awfully guilty that her son had seen her in this state. She also felt that he was angry with her for letting his father leave when he was only two years old. She attributed the distance in their relationship to these experiences.

Beryl said that she found being a new mum difficult and needed support and was put on Valium. She said that her first born son Martin had a piercing cry which was intolerable. Martin was later discovered to have had a bleed on the brain when he was four months old after having had convulsions. The doctors said that the bleeding had occurred when he was two months old but, because she was on Valium, she did not register that he needed medical help. When he was nine months old, he was diagnosed with infantile convulsions.

Now, she said, Martin had accused her of dropping him on his head when he was a baby. The doctor had questioned whether he had been shaken as a baby, which Beryl denied. She found these accusations by her son very painful.

She struggled with constant worry about her health, as she had to see the consultants for regular check-ups for her lungs. They were unaware of the fact that she misused alcohol and which led to her frequently forgetting to take her night-time anti-rejection medication.

Another painful memory she recounted to me was about her move to where she now lives from up north during her secondary school years. She felt that she did not fit in with the other school girls as her mother made her wear the uniform from her previous school. She felt self-conscious about her appearance and her accent for which she was teased. She said it was devastating for her but her mother did not think this would have affected her.

Another huge loss for her was when she was forty, her mother decided to move back to Ireland. She said that she could not cope with this and felt that she needed her mother, and was also angry about the separation from her mother.

Her attendance was good, and Beryl eagerly made use of the therapeutic space to explore her difficulties. She said that she looked forward to the sessions and felt that the fifty minutes was not enough. She often told me that she benefited a lot from our sessions and felt very early on that they may have helped her to invest in relationships/friendships. However, although she was extremely lonely, she was scared to invest in relationships, "in case they let her down". Beryl frequently discussed her use of alcohol and sometimes doubted that she was "really alcoholic". The fact that her uncle was an alcoholic made her wonder whether her habit was genetic.

By the thirteenth week of therapy Beryl told me that she had started drinking again and that she felt very disappointed in herself. Her drinking escalated quickly from one to two bottles of wine per day. Her drinking exacerbated her feelings of loneliness. During our work together her daughter moved in with her and this caused Beryl huge anxiety as she believed that they "are not compatible". They had heated arguments and neither was able to listen to the other.

She eventually owned up to realising that she "was alcoholic" and decided to go for another detox. However, Beryl was soon drinking again because she felt so lonely and disappointed with people who were not caring for her enough. This led to a third detox about two years into our work and she resumed drinking the very same day she left the rehabilitation facility; she felt a huge sense of disappointment because she was initially meant to be there for ten days, but the detox was cut short and on day six she was told that she had had all the available medication and, due to a lack of funding for the group therapy and other activities, these had to be cancelled.

This was a huge blow that was unbearable for her and was very hard for me. At this point I felt hopeless and really wanted to give up working with her. For the next few weeks, I wished that she would give up and just send me a message saying that this was too much for her because by now it was getting too much for me. Month after month, my hopes were dashed. She broke all her promises to me that she would give up drinking.

I wanted out! I had a very honest conversation with my supervisor, telling her that this was not for me: "I just cannot sit with this hopeless scenario any longer and am ready to throw in the towel."

My supervisor was very understanding and being, also, very psychodynamic in her thinking, she pointed out that these emotions could very well reflect what Beryl was feeling. I knew for sure that some of them were mine in response to just how unproductive the therapy felt. However, she then said something to me that will remain with me forever: "Somebody has to hold the hope." This really got through to me. It was my job as a therapist to hold the hope. This is what I was here for. This was a turning point in our therapy.

I thought at this point I would undertake a TAIP, to unravel the *traumatic attachment* so that Beryl could make sense of her dependency issues, her difficulties staying with her uncomfortable emotions and possibly why she has always felt let down by people.

Ten minutes into the session, I brought up the TAIP when she was telling me how much her mother had wanted her children to be dependent on her. This is quite common in people who have developed a traumatic attachment.

(B is the client; M is the therapist)

B: I know but do you know what, well I have been thinking for many years that she wanted to make us all dependent on her.

M: Who did? your mum?

B: Mum, so that she could kind of be in charge, do you know what I mean? And we all had to please her so she would help us.

M: How does that feel?

B: Feels like she was quite selfish really to do that.

M: And keeping you in a needy position.

B: Yeah, keeping me dependent on her and so when she did leave, I was absolutely devastated and my other siblings weren't so much because they had partners, but I knew that if she left when she said she was going to leave, my partner would be ten times worse to me and he was so …

M: I think this is an ideal time to do this, you know the test I have spoken to you about and it's just to imagine that now, as an adult you are, how old are you? Fifty-eight?

B: Yeah, nearly fifty-nine.

M: Nearly fifty-nine, you have got three children, you are an adult in your own right, you have achieved so much with your life, you run your own household. Imagine that your mum walked into this room now, with you being the fifty-nine-year-old woman, and I am going to ask you to repeat something after me that you will say to your mum, and just note how it feels for you to say these words. You might feel it somewhere in your body, take notice of where you feel it … In she comes, she sits on that chair and I want you to say to her: "Mum, I am fifty-nine years old and I don't need you to care for me anymore like I did when I was a child."

B: I couldn't, I couldn't say that. I still need her to be there for me.

M: You do, I thought you would say that, what would it feel like to say it?

B: Well, I wouldn't say it, I wouldn't because I do need her to be there for me, you know as a person not so much as a child, yeah you know.

M: Yeah, as an adult

B: Yeah, she has been so close to me and been through so much with me that I still need her to be around, but you know when she left when I was forty (to go and live in Ireland), no a bit older, that's when I was just devastated because I still needed her so much.

M: What did you need her for?

B: For everything, for moral support, for comfort, for listening, for back up. I mean she was always the one that if people hurt me, she would go out and fight the battle for me do you know, like my father wouldn't.

M: So, at the thought of saying that to your mother do you feel anything?

B: Saying what?

M: If you would be able to say to her, "I don't need you to look after me anymore", what feelings does that bring up for you?

B: I couldn't say it, it makes me feel really empty, I couldn't say that!

M: Do you feel anything in your body?

B: Yeah I can feel it in my stomach, you know, hurt, I know I can't feel like that.

M: What would the feeling in your stomach be?

B: Awful. It would feel like *a big empty hole* because I do really need her and you know, I know I am a grown-up and I am sixty and I should be able to get on with my own life, maybe I could be if I had a caring partner, but I've never had a caring partner.

M: Do you feel unable to get on with your own life?

B: Well in a way yeah and I do get on with my own life, I do it, I do manage.

M: But you feel that that care is missing.

B: But you know I know on the other hand I can't blame her for trying to make things better for herself.

M: Do you imagine that your children feel like that?

B: I don't know because I consciously brought my children up not to be dependent on me.

M: Andy leads an independent life, so does Sarah, so does your oldest son.

B: Yeah.

M: So, what made you consciously decide that you definitely want them to be independent?

B: Because I didn't want them to be reliant on me.

M: Like the way that you were reliant on your mother.

B: Yeah, because it would ruin their lives, you know when I wasn't around anymore.

M: So are you saying that by your mother dying that it has ruined your life or before that when she moved to Ireland?

B: Before that, even before that for years when we moved to Harlow when we used to live in Cheshire. I had just started at this all-girls' grammar school, I have told you all this before and I was so proud you know to be in this posh uniform with a leather satchel and … no consideration for our feelings, they moved down to Harlow in a terraced house where we lived in a semi-detached Victorian house you know in Cheshire.

M: So, you feel that your parents didn't give any regard to your feelings.

B: No, not at all, they just wanted to shunt us off.

M: What does that feel like?

B: Awful, awful, dreadful, I mean there are girls' high schools admittedly not in here, you know, why couldn't they have took a bit more interest in finding out you know what would be more suitable for me instead of shoving me into you know a great big comprehensive school with great big sixteen-year-old boys like six foot tall and I was eleven years old and I was only little and I had to wear a different uniform to everybody else, had a different accent to everybody else, and that was for, I don't know, about six months until they bought me the proper uniform!

M: That was a long time.

In the weeks after we completed the TAIP, Beryl was diagnosed with pancreatitis. She was extremely fearful for her health at this point. We discussed her anxieties around this. We also discussed her anger and for the first time she admitted that she was angry with her parents, and she wanted me to help her to forgive them, as the anger was too intense and she was unable to hold it in.

She also admitted that she has now owned that her alcoholism was her own doing and that up until now she had blamed, "everyone else".

A few weeks after we had done TAIP, I asked Beryl to reflect on what came up for her. I questioned what she made of the emptiness that she had felt in her stomach at the idea of saying to her mother that she did not need her anymore.

Reflecting on what she thought the "emptiness" might be, Beryl said that she felt that there was something missing in the relationship with her mother. The hole she felt in her stomach she said she had tried to fill with excessive consumption of wine every single night. I was quite surprised when she brought this up as I was not expecting that, so many weeks later, she would still have been thinking of the TAIP. It seemed that she had been unconsciously working on it all this time.

We had about twelve sessions after this, working towards an ending, as my work with the agency was coming to an end. She was very apprehensive about our work ending as she had become so reliant on her sessions as a way of making contact with another human being and also attending gave her a purpose in her week.

We explored how she could use what she has learned about herself to help her with forming more meaningful relationships. During our work she had often complained that people did not return the kindness that she had showed them; she felt people took advantage of her and couldn't understand why she kept going out of her way to be kind to them. She benefited greatly from the idea that she was treating them, the way she had always wished to be treated. In one of our ending sessions, she said "I was being mother to them, you know, the way I wished my mother had been to me. Well, I don't have to do that anymore."

In those final twelve sessions, she was able to mourn the loss of her mother, overcoming her unresolved grief. The integration of her dissociated self, triggered by the experience of the TAIP, meant that her addiction could finally end.

A few years later, I contacted Beryl and learnt that she was still not drinking alcohol.

The use of the TAIP in this case revealed that Beryl's previous inability to make use of therapy was the result of the unconscious traumatically attached IWM of her child-Self attached to her idealised mother.

A few months ago, I wrote to Beryl in relation to my chapter in this book. I never received a reply from her, but I received a call from her son: he told me that he had received my letter, as, sadly, his mother had died a few months before. When I explained to him who I was, he told me that from the time that she had ended her work with me, she no longer rang him being intoxicated and abusive. He added, "You gave her some good years and we had an ok relationship after that."

Unresolved grief: "the huge hole inside of me"

Claire came to see me in the summer of 2012. We worked together for nineteen months. This was her first time in therapy. We met weekly. Her response to my query of why she had come to see me was, "I have had so many losses that I have not processed". Her mother had died from Hodgkin's disease when Claire was twenty-one.

Her first husband had died of a brain tumour within their first year of marriage. She was forty-one at the time and living with her second husband, with whom she job-shared as a priest, and her son who was two years and three months old. She has a twin brother to whom she is close and has a good relationship with her father. She described her early life as having felt loved by her mother. As a young child there was an ever-present and intrusive grandmother who, her mother told her, would enter her mother's bedroom to rock her brother and her while her mother slept. She said that she was not able to voice her anger as a child to her mother. When she became a teenager, she can remember her mother saying, "My mother is killing me." She later found out that her mother did not want to have children. How did she feel about this? "I am very proud of her," she said. This kind of idealisation of her mother was very pervasive throughout our work. She was often very physically tired, which she put down to not sleeping well

Claire reported having low moods and struggled with getting up in the night to breastfeed her son. She found breastfeeding depressing but felt that she had to continue doing it as a way of keeping her son safe. She desperately wanted to give up. She said, "I know it is stupid, but I feel like if I don't breast feed him, he will die." She lived in constant fear that her husband and her son would die.

As a priest, a major part of her job involved conducting funerals, visiting the sick, and supporting bereaved families. Claire was very in touch with her love for God and felt ungrateful for feeling down. She often commenced our sessions saying that she had had a bad week of feeling down and being tearful. She also spoke about feeling like a failure to be back in therapy as she had previously had bereavement therapy after her mother died. She felt a huge lack of family support around her as there were no family members who lived close by. Claire often described being overly angry with her husband and that she did not want to be like this. She described feeling worthless and acknowledged that her emotions were often "disproportionate", going from being extremely angry to extremely joyful or sad.

She described the first two years of her life with her son as being sad and miserable. She would say to herself in the middle of the night while she fed him, "you are horrible, you are horrible", over and over again.

Claire expressed much gratitude for the sessions and said that she found silences very difficult because when she was a child, whenever her mother was angry, she would go silent.

A few weeks into our sessions she reported that her son was now sleeping through the night. She still found it challenging to continue breastfeeding him.

Another important goal for her was to understand and then tackle her extreme hoarding. She described finding it extremely difficult to dispose of items that she considered had emotional value. I was eventually made to understand that these items included everything that belonged to her mother and to her late husband in their small accommodation. She described her house as being so cluttered that one was unable to see any of the floor.

Nine months into our work, as Claire struggled with her unresolved grief, I decided to carry out a TAIP with her. I could see that she that she had been unable to mourn for her mother by the way she presented her relationship with her mother and by how difficult it was for her to come to terms with her mother's death.

By this stage, I had also noticed that her history fulfilled the three criteria (highlighted in Chapter 4, p. 75) that indicate a likely *traumatic attachment* to at least one of her caregivers:

1. A strong moral defence expressed by feeling to blame.
2. Idealisation of the parental figure.
3. A history of resistance to change in previous therapies.

My hope was that by using TAIP she might be able to examine her Child Self's idealised relationship with her mother and, in so doing, begin to integrate her divided Self and work through her loss.

(C is the client; M is the therapist)

M: I suppose we could think about the test at this point, um, what the test requires of you is to think of yourself as you are now, an adult, a mother, and the achievements that you've had in your life; you've got a very important job. And what I'm going to ask you to do is repeat a few words after me.

C: Can I refuse (laughing).

M: You can if you want …

C: Are they positive words though?

M: It is something to work with. It can be quite meaningful for you.

C: I felt quite excited today thinking is it going to start today.

M: So, what's required is that you think of yourself as you are now, what we're going to do, as you say the words, I want you to note where you feel it in your body, if you feel anything in your body, or any feelings emotionally, so what's going to happen is I'm going to ask you to imagine that your mother walked into this room now, she sat there across from you, and I'd like you to turn towards her and say "Mother, I don't need you to look after me anymore as I did when I was a child."

C: OK. Could I call her what I normally would, "Mummy"?

M: Yes.

C: OK, Mummy I don't need you to look after me anymore.

M: I'm an adult and I'm in charge of my own life.

C: I'm an adult and I'm in charge of my own life.

M: And that's it.

(Long silence …)

C: I feel a sense of her joy, you know, her saying, um, I can hear her laughter, actually, and her joy for me actually, that's what it feels like.

M: Her joy for you? What do you feel?

C: I feel loved, I feel her love.

M: Do you feel any anything else?

C: I feel a sense of pride, reminds me of the time when I had to, when she saw me being an adult, when she was ill and she wanted to carry on working, and basically I came and said that they would wouldn't want her to work anymore because of her illness, and I basically defended her and spoke, and she said to me afterwards "I'm so impressed by how you were, I was so impressed by how you, I never knew you could argue and speak so well" and it's that kind of feeling I'm getting of um, her pride for me, my pride in all that I've, yeah, all that I have achieved, and a sense of sense of standing alone. I feel that I'm standing alone in a powerful way, a bit like, I love that that feeling of being on holiday, and standing at the edge of a cliff and feeling all the air around me and sort of having space, so feeling strong actually, yeah.

M: And you had tears?

C: I think I was missing her, but recognition of her, her saying you can do it, you are doing it, you have done it, you are doing it without me, and you're doing it well I think, but just joy and love actually. It felt as if she was listening to me very seriously when I was saying that, with respect, but there was also a sense of a kind of joy for me.

M: So, you feel like you got her approval.

C: Completely, oh yeah, completely.

M: What do you make of all this?

C: At the moment I'm just slightly psychoanalysing it myself, because I remember when I was having counselling after she died, it might have been after my first husband died, you had to reach a stage where you can say after a person's died, "I can actually go on without you". I can do this, and even, which I find still slightly difficult, even there are things that are better now because you're no longer alive. That's something she'd, maybe I misunderstood that.

M: Do you find that difficult?

C: Yes, very difficult.

M: I wonder what she meant?

C: Maybe it's how I misinterpreted it, or misunderstood quite what she was saying, but I'm feeling slightly uncomfortable with that, that you can see there are thing that are better almost, I don't … but I suppose notes towards seeing the positive things you've achieved.

M: And maybe to be able to see how you've moved on with your life in a positive way?

C: I do feel a real sense of her, her love and her … A real sense of pride actually. (crying)

M: Do you feel that she's always been proud of you?

C: Yes, I've always felt that, yeah, yeah, and sometimes I feel it when I'm with my son, getting a sense of her love for me and that I'm doing a good job,

M: Which is important for you because you …

C: Yeah.

M: Did you have any bodily reactions? … Anything in your stomach? …

C: Well, I suppose I had tears welling up in me, I dunno whether that counts … I don't know. I've got quite a vivid imagination, so that kind of thing I find I can get into it quite quickly, it's quite emotional, I didn't expect it to be instantly quite so emotional. I wasn't prepared for you to say imagine your mother coming in … so that was a bit shocking in a way.

M: Shocking?

C: I think so.

M: Scarily so?

C: No, it felt perhaps surprising but normal in a weird kind of, cos when I sense my mother it's like that its surprising but feels totally normal as well, sort of a weird mixture

M: Like tears welling up.

C: I feel deep joy, love, a really strong sense of her presence actually, very strong, I could see her very strongly then, in a quite professional way, because she was a medical-social worker, so she was being very attentive, she was doing what you'd asked her to do—sit there and listen, so I felt as first she was being very professional, then she just wanted to giggle, and laugh and tell me how wonderful I was doing, I didn't feel, at first it was her listening and then it was an overwhelming sense of love and joy, but I felt she was holding back to start with, that's what it made me feel, I had to do it first, and then she'd respond I think … It wasn't at all her being, she wasn't being dominating at all, it was very much she was listening to me and respecting. It was very much as I remembered her when we were older, and adult, I felt very much an adult with her, an adult relationship. Not I was a child, I was her daughter …

M: You didn't feel like you were being a child?

C: No, that's why it reminded me of a time being an adult and defending her.

M: I wonder what it would have been like if it was your Child Self?

C: I don't know, yes it so wasn't my child self as you asked me to imagine me as I was now.

M: Yes.

C: If you'd asked me to imagine if I was a child, cos I wouldn't have been able to say it as a child because I wouldn't have wanted her to not be, I'd still need her here, but I wouldn't have wanted to say I've grown up because I wasn't grown up, but I didn't feel any sense of being a child. I suppose a lot of it depends on when you do that test, depends on what mindset you're in.

M: But for a long time, you've been working very hard to process the loss of your mum.

C: Anymore? Is that it? It's very stressful … gosh, amazing yeah, and now we need to do three months of therapy after that to potentially deal with it, it's quite interesting that, not necessarily, that it's how long you could bring things up that needed attention. So, I can't even remember now what I've said to her.

M: I don't need you to care for me anymore as I did when I was a child.

C: Is that what I said? I don't remember anything that I said, I probably do need her to care for me still.

(It appears that at this point during TAIP she had dissociated as it might have been in reality too difficult to say the words when she felt that she still needed her mother.)

M: It may be that you still do need her to care for you.

C: Well, I need people to care for me, so if she was still alive, I'd be wanting her to still care for me, just as I want my family to care for me.

M: In what way?

C: Well, I think when I'm sad I find it very comforting to tell people, so I'd tell my father, my brother Bob, if I'm feeling low, and they're very comforting so if she was still alive, I'd definitely still say to her, oh gosh, or if there's a problem or have you got any good advice about how to start potty-training Larry, you know, all those sorts of questions, I mean I would still, do still need her, to do … but is there something about saying that you don't, that frees you, doesn't it? In some way?

M: Different people have different reactions.

C: My emotional response was one of empowerment during that definitely, but as I'm analysing it now, I'm thinking I do need her actually, saying what I felt when I was doing that felt her sense of, just a real sense of her love, and her absolutely wanting the best for me, and completely understanding that this is helpful; I felt that she had a sense of course, this is what you need to do to help you sort things, but I do need her still, I do value her still to care for me, you know it's funny.

M: Do you mean emotionally?

C: I wish she was here, I suppose, you know.

M: It's really sad to have lost your mum so quickly.

C: I feel now that I feel slightly guilty actually (crying), I think by saying that I don't need her when I do need her, I think I see this as a huge hole inside of me, feels like there's still this massive whole inside me, so it is still quite physically here (indicates top of her chest), a huge gap where she's not.

M: Yeah, so difficult isn't it.

C: And I know she'd want me to live with joy, that's what she wants for me.

M: So, do you feel like if she was here, that gap wouldn't be there? She'd be able to …

C: Yeah, she wouldn't be able to support it all, there's always going to be problems in your life which you can't rely on your parents for or you know, but yeah a lot of the pain I think, yeah, which is quite interesting I think because I really thought I'd dealt with it you know that's the weird thing, I really thought I'd dealt with it …

This is a demonstration of just how effective the TAIP can be to elicit a traumatic attachment that has manifested in unresolved mourning. She reported experiencing bodily sensations.

M: What, losing your mum?

C: Yeah, I really thought I'd sorted it.

M: Remember when we discussed when you have a child it brings up so much, all the unconscious processes of your own experiences with your own mum and it is nice to have your mum when you've had a baby.

C: Yeah, I just think it's so weird because in both my weddings, I didn't feel that terrible sense of missing her, I felt her love, her joy around me, didn't get that agonising sense of where is my mother, I felt her presence spiritually with me, didn't feel, and I remember the counselling I had after she died, she said this will be a key point of your life, there'll be moments where you find it very hard, and I'm thinking yes it will, and then it wasn't, but either way. And when I was priested another important part of my life, I didn't feel her absence I felt her after Larry was born, actually I mean.

M: Also having a child brings up lots of unconscious conflicts, unresolved conflicts that there were in the relationship with you and your mother. What else can we make of this emptiness that you feel, how did you describe it …?

C: Huge hole.

M: Oh yes, what else can we make of that?

C: Its quite draining, and it gets in the way of a lot of stuff, it's a bit like after I broke my ankle I was still limping and now I, cos I've slipped my disc it's still sore, its constantly sore, I'm sore all the time, but I don't always notice its hurting, then I think oh yeah it is, like today has been really busy and I wanted to lie down then someone would summon me to hospital and I'd have to rush off there, I've just come from hospital now, its sore now, I think it's just that feeling of I'm always slightly sore, this feeling (indicates chest) it's there all the time actually.

M: So, it's an emotional soreness.

C: Just pain I think, just pain, yeah pain

M: And do you know exactly what causes this pain?

C: She's dead, she's not here (crying) so nothing's ever quite right, I mean I remember thinking after she died just nothing is ever going to be quite right again, maybe that's it, even now I've got a lovely husband, the job that I wanted to do, gorgeous son, nothing is quite right.

M: Because your mum's not here?

C: And no matter how I try to be thankful for all the good things, it's never going to be right is it, it's not right.

M: And that hole has always been? What would you like to do with that hole?

C: Of course, I'd love it to be healed, its much bigger than I thought it was.

M: It's almost as if it's incompatible with life?

C: It's definitely stopping me living fully, it's definitely stopping me, it's like my mother would have hated that, she would have you know, she would have hated the fact that her death would have hurt me so much I would think.

M: And that's the difficult thing about it, she had no control, you had no control over it. I think that's why it's so difficult, there's nothing that anybody could have done to prevent it.

(Long pause …)

M: And when you said you didn't realise how big the whole was, what made you think that it was bigger than you thought it was?

C: I was just visualising it, when you were saying how you feel and how does that manifest itself, I see this quite strong picture of this big gap in me,

M: And you wanted to heal the hole, what do you think it would take to heal that hole?

C: No idea, I think its somehow being honest about the joyful things and allowing myself more joy probably, not feeling guilty about forcing myself to do all the stuff I find horrible or hard work, allowing myself to just celebrate, I do that anyway, but to do more of just enjoying being with Larry and John, I think, just enjoying myself with them, not feeling constantly guilty doing the hard stuff, there's always hard work to do, but I don't have to always.

I think I'm making more of a conscious choice now with my friendships, there's a couple of friends that I've found deeply difficult, and you know what, I'm just not going to contact them; they are kind of more through friends of other relationships, and whenever I see these people they just drag me down and make me feel alone … so I think that while I'm caring for people, and particularly my friendships, I'm consciously much more aware of the cost it has I think, the emotional physical cost on me, and there was one evening when I was mean to be ringing a girlfriend but in the past I would have just done it, if I've said it I will do it, I was just too tired so I texted her and said sorry I'm really tired I'll ring you another night, so it's about, I think it's about self-preservation, about caring for myself.

M: And putting your needs first.

C: Or at least the same level as the other person but sometimes before them. It's about sustaining your own relationship and yourself.

M: Yes, and it is what we discussed before, about why, how did you develop this way of relating, about always putting the needs of the other person first.

About twenty minutes later in the session she brought up the TAIP.

C: So when we did that thing about my mother saying about how I am managing, that's quite timely actually but I can't say that I don't need her because I do need her, but

I said it. I can say it when you ask me to, but since then I want to take it back, I wish I could almost take it back and say "I need you. I really do need you; I need you and I wish you were here", I am being an adult and I am managing. I think that's it.

M: Yeah, at the moment (pause).

M: How would you describe the overall experience of having said that, or this session actually?

C: I feel like I have, it's always releases after you have cried. I feel relaxed I suppose, it does remind me of grief in a way. I feel bereaved quite badly now, but I feel bereaved but drinking champagne (laughs). It's that sense of my experience when people have died. You are really missing them but there is also massive sense of joy, that's what it feels like as well. So, if I look back over the times of acute bereavement there's been moments where it's really been. I really felt terribly sad for missing that person, but also, I suppose I felt hope for the future as well. So maybe that's what it is. Bereaving but also the hope and belief that there are good things to come, that life is still good, and can be good again. Even though it's awful and I am missing them, there are still good things to come.

(This demonstrates the start of her grieving process for the loss of her mother and as she processes this loss, she will be able to free herself of the traumatic attachment.)

M: Which is positive because you are holding out hope.

C: If I look at the future, I feel excitement actually and I feel hope.

The following week she came uncharacteristically late for our session and said that she did not want to come today because after the TAIP she had felt sad for the entire week. She reported having had a panic attack, something she had not experienced for years. She said she has been riddled with guilt for saying that she did not need her mother. She spoke of her anger towards her unsupportive boss and about feeling dishonest for not being able to say what she really wants to say and that she feels that "there is a horrible person underneath all this falseness".

A few weeks after carrying out the TAIP, we looked at the recording together, and she initially did not recognise herself on the recording. She asked me, "Is that really me?" It seemed that she had been so deeply affected by the idea of speaking to a mother with whom she had had such profound unresolved issues that she somehow had assumed a different state, that on reflection she could not recognise herself.

We carried on working for another six months, during which time we discussed her death anxiety, her relationship with her mother, and her anger and how important it was to her for me not to think badly of her. Her anger was mostly directed at her boss who was never around and therefore left the huge burden of the work for her and her husband.

We had to end therapy as she was moving away to another assignment. Towards the end of the work, she was able to sleep better and said that her low moods weren't as frequent as she was able to embrace the positive things and people in her life. Her parting words to me were, "thank you for holding my difficult feelings."

Approximately three years after our work had ended, Claire reported being in a "better place and feeling more in control of my life". She has moved away and is even enjoying her new job.

Eight years after work ended, I spoke to Claire. She was working as a chaplain in a school and was "happier in her life". Doing the TAIP allowed us to explore her unresolved grief for the loss of her mother, her feelings of grief; her anger and her own death anxieties and her fear of losing her loved ones. She was able to move on to a job that was more comfortable for her and be more fulfilled in her life.

Complicated unresolved grief: "the concrete in his chest had moved down into his stomach"

In the autumn of 2019 Peter, a fifty-year-old man was referred to me via his job's employee assistance programme for six sessions initially. He arrived five minutes early for his first session. He reported living with his wife and his now fourteen-year-old daughter. He was fourteen when his mother died, the youngest of three brothers. His brothers are seven and eleven years older than he is. They have a close relationship.

He said he worked at the railway and was finding it very stressful there. He had been having low moods over the last two years at least. He would sometimes find himself in tears, not knowing what prompted this. He said that his wife and his supervisor at work were very worried about him. He reported being anxious and depressed over the previous year.

His mother had died of cancer when he was fourteen years old. He said that she had been in and out of hospital and then she came home one weekend and that was the last time he had seen her.

In this first session he fluctuated between talking about his mother and the difficulties of his job. He described his job as being a "threatening environment". He worked as a ticket clerk at a railway station. He said that years ago he had seen a dead body on the tracks and though he found the experience distressing, no one offered him any counselling or any support. He found the schedule quite gruelling with not enough time off to be with his family. This was his first time in therapy.

In subsequent sessions Peter described experiencing low moods and wanting to just "drive away" and thinking, "Where is the rope?" He had lost interest in hobbies and had not been on a holiday for over ten years.

My thoughts at the time were of desperation. What we are dealing with is very serious and with only six sessions I felt pressured to do something for this man. By session three, the GP had signed him off work with anxiety. I offered to do the TAIP with him. This was evidently a case of unresolved grief, possibly due to a *traumatic attachment*.

The session started with him talking about going into head office for a discussion about getting him to return to work.

(P is the client; M is the therapist)

P: I think they are going to try to get me to come back to work on a phased return. I said to her that I had been bad last week, which I have been.

M: What's the reason for this?

P: I feel sick a lot, my heart is up in my throat, my chest tightens up now and again.

M: Oh dear.

P: I have been more teary than I have been for over a month. I have been crying (nodding in a matter of fact way).

M: What's the feeling?

P: A few times I have felt like just getting in my car and going driving and not getting out again.

M: So, when you are crying, what emotions are behind the tears, do you know?

P: No, I said to my wife yesterday, it's like being sick without feeling sick first. It's like feeling nausea. Its emotion, as I have said, I had this last year. I did have a spell when I was waking up in the mornings. I have not been sleeping and eating properly, especially last week.

M: You are not in a good way, are you?

P: No, I could be sitting there, and you could just feel it, like a gush of water coming up. Sometimes, it's not even there and then woosh, sometimes there are not even tears. I remember having it last year as well. I had to wake up and grit my teeth. And then I think what's all that about?

M: What is it about?

P: Maybe it's just tensions, I don't know.

M: If we could try and put that into perspective today. The little test that I was telling you about. What it entails is you saying some words after me. So, you think of yourself in the present as you are now. Peter, fifty years old, you've got a job, you are married, you've got a beautiful daughter. What I would like you to do is: imagine that your mother came into this room now. And I want you to repeat some words after me to her.

P: (nodding enthusiastically to show that he has understood)

M: So, she sits in that chair, I know it's a bit weird as she is not here anymore, bless her. Say, she appeared in that chair, I would like you to say to her, "Mother, I am an adult now, I am fifty years old, I have got a job, married, I have got a child. I don't need to be sad about losing you anymore." And note what it feels like in your body.

(These words are a variation from the usual words of, "I don't need you as I did when I was a child". With unresolved grief the individual's attachment is still intact and the longing for and idealisation of that parent is still at play even though that parent/caregiver is dead.)

P: (long pause) I am building up to it.

M: Take your time.

P: (sits forward in his chair and throws his arms helplessly in the air) Mum, I am fifty now, got a wife, lovely daughter, I am working, got a house, I don't need to be sad anymore.

M: I don't need to be sad about losing you.

P: I don't need to be sad about losing you. I have always felt that you are there, you are watching me. I have always felt your presence.

M: What does it feel like in your body as you said those words?

P: There is a tension.

M: What is the tension. Describe it. Where in your body is it?

P: (puts his left hand over the left of his chest) It's here.

M: What's it like, this tension?

P: When I said that I don't need to be sad anymore, it felt like it loosened, it moved (a long contemplative pause). It's like something opened.

M: What are you feeling now, in this moment?

P: A bit numb, in a way. I am really trying to get it into here (points to his head) that she is sitting there.

M: And into your body as well. That is where we have our feelings.

P: It felt like a balloon had inflated and then went down again.

M: Hmmm, what do you make of that?

P: Now I feel a bit numb, I can't describe it.

M: I wonder what the numbness is doing. You did have a sensation there before.

P: I feel like I never lost her. Feels like I have opened a scar.

M: Oh? (At this point I was feeling desperate for him to be able to hold on to his bodily sensations so that he might be able to interpret them.)

P: At the moment, I am trying to access that emotion, imagine that she is here. If she was, I would be over there giving her a hug (sits up in his chair, rocking backwards and forwards). You know, as I have said before, I have always cried like the weather out there but deep down. But last week my wife said to me, "Peter, you have never opened up about your mum." And she said ever since I have known you, I don't think you have ever got over it. She never knew my mum. I don't think that I have ever really properly … I thought I had.

M: Why haven't you got over her?

P: I don't know. It's like, I met a cousin last week and we spoke about him and when he lost his mum. I said to him that I used to always think I have overcome it, but, as you do, I just got on with life. You know, what's done is done. You can't bring them back, you just get on with it and maybe that's the mindset I should not have had, I don't know.

M: Well, it's not been the mindset you've had, and we feel about things the way we feel about losing people. So, it might be worth thinking about why is it that, I am not saying you should or shouldn't, but why is it that you, Peter has not got over the loss of your mum.

P: I don't know, I thought I had, always thought that I had but I don't think I really have properly, not deep down.

M: So, on the level that you have managed, what would it mean for you to go deeply into acknowledging that loss?

P: The way I see it, it's like a scar but it like its many years ago and it healed over.

M: Can I tell you something? The feelings are timeless, they are stored unconsciously, and those feelings can be as though you have just lost her two minutes ago or two years ago.

P: (nodding enthusiastically) I get that.

M: If we focus on how it feels, what would it feel like to go deeply into that loss?

P: I don't really know what it feels like.

M: What do you imagine? What would it mean for you?

P: I don't know how I would react (in a very subdued tone). I don't really know. I often felt that there are emotions there that I have never opened up, only to my wife, where she has said I've never seen you like that. She said, "Peter, you spilled your heart out like I have never seen when you spoke about your mum. I have never heard you speak like that." But I don't remember it. She said, "You were away. You weren't with me."

M: You didn't realise what you were saying?

P: (Shakes his head) She said, "I have never known you to speak like that. You were on a different planet. You were just away, and I let you pour it all out." There were tears.

(It appears that his grief poured out in a dissociated state with his wife, a state which he cannot access now.)

M: I suppose it was the depth of sadness.

P: As I said, in the last few months, I seem to be focusing a lot more on that. Not many people have their parents when they are fifty.

M: Would you say that you are missing them?

P: (Nods)

M: So, you wish that they were still here?

P: Yes.

M: Why?

P: I know they would be nearly eighty-odd now but I think I lost them too soon as far as I was concerned (holds his chest and stomach as though hugging himself) and I believe when your time is up your time is up and there is nothing you can do about it.

M: But what's important is how you feel about that loss.

P: And I said before, I have had a good childhood, very close to both of them. I was the youngest by seven years. My oldest brother was eleven years older than me. And I have always said that I have never been the same. I was punch-drunk, and I am still punch-drunk.

M: I don't suppose it can ever be the same after losing your mum that early. Its huge, you know, it's a big thing.

P: My mate said, "You lost your dad, but I don't think you were that upset." I said to him, "You've still got your parents, but you don't know what it means."

M: This is probably a good way of exploring it. What has it meant to you to have lost your mum when you were fourteen years old?

P: Well, it's things like, I have learnt a lot looking at other people, for example, when sons have fallen out and I look at the importance of, for me I always said that a boy and a mum is different to a boy and a dad. Like my daughter, she is all for me. My mum never got to see my daughter. It's frightening how alike she looks. I think that's another step as well. My wife even talks about it. We looked at photos, I have a picture on my living room wall with my mum when she was eighteen. She looks just the spitting image, just everything (uses both hands to cover his face, rocks back and forth in his chair). I think the best one was when she was thirteen, last year she was thirteen. I got a picture of my mum at age thirteen and I have caught people out showing them the photo of my mum and they think it's my daughter ...

(Peter's hitherto dissociated experience of his mother's loss was reawakened by his daughter reaching his age when his mother died. Children often trigger unconscious painful parental memories when they grow up.)

(Peter spoke about how quickly his mother died from the time she went into hospital.)

M: Oh no. You didn't get to say goodbye.

P: I did and I didn't. The reason I did was when she was in hospital having tests, dad was breaking down a lot and I comforted him. I remember living on Ambrosia cream rice. She never used to eat that because she was anaemic. And then they let her out one weekend to come back; I think about this a lot. She spent a day or two, but I remember going, "Alright mum" as they came to take her back to the hospital. What I do remember, as you would do as it was the last time, I saw her was when she stood at the doorstep, she stood back off the door, she stepped down, my dad was behind me and I was holding the door. The car was waiting for her. She said, "You take good care of him. You take good care of him."

M: And that was the last time you saw her.

P: That's the last time I saw her.

M: What are you feeling now, as you are saying that?

P: Sadness, I didn't know then but now it's heartbreaking.

M: Are you feeling anything in your body?

P: (puts his right hand to the left side of his chest and scrunchies up his T-shirt). Crushing.

M: I wonder if that's the tightness that you have been experiencing, the sadness. What do you want to do with that sadness?

P: (Shakes his head) I don't know. I don't know what I can do. The fact that she died in the ward next door to the ward I was born in, that I often think about.

M: Yes, what do you think about it?

(He did not respond to this as it might have been too painful, or he was unable to think of what he would like to do with the sadness. I prompted him to talk about the feeling he had in his chest.)

M: So, what is this concrete then?

P: I don't know if it's ever something I have ever let go. I always thought I did. Someone said to me, not sure if it was an aunt or uncle, but they said, "Your mum never let it out, she never grieved. She bottled it in, she bottled it in" (Slapping at his stomach). They said, "Learn from that, don't bottle it in." I would say, it hit me at an age, where I did not do exams, it completely messed me up. I never got in trouble with the police or anything, didn't go with bad crowds or anything like that. I think more than anything it put me in a shell (squeezing his palms together). It's clammed me up. It's made me sort of, more cautious with things.

M: Cautious with living?

P: Yeah, yeah definitely. And thinking, I have let it out but over recent times I am wondering if I have. I am wondering if I even know how to. And there is a part of me that thinks that, crikey you are fifty, you should be letting go what happened to mum, it couldn't be helped, she was taken, that's the end of it!

M: In a way, we could say it happened to you because you lost your mum.

P: I would say it hit me for six. I have always said that. My mum's best friend, growing up (points to his chest) I can feel this really tightening up.

M: What's that?

P: Something is trying to come up (rubbing his chest) It's like anxiety. I have had it all last week.

M: What's the function of the anxiety?

P: I have felt sick sometimes, I have had lots of headaches this week. Pressure on this side (grabs the right side of his head). This is what I used to get when I had that balancing thing.

M: What's the purpose of the anxiety? Because all these things serve a purpose in us. What is it for you?

P: I have started to feel now that maybe it's stopped me from living how I should live, sort of, not freely but, I don't know how to enjoy it. I don't know how to relax. I used to love listening to music. I have hardly listened to music for months. Don't feel like it.

M: Would you say that's you grieving?

P: I think that it has been going on for some time without me realising it. Looking at it now because all the situation with the work thing, it's been like it my wife wants nothing more than for me to get out of it. She doesn't want me to go back. She says, "Peter, if you go back, you will be back to square one." But I think all this is built up and then the changing things with work. I don't get time for anything else. Only living to work. That's my life and I am still thinking, how do I get out of it? And all this week I sit there thinking, "Do you know what? I am fifty I need to get this sorted."

M: Yeah. How can it be sorted? How do you see it being sorted?

P: As for my life at the moment I need to move on to get a bit of a life back. My wife has already noticed the difference in me. I am very snappy, irritable. But I feel more that although this situation at work isn't ideal for me, all the years I have been bottling up and maybe I need to sort what's been there over the years with the loss to then channel that into my modern life now.

M: That sounds reasonable.

P: (Turns round to look at the clock)

M: We have five minutes left. So, what do you make of what we said earlier, saying to your mum "I don't need to be sad anymore?"

P: I want to try to lay it to rest.

M: What do you think of me asking you to say such a thing?

P: I think that's fair. Because I certainly felt something. It took me a while to try and build up the emotion that she is sitting there. I find it difficult to come to terms with. It's like someone smacked my head and the ringing has never stopped.

M: It has had a resounding effect? That must have been so hard for you though.

In the last five minutes of this session Peter said that the concrete that was in his chest earlier has moved down to his stomach. He decided to ask his insurance company for another twelve sessions. He felt that the sessions were going too quickly.

I waited expectantly for the next session. He spoke about his mother. He often wondered whether they had wanted a girl and that's why they had him, a third boy.

We decided to put the extra twelve sessions to good use. He engaged fully, using the space to explore his feelings and experiences. During this time, he was actively trying to find another job, but he was struggling with his confidence at interviews. He felt hopeless when he was rejected for someone else with more experience. He said that the rejection felt like a rejection of him personally and that they did not like the look of him.

As time went on, Peter said that he could feel a lightness in his moods. He reflected on the TAIP that we did and said that losing his mother felt like he had lost a limb and that the wound had never healed.

Doing the TAIP gave him permission to grieve and to express his sadness about losing his mother. He felt that he was slowly processing the emotions and wanted to live his life to the full.

By the end of therapy, he said that he was feeling at peace with going back to his old job but had the confidence to keep looking for a new job. He had booked a family holiday and was looking forward to it. He said that the therapy had helped him to be more hopeful and to be able to confide in people about his feelings.

I spoke to him three years after we had completed therapy and he said that he was more content in his life, he is not as irritable and sad anymore. He is also sleeping much better.

This case is an example of how the TAIP can be effective in short-term work. We had only eighteen sessions, but Peter was able to use that time to process his unresolved grief over the death of his mother. The TAIP, with all its attention to his bodily response, had informed him that he was carrying heavy feelings about the loss of his mother. The TAIP helped him to identify this and to go on living a fuller life.

CHAPTER 8

The visceral impact of the TAIP: what could not be expressed by words is expressed through the body

Jayshree Unadkat

As human beings we have an inherent, intrinsic need to connect with others. From before birth, we are attached to a human through a cord in our mother's womb, which provides us with the sustenance required to grow and, indeed, stay alive. Thus, attachment does not only begin when we come out into the world, it is present well before that time. There has been much research carried out showing that how the mother behaves, what she does and does not do whilst pregnant, has a profound effect on the child she is carrying (Sadeghi & Mazaheri, 2009; Ustunsoz, Guvenc, Akyuz & Oflaz, 2010).

The world of unconscious attachment—how we are emotionally responded to and comforted by our primary caregiver—and its impact on our lives is fascinating to me as a counsellor, in both personal and professional ways. As I work with people to understand how we connect and maintain relationships, there is no way to avoid the expression of these unconscious experiences. This is especially true when early wounds cause present distress.

I attended a lecture delivered by Felicity de Zulueta on trauma and attachment whilst I was training to become a psychodynamic counsellor/psychotherapist. Felicity's lecture connected the dots for me in a way that made sense of my own attachment pattern and how this affects my relationships. Following on from this, the opportunity to work with Felicity on a clinical research project focusing on the *traumatic attachment* has proven to be of great value to me professionally.

In response to painful and frightening experiences, some clients deal with their attachment distress by self-sabotaging relationships or by using anger to maintain a distance from the other. Others turn to alcohol in times of stress and pain. Clients' negative emotional experiences and resulting defences are also acted out in sessions in the form of lateness or erratic/non-attendance.

Working with these individuals, I began to understand the intensity of the distress and pain they face in acknowledging their need for professional help.

It also became important for me to be aware that clients, by coming to therapy, are looking to make sense of their distress, and to work through their feelings to gain a more positive experience. In an ideal world, we hope that working through these difficulties may lead to acceptance and understanding as to their origins and growth. However, in order to get to this point, therapy must enable the expression of a full repertoire of emotions, even when a particular emotion is vigorously denied or defended against. During my work with clients, I have long noted the way that emotion is expressed not only verbally, but physically. Indeed, when a person could not verbalise an emotion, their body state would hold the clues.

I am painfully aware of the emotional resistance and challenges that clients present in therapy. Each client expresses a different narrative of their childhood experience, which may explain the journey to their present addictive or "anti social" behaviour. For example, the degree of alcohol dependency is almost always psychological but, at times, physical too.

Each story speaks of the deficit in parenting—whether through some form of neglect or abuse. Depending on the intensity of the deficit, the felt emotion or lack of it would be revealed in the response. A child who has experienced emotional neglect may learn to create a sense of personal safety by not expressing or withdrawing from particular emotions. Equally, a child who has experienced both physical and emotional neglect, can be triggered into re-enacting their past dissociative defence in therapy.

The impact of trauma and its dissociative effects have been increasingly recognised over the last thirty years, particularly in relation to trauma experienced in infancy and early childhood (Van der Kolk, 2014). I have been able to recognise this during my career.

As I continued to work in the research group with Felicity and other therapists, I began to appreciate the effectiveness of the TAIP in giving clients access to their unconscious traumatic attachments, and I began to use this protocol with some of my clients. Their responses are described below.

Larger than life with an internal shell: addiction and unresolved grief

Greg entered the therapy room with a huff and a puff, like an exasperated bull going into the bull ring. His face was red and flushed, his body round, giving me the sudden impression of a rather gruff Father Christmas. I was working as a trainee counsellor in an addictions service, and I was taken aback at seeing this larger-than-life client. My presumptions (unconscious in the moment), from having worked with other clients who showed the physical ravages of h cocaine, morphine, crystal meth, and many other concoctions to help them make it ough another day (Maté, 2008).

Greg expressed difficulty in thinking clearly and in considering his own feelings. He spoke f having to put up a front and to appear confident, but he also stated that he found it difficult o connect with his own feelings and who he was.

The need to avoid confrontation seemed to be the main response that Greg was familiar with. He recited, almost in a monotone voice, his early experience of abandonment, when his mother walked out on them when he was six. He was not sure how long she was absent, whilst his dad was either working or sleeping.

Greg left home at the age of seventeen and stated that he "did not look back", only returning when his dad passed away, when he was twenty-one. "Do you know what, I didn't cry at the funeral. I remember driving back from the funeral emotionless."

Grief from loss or death is recognised and understood, yet what seems less obvious is the grief of what could have been or what was not possible or was absent. "My mum got married so soon after dad went. How could she do that?" Greg's face at that point showed a flash of anger that I had not seen previously. "I was so angry that she could do that again to us." By "again", Greg was recalling mum leaving them when he was six and not knowing if or when she would be back. Greg spoke of being angry with her and not speaking to her for many years. She died in 2007.

Greg had a passion for horses, having been a trainer and a riding instructor for many years. He would often say, "You know where you are with animals, I love working with my horses, and I can feel that they love me back."

He frequently stated in sessions: "I don't keep in touch with anyone that has gone from my life" and "I prefer to walk away and not look back". Greg shared with me that his relationship with his wife was tumultuous; he experienced anger at the lack of forgiveness from her.

Reflecting on our sessions, in my countertransference, I frequently felt the mixed emotions that Greg was dealing with: disappointment and sadness as well as a need to keep me at a distance in the sessions. However, as we worked together, we began to develop a therapeutic relationship; Greg attended more regularly, but always a little late, which meant he would not receive the full hour or fifty minutes.

During our sessions, he often found it difficult to engage and would fall asleep for a few seconds. Exploring the momentary "falling asleep" felt challenging as he would brush it off as being tired, having had a long day, and stating that as he sits down he feels relaxed and that he is also of that age where he does tend to "doze off".

Noticing this lapse in concentration, I would wonder what might be causing this, and I bega tracking what was going on when it began to happen; painful recollection of the empty feeli' when growing up and the absence of emotional connection with his parents appeared to e this disconnection, triggering this momentary "dozing off".

As discussed in previous chapters, the body's autonomic defence mechanisms of th flight–freeze response can come into play when a past traumatic experience or s'

alcohol addiction, did not fit the person I was seeing in front of me. I we.
room, poised for the story that might unfold.

> Greg, a sixty-eight-year-old male, had been drinking for over thirty years, t.
> age of fourteen, as a way of "belonging" to a group. Having left home at seve
> of finding a group that understood him and the feeling of belonging with his d.
> meant that he could begin to form a sense of self-acceptance. He worked as a
> stating that he felt at home with his horses and loved what he did.
> Greg had been married for twenty-three years to a wife twenty years his junior.
> to two children aged twenty-one and eleven. He described his relationship with hi.
> as being "absent for the best part of her growing years" and expressed "regret and a
> responsibility for her distress". He experienced his relationship with his son (eleven yea
> the time) as being more connected and he identified with his son's way of being.

In one early session, Greg announced that he would need to leave early as he was taking a ri.
lesson. He would often be late but apologise profusely. This resistance to attending compl
sessions would manifest itself in a tension between providing for himself and the need for tl
approval of others, an issue that would frequently emerge in the sessions.

I grew fond of Greg, forgiving the absences and lateness, with a short reminder each time;
he would apologise, and we would carry on with this dance of push and pull, of presence and
absence.

His life story would unfold as a conflict between how he saw himself vs his fears of disap-
pointing his family and friends; he would prefer to walk away from confrontations and, indeed,
from his anger with how life had treated him. Drinking, he stated, became his ally and made
him feel better.

Working with clients who were dependent on alcohol reveals how, when things are
emotionally difficult to handle, they deal with their inner turmoil by drinking, which can also
be seen as self-medicating.

Greg would enter the room, a large figure physically, but *as* a shell of a self internally. Initially,
he presented as carefree and humorous, joking and making light of his situation. However, he
would often struggle to communicate his feelings, and would repeatedly say "yes that's it, that's
how I feel" when I was able to vocalise what might have been his experience. Greg's inability to
articulate his emotions could be traced back to the emotional absence of his parents; he would
say: "Oh, me and my sister wanted for nothing, mum and dad made sure we had everything
we could want whilst they carried on working long hours, as landlord and landlady of a pub."
Recalling this, Greg looked forlorn and almost dreamy, but at the same time a shadow of sadness
would develop.

In his book *In the Realm of Hungry Ghosts,* Maté paints a very rich picture of troubled souls,
his patients going through life self-soothing the pain of abandonment and rejection by abusing

threatening emerges. There is a wealth of evidence that shows how this can be triggered by a memory or feelings related to a specific event or a difficult experience. Felitti's 2003 article on addictions and ACEs highlights the connection between the two and the unconscious maintenance of the addiction as a defence against the emotional trauma experienced in early life.

I had been working with Greg for nearly two years, as we struggled along with the cycles of drinking and disengagement in his relationships, it felt appropriate to introduce the TAIP as a way of breaking the deadlock. The TAIP, I felt, would perhaps enable us to look at the defensive emotions that had enabled Greg to manage some semblance of a life.

In the session before introducing the TAIP, Greg started talking about his regrets as well as saying "not enough fuss was made of me". He communicated a lack of concern from his parents in his younger years and a longing for that which was reflected in his lack of confidence and belief in his abilities.

The TAIP began with me bringing the adult self into the room by saying "Greg you are a sixty-eight-year-old man who has a family, work that you enjoy and have made a success of. You are respected and liked by your clients." I then asked Greg to repeat the sentence, "Mum, I am sixty-eight years old, I have a family of my own and a successful career. I am respected by people around me and I am good at what I do … and I don't need you like I did when I was a child."

Greg heard this last statement and hesitated a little.

(G is the client; J is the therapist)

G: I can't do it.
J: What are you feeling?"

(silence)

J: What are you feeling?
G: Can't say, perhaps it is too near the truth.
J: Too near the truth?
G: I don't know. Why I am feeling like this, it's genuine?
J: What do you notice in your body?

(Greg at this point began to play with his fingernails and became tearful.)

We sat in silence for some time, and then Greg began to talk about his wife and children. As the session ended, there was sadness in his voice.

Greg's difficulty in repeating the sentence shows the power of the unconscious traumatic attachment. Whilst he was often able to talk about his anger towards his mum, the pain of loss lay in the unconscious denial of the need he had for her.

Bessel van der Kolk, states in his book *The Body Keeps the Score*: "ignoring the reality also eats away at our sense of self identity and purpose" (Van der Kolk, 2015, p. 233). Van der Kolk looks at the connection between mind and body, stating that trauma manifests itself in the body in different ways, and it is held within the body as a way of expressing what cannot be spoken.

Following on from the TAIP session, we continued having our weekly sessions. Whilst we did not revisit the TAIP, or refer to it, there was a noticeable change in this man who had been drinking for over thirty years; there seemed to be a shift in the way Greg presented himself in the sessions. About six sessions after using the TAIP, Greg said that he was trying to abstain from drinking and felt that he was beginning to connect more with his children too. As we continued with our sessions, Greg spoke of trying to engage with work and at rebuilding his relationship with his wife. In further sessions, he tended to be more subdued and quieter, not deflecting with his jokes and making light of his distress.

As my time with the addictions service came to an end, some six months after we had carried out the TAIP, saying goodbye to Greg felt hard. We had begun working on Greg's feelings about ending therapy for a couple of months. Greg shared that he had started to attend AA (Alcoholics Anonymous); it took place in the same building on the upper floor. He spoke of feeling a little anxious about ending therapy but felt he had started to develop connections in the AA group which helped him to feel a part of that community. In our last session Greg acknowledged his journey in therapy; his dependence on alcohol had begun to lessen, his sense of acceptance of the life he had lived and the losses he so furiously defended against seemed to feel less of a struggle. Anger that would have been manifested in drinking, to squash down the feelings of rejection and loss, felt more manageable. Greg started to share his emotional presence with his children, and a sense of being able to care for himself and his family began to emerge.

It can be concluded that by using the TAIP, Greg found himself able to speak about his hitherto unconscious unresolved grief and his experiences of neglect in childhood. Finally, his reliance on alcohol could be made sense of and was no longer needed to avoid or defend himself against what he felt was unmanageable.

Ravages of time and fear of the unknown: anxiety and alcoholism

On the other hand, the ravages of time had affected Harry, a man in his late fifties. Meeting him for the first time, I was reminded of Skeletor (a fantasy menacing figure in *He-Man*—a children's cartoon programme in the 1980s depicting the hero, He-Man, and his rival, Skeletor). Not that Harry was menacing—on the contrary he presented as a gentle unassuming man riddled with anxiety who struggled to accept himself.

> Harry had abstained from drinking for eighteen years but struggled to manage anything that was not planned or familiar to him. His parents divorced when he was eleven after which his father started to gamble. Mother left and Harry was given a choice between Mum or Dad. Harry spoke of this in many sessions saying, "I chose the place not the person", and he stayed where he felt most secure, which was at his old home. He then spoke of this meaning losing the chance to be with his mum who rejected him for not living with her.
>
> He also told me that from the age of thirteen to seventeen/eighteen he was mostly alone and turned to a life of prostitution to earn money and become independent. He had begun to

drink from the age of fifteen. He also spoke of his time as a teenager, when he felt completely lost and turned to the gay community, where he spoke fondly of a couple who took him in and looked after him while he was a "rent boy".

Whilst Harry had managed to abstain from drinking, he presented with an overwhelming sense of anxiety about day-to-day life. Even the simplest need to make a choice sent him into a spin, unable to relax, and a sense of fear appeared to overshadow his ability to manage. He would often talk about being a good AA member, of feelings of pride that he was entrusted to open and lock the room and manage refreshments, and of being given respect by other members.

In our sessions, Harry was always polite and warm, communicative about his life in the past and present, expressing a long-standing feeling of anxiety that he wanted to manage and understand. We had worked together for one year. His struggle and anxiety over anything unplanned or spontaneous continued.

Feeling that there was no way to resolve it, at this point I felt that the TAIP would enable us to break through this impasse. I inquired if he would be willing to do the TAIP, which I felt could aid him to connect to his unconscious feelings of abandonment and isolation and the trauma of neglect from his parents that could not be expressed.

Harry consented to do so. The session began with him expressing concern about his wife, that she was doing too much, and he felt that he needed to be more present in the relationship. Harry spoke of his reluctance to take time off from work, or to plan time off to go on a break, as he found planning anything that was not structured so anxiety-provoking.

As we prepared for the TAIP, I could see Harry becoming nervous, so we slowed down and I checked with him if he felt OK to go ahead with the procedure. I began with bringing the adult Harry into the room, by affirming that he was a fifty-five-year-old man who has a loving wife, friends, a good job and he has been successful in this. I then asked him to imagine that his mum was in the room and asked him if he could repeat the words: "Mum, I am fifty-five now, I have a loving wife and a good job, I have many friends, I am successful, and I don't need you like I did when I was a child."

Harry took a minute to compose himself and repeated the words slowly.

(H is the client; J is the therapist)

H: Mum, I am fifty-five, I have a wife and good job and I have friends and I am successful. I don't need you like I did when I was a child.
(After a couple of minutes of silence, I interjected.)
J: What is going on for you?
H: I said the words, but it felt callous.
J: Callous?
H: Yes, it felt like I was abandoning her.
J: Can you say more?
H: Ummm … it felt like I was taking revenge. I do want to look after her, and by saying I don't need her, it means I am rejecting her.

(Harry sat in silence.)
J: How are you feeling?
H: Okay I think?
J: Could you tell me if you feel anything in your body?
H: I feel numb, I find it difficult to say.
J: You feel numb? Where do you notice this?
H: I guess it's in my stomach? But I am not sure.

In the rest of the session, Harry was quiet and reflected on his life so far, his affection for his wife, as well as feelings of guilt that he was not able to be as spontaneous as his wife and be a bit more carefree.

Fairbairn introduced the term "moral defence" (1952), and in simple terms, this relates to the child who, to protect the idealised image of his attachment figure, would prefer to become the "bad/rejecting" person and thereby defend against the reality of having been rejected by his attachment figure.

What is communicated by Harry in the TAIP points not only to the *traumatic attachment* but also his IWM of an idealised mother that his embodied Child Self was fearful of abandoning. Harry appears to have been using the "moral defence" in his attempt to maintain the image of his mum intact.

By using the TAIP, we elicited the Child Self's idealised mother and then encouraged his Adult Self to verbally override the Child Self's fear of losing her, a fear which he felt in his stomach. In so doing, the fractured Self could begin to heal as the two split Selves come together.

As we carried on with the sessions, Harry began to express emotions of anger, projected into his work situation, and feelings of being undeservingly punished. He also began to express anxiety about his failing body and fear of illness, questioning if he can rely on others. Harry began to connect little by little with his physical presence, his body, and emotions that he may have distanced himself from over so many years of neglect and abandonment. He portrayed a need to see his body as being separate from himself, and that this was perhaps an important defence that he had developed to be able to "use" his body to survive as a teenager.

The expression of anger, perhaps, was the turning point for Harry, as he had held the rage of being abandoned by both parents, and while not being able to express this directly, he was at last able to connect to it and find a way forward.

Then, over the following three months, subtle changes in Harry's presentation began to emerge. He started to talk about taking time off from work, trying to plan short breaks, and he communicated that he had begun to express his anxieties to his wife. Harry was able to complete therapy and stated that he felt able to communicate with his wife much more and, most importantly, he was able to tolerate uncertainty and be more spontaneous. He had begun to plan time off from work and expressed that to his surprise he was looking forward to it, being able to relax and sometimes just do nothing.

This case highlights the emotional neglect Harry experienced, and the lack of safety that caused him to not trust anything that was out of his control and, thus, his struggle with being spontaneous. He had been able to stop drinking over the many years of attending AA groups but had not been able to conquer his anxiety.

The TAIP enabled him to get in touch with his internal fear of abandonment and, by expressing this through words and reflection, he was able to mourn the loss of his mother and the security that he was not able to have as a child and subsequently overcome the anxieties about anything that threatened it.

The lost child: anxiety and substance abuse

Alex waited patiently at the front door for me to let him in, his slight figure in baggy trousers, hair long and tied back in a bun, his face gaunt. He beamed, giving me a big smile as we entered the room. He appeared hesitant as to where he should sit, taking a few seconds to settle down; with a nervous smile as he looked around the room. Alex, aged twenty-seven, had contacted me for therapy to work on his anxiety and panic which he wanted to address as well as the need to be able to feel "better".

> Alex sat quietly still holding his heavy rucksack and a coat which he kept close to his body. "I feel anxiety and I panic a lot. I can't seem to relax but at the same time I feel numb, not able to feel emotions". Alex lived alone on a boat (a barge), preferring to move around and not build close relationships. He had been on antidepressants for the best part of ten years, smoked weed, and drank to calm himself down and relax in the evening. A "ritual" he stated was the one thing that kept him going.
>
> At the age of nine his parents separated, but they stayed in the same house, which Alex found "difficult" as he would often hear them arguing and recalled "at times dad would storm out of the room shouting and then tell us there was nothing wrong". Alex recalls memories of his dad sleeping in the hallway, and both he and his sister would have to shut themselves away so they could not hear the shouting. At the age of eleven, Alex's parents divorced: his dad stayed in the house whilst his mum moved out with the children, and "no one talked about what happened or why things were the way they were". Alex lived with his mum until the age of sixteen and then chose to live with his dad and his partner, whom he describes as "evil"; she did not want him there and would "pick" on him for the slightest thing, and his dad would not "stick up" for him.
>
> As soon as Alex was able to get a job working as a grave digger, he began to live on a boat that he had bought and repaired to make it habitable. As a young man, Alex felt he had a community on the water and spoke of being able to socialise with fellow "boaters", which would lead him to take drugs and drink as a way of connecting with them, feeling accepted and included. However, Alex said that this was not sustainable for him, and he became unable to manage and would suffer bouts of panic and anxiety that would debilitate him. He began to recluse himself more and more and felt socially anxious.

In our sessions, when Alex talked about the divorce, his body would stiffen, and his facial expressions would change to almost nothing; a blank look in his eyes would be present. Alex often stated, he did not remember much of what happened, saying "there was an Alex before the divorce and Alex after" his parents divorced.

Alex also struggled with maintaining romantic relationships; he often said: "Anne is not good for me, but when I can't be with her, I am a mess; if I don't get a reply from her, I become very anxious and I cannot do anything. I would send her lots of texts one after the other, and my anxiety would hit the roof."

Alex often came into the room stating, "I am exhausted, as I have ridden my bike for thirteen miles to get to therapy." I often wondered if this was his way of showing his commitment and perhaps looking towards me to feel that I was committed too, and to be trusted. In countertransference I would often feel fearful about taking time off or letting him down in some ways. Whilst working with Alex, we were hit by the pandemic, which meant that we could not carry on with the sessions. He did not have a stable Wi-Fi connection or a reliable computer to work on remotely.

Whilst Alex stated in our last session (before we had to isolate) "I understand, it is what it is", his tone was flat and resigned. He said "see you on the other side" as we parted. Sadness and resignation seemed to be palpable in the room; after all, he was being abandoned again.

Alex had often uttered, in one form or another, his thoughts about the unfairness of society, the government, and legal enforcement, as well as his frustration towards his family. He would say "Mum doesn't make any attempt to understand, Dad is not able to." His answer, or indeed avoidance of this, was to live on a boat and move around.

Alex struggled to manage the isolation and loneliness during the pandemic. He often asked by text when we would resume our sessions. We had kept in touch, (due to my concerns about the severity of his anxiety and isolation). He had communicated to me that he did not always feel safe and so I had suggested to him to go to the accident and emergency service in the local hospital, which he duly did, as that was the only place where he could get some support during the pandemic.

Alex's need was so present that we agreed to carry out the first few sessions outside (as we were not completely out of full lockdown) in a quiet place without being overlooked; and as our sessions were during the evening, we had privacy. We subsequently moved back into the office, where Alex complained about no one understanding his need; the absent doctors and lack of mental health support. He felt abandoned. His anger was palpable and flashes of this were aimed at everyone, including myself. Under the anger hid the vulnerability of a lost and frightened child, who had no one to turn to—a reminder of the childhood that he had spoken about in our earlier sessions.

As we worked together, Alex would come to the sessions on time and was always able to express his feelings about how others did not understand, how the world is not a "nice" place and the contempt he felt for rules and regulations. He would often say, "I do not belong", or "I find people difficult", or "I avoid talking to people and feel irritated if they approach me."

Alex would speak about his relationship with his mum as "she does not understand, she is more interested in reading the *Daily Mail*". He would also often relay the need to take care of his mum, while at the same time finding her annoying and stating, "she does not get it". He spoke about his father, as "a figure who was now old and has Parkinson's", and that he was worried about him. Alex stated that he did not have a relationship with either parent, but that he "tolerates going to visit them". He did not like them coming to him on his boat; he would often say, "Mum and my sister came to see me, it was difficult as I did not want them to stay too long, as they stress me out and I get very anxious."

"I feel like nothing is changing, I am not making any progress," Alex said in a dismissive way during our sixth session after the lockdown isolation, his shoulders slightly hunched, his gaze averted. I acknowledged his concern and wondered about his disappointment, staying quiet for a few minutes. Alex continued by stating that he was still anxious, has panic attacks, and did not seem to be able to deal with things.

At this point we had been working together for a period of one year with the break in between of six months due to the pandemic. I felt that we might be able to think about trying the TAIP and began to explore this idea with him. Alex listened to what this would involve and agreed that if it would help him to feel less anxious, to understand things, change how he reacts and not panic the way he does, then he would give it a try.

In the following few sessions Alex talked about his relationship with Anne, the tumultuous nature of it, and stated: "She is not good for me, and I have been trying to distance myself from her but am not able to." He seemed emotional and distant at the same time, the conflict present in his body tensing and shifting in the chair. "Have you experienced these feelings before, Alex?" I asked. Alex was silent and thought for a while before replying, "What do you mean?" "These feeling of someone not being good for you but also feeling wanting to be with them?" Alex thought again and spoke about a time when he had some homework to do and it was late, he was asking his mum to help him, and something happened, he could not recollect what, but his mum just walked away and said, "Do it yourself, I am not helping you, I am going to bed." Alex went on to say that he felt very upset, anxious, and alone, as a result of his mum turning on him the way she did.

The sadness and fear he may have felt were less present and instead there would be contempt and anger towards his mum and at the same time some sense of responsibility for her.

Alex would often talk about reaching out to her, and she trying to ask what he needed, for example, what he would like for Christmas. In one session Alex spoke about this with anger as well as resignation stating, "What is the point of my mum asking me what I want for Christmas and then just getting me any old toot; she knows I don't like those things she buys; they are of no use to me. Why do I bother, as it's the same every time?"

The struggle Alex experienced with his mum and an absent dad (who was both physically and emotionally absent most of Alex's growing years) came into the room many times. I felt that the absence of a strong male role model and the abandonment Alex experienced could be the basis for using the TAIP in relation to his dad. I enquired again in our ninth session (after we had recommenced) if Alex remembered us taking about the TAIP. Alex did remember and agreed to try in the current session.

Introducing the TAIP, setting the scene so to speak, I began with reaffirming Alex as the adult in the room by stating that he was a twenty-seven-year-old, living independently, holding down a job, making some friends and managing his life. I then asked Alex to imagine his dad was in the room and to say to him: "Dad I am twenty-seven, independent, have a job and manage my life OK, and I don't need you like I did when I was a child."

Alex was silent for a couple of minutes and then said, "Well, I have an issue with saying that." I asked, "Are you able to say what that is?"

(A is the client; J is the therapist)

A: Ummm, well I guess it's the word "dad".
J: The word "dad"?
A: Yes—you see I have never seen my dad as my dad, I never call him that.
J: You never call him dad …
A: No I call him by his name and so can't connect to the word "dad".

(This statement seems to be so powerful in its force that Alex not only struggled to connect to his dad but also to the role he would have had in Alex's life.)

J: What is going on for you, do you notice anything in your body?
A: I feel a bit uptight, you know not at ease.
J: Can you say where you feel this?
A: I guess my chest feels tight and I feel a bit panicky.
J: So your chest feels tight, and you feel a bit panicky.
A: (nods)
J: Do you notice anything else?
A: Just weird really, kind of funny feeling in my stomach?
J: Funny feeling in your stomach, perhaps like a drop in your stomach?
A: Yes, I guess so, I feel a bit blank too.

We sat for a while in silence. Alex seemed to be subdued and still in his chair, his eyes averted, downcast, his body slightly limp. Alex's physical responses to the sentences spoke volumes—drop in the stomach, tight chest, and feeling a bit panicky—all pointers to the *fight–flight* response of the defence system of the ANS (described in Chapter 3). Alex had described his panic previously as being a "caged animal" not able to escape as well as needing to curl up in a ball and not speak to anyone, hiding away in his boat, smoking weed and having a drink, the two being his companions to manage his distress.

Following on from that session, a few weeks on, Alex began to speak of some sporadic memories when he was a teenager as well as before the divorce of his parents. He spoke of being close to his nan and how he would turn to her when he wanted to have company as an adult, expressing his fondness for her. He would say, "She didn't stand for any nonsense and would say it like it is, but I knew where I was with her." He would recall the times he spent with her and the warmth he felt towards her compared to the feelings of being emotionally abandoned by his parents. Alex had lost his nan a couple of years before he began therapy. Alex also spoke of his cat, who he also had lost a year after his nan passed away.

In one session after we had used the TAIP, Alex shared that he had given his mum a Mother's Day card saying, "I don't normally believe in these things, but I gave it to her as that might be nice for her."

As we continued therapy, within three months Alex began to drink less and gave up weed. This seemed to be a major turning point for him because when we had talked about his dependence on these substances, he would throw a steely stare and state, "No one can tell me to give that up, no one would dare!" This defiance spoke perhaps of how much pain he was defending against, which began to surface as he limited his drinking. Alex began to express sadness about his failed relationships, friendships that had gone, connections lost, as he also became more present in the sessions. His eyes looked clear and vibrantly blue, his skin losing the ashen tinge, replaced by a new glow.

He also shared that he visited his dad on his birthday and spent some time with him too. While these were very small steps, they seemed to convey some reconnection. Alex began to think more about his tumultuous relationship with the on-and-off girlfriend, Anne, recognising the pattern of push and pull that there had been, and his huge fear of being abandoned.

Alex decided that he wanted a break from therapy and began to withdraw from the sessions slowly, by attending every other week for a few weeks and then finishing by sending me a message stating that he was not able to attend anymore due to commitments that made it harder to meet. He ended the message by saying that he knew where I was and would contact me if he needed further sessions.

Alex did contact me, wanting to start again. He asked for a session the following week; however, as I was on annual leave, I offered to see him once I was back from my break. Alex decided not to re-engage. We did arrange one more session as we had not formally ended therapy and to touch base on how he was doing.

Alex attended that session; he was still not smoking weed and was drinking a minimal amount. He was engaging with his mum and dad and sister a little more, keeping some distance. Alex shared that he was feeling much better, had not had a panic attack in ages, and that he had made progress in his relationship with his ex, establishing clearer boundaries and managing his emotions better. He was still on his antidepressants but felt less withdrawn.

At the end of our last session Alex said, "This is not goodbye, it's just for now, as I know you are here and if I need to, I will come back again."

As we ended, my feelings of pride were mixed with a tinge of sadness, almost like letting go one of my children as they became independent and flew the nest. Alex had tapped into my motherly emotions, as I reflected to myself on how much he reminded me of my son; not in the same emotional way, but in other ways that sit in the realms of the unconscious.

The TAIP is a powerful way of acknowledging the connection between the emotions and how these appear in the body. Although we did not revisit the TAIP again, changes in Alex's behaviour and his ability to cope without needing to self-medicate through alcohol or drugs speak volumes.

I will end this chapter by going back to the beginning, as we all have a need for the "other". With the clients I have presented in this chapter, what comes through in each case, is that carrying out the TAIP connects them to the unconscious *traumatic attachment* regardless of their ability to say the words or not. The TAIP is a psychotherapeutic tool that enables therapists to access the fractured Self and to heal it by giving our adult patients the empathic support that they need to overcome their Child Self's terror of losing their idealised parent.

In my view, these case study examples show how clients can start to free themselves from the terrible negative emotions and physical constraints resulting from their ACEs and begin to re-engage with their loved ones in a more normalised and constructive environment.

The importance of integration in healing traumatic attachment: case studies using Lifespan Integration therapy and the TAIP

Leonor de Escoriaza

One day, my supervisor compared me to Obelix, the French cartoon character: "You fell into the magic potion when you were small," she said. I indeed fell into the potion of Lifespan Integration (LI) therapy, a body-based therapy that heals going to the root, able to treat complex trauma and insecure attachment (through neural integration and attunement mainly). Accordingly, I also fell into the trauma and attachment world, when I was still a student. I was struck by the efficiency of LI with "durable" healing, but also by the concepts of dissociation and integration and how helpful they are in my clinical work with all sorts of patients but especially for patients suffering from complex trauma.

I never stopped looking for truly efficient ways to work with my patients and one day at a conference, I heard Felicity de Zulueta talking about the TAIP. I was new in the UK and went directly to ask her if she could be my supervisor, as I admired her curiosity, the way she thinks outside the box, and her powerful clinical perspective, as well as her multicultural open-mindedness. Felicity laughed and explained she was retired from clinical work but told me she was running a clinical-research group around the *traumatic attachment*. It sounded so interesting that I kept in contact with her, and I finally joined this interesting research group! It is formed by a variety of friendly and talented psychotherapists from a variety of backgrounds (systemic, EMDR, LI, psychodynamic, etc.) and has been an enriching environment. We all gather regularly to share our clinical experience with the TAIP and how it unlocks the *traumatic attachment*. This work is very coherent and complementary to my work with patients suffering from complex trauma.

Love is repetition: about integration and dissociation

"The sheep story please"—"Again?"—"The sheep!"

My two-year-old niece asks once again for the same bedtime story. How many times will a parent/caregiver repeat the same bedtime story, play the same game, and repeat the same routine? How comforting it is for the infant!

Repetition and routine can serve many purposes: in LI therapy the repetition of the timeline of the patient is used to restart the natural integration process in the brain "by restructuring and integrating neural systems in the body-mind" (Pace, 2003, p. ix) to process trauma, integrate the Self, and thereby offer a way to heal the effects of insecure attachments. The LI timeline comprises a list of the patient's memories from his or her earliest memories to the present time. During each LI protocol the therapist needs to remain attuned to the patient whilst repeatedly leading him or her through the timeline. Repetition is one of the keys to integration in the brain: it fires neurons and helps interconnecting memories with emotions. It brings chronology and predictability as well as a more coherent narrative. As Siegel wrote: "The way we make sense of our lives and free ourselves from the prisons of the past are an important predictor of relational health" (Siegel, 2021).

Repetition is one of the many ingredients that stimulate integration, the body's natural way of organising what happens to us and the body's powerful self-healing tool. "Integration is the fundamental mechanism of health and wellbeing. Integration is the linkage of differentiated parts of a system" (Siegel, 2012, ch. 16, p. 1).

It is now largely agreed that infants thrive with a loving, coherent, and predictable attachment figure who can be emotionally available to attune to their needs and restore the child's psycho-biological equilibrium by regulating their emotions when necessary. As we saw in Chapter 3, that parental capacity can be disturbed by environmental stress, health and mental health issues, particularly when the parent suffers from the effects of PTSD (post-traumatic stress disorder).

We need to feel attuned to a significant "other" or to be part of a close-knit community throughout our lives to be able to integrate overwhelming adverse experiences. Loneliness and isolation have a big part to play in the current rise in levels of PTSD and trauma-related mental health issues. Attuned emotional support can allow emotional regulation and integration to take place, even after some time has passed, as has been demonstrated in the preceding chapters.

Before the age of two, the infant registers most experiences in the right hemisphere of the brain, the "emotional brain", as implicit or unconscious memories or powerful emotional sensations which play an important role in the making of the child's IWMs and the development of its sense of Self; these will determine, to a great extent, how they expect to be seen and treated by others and thereby what to expect from life. Those first impressions of the world are usually imprinted in their body and mind for the rest of their lives in the form of secure and insecure attachment patterns, one of which arises out of terror and is referred to as the disorganised attachment (Chapter 3). This is very much the subject of this book since it is at the origin of the *traumatic attachment* and the TAIP.

Our interest in the *traumatic attachment* stems from the fact that up to now it has proved very difficult to treat people suffering from the effects of a disorganised attachment and the general consensus is that "Although the manifestation of trauma in the body is a phenomenon well-endorsed by clinicians and traumatized individuals, the neurobiological underpinnings of this manifestation remain unclear" (Kearney & Lanius, 2022). On the receiving end of a terrifying experience caused by his or her attachment figure (usually but not necessarily the mother) the parasympathetic defence system of the child's ANS comes to she rescue as the child is in what Felicity calls the Red Zone. Unable to fight or flee, the now-helpless infant freezes (as mammals do in such states), and numbing, immobility takes place as endogenous opiates are released.

It is at this time that the desperate yearning for a protective mother to attach to, results in the creation of an IWM of the child clinging to an idealised version of mother. This indirectly ensures his or her survival, since it enables the child to reconnect with mother when she is no longer terrifying. However, it also has a major consequence: to preserve mother's ideali-sation; all those terrifying IWMs and associated memories of "me in relation to a screaming or hurting mother" must be kept apart. This leads to the first structural dissociation of the Self as detailed in Chapter 3, a dissociation that will have a long-lasting effect on the child and future adult's capacity to integrate. The result will be the loss of the capacity to integrate leading to the inability to regulate emotions, poor health and well-being unless this effect can be reversed.

This is where LI comes into play since it is designed to restart/potentiate integration, and this is also where the TAIP comes into play since it is designed to reverse the effects of the autonomic defence system and thereby remove the need for the *traumatic attachment* to the idealised mother.

The following two examples of my work illustrate the use of the TAIP following an initial period of LI therapy. This describes how I gradually discover the potential use of this procedure and integrate it into my LI practice. We have changed names and some details to protect the anonymity of the clients in this chapter.

Promoting Integration through the use of LI and the TAIP to treat unresolved grief, anxiety, and attachment

The TAIP is a technique that can be integrated with many therapies, especially those that promote integration. In this section, I will describe Ali's case and how the theory and practice of LI combines with the TAIP to help a client.

Initial stage of LI therapy

Ali first came to see me in October 2018 because of her anxiety. She said that she could not relax and had had anxiety attacks since she was eighteen years old, but she also experienced a lot of sadness, due to an accumulation of losses. Ali had lost her mother the previous year to a long illness. She had found it impossible to go and look after her during her illness and Ali had got married far away from home at that time.

Sometime after her mother's death, Ali left her second husband. Her difficulties in sleeping started around that time. She explained that she felt very anxious breaking up that relationship. She had married twice, mainly for her foreign partners to get residency documents. Ali was afraid that her ex-husband took the marriage more seriously than she did and she felt guilty about that. She explained to me that she felt "weird", as she didn't feel like she "was herself lately" and didn't "want to be in her head".

This confusion still had to be explored but I thought that it sounded a lot like a dissociative reaction which had arisen after two major separation events, her mother's death and her second divorce. Whilst a secure attachment provides the appropriate resources to overcome these life events, Ali's inability to look after her mother when she was dying, her difficulty to grieve her loss, and her somatisation were clear signs of an insecure attachment probably due to a traumatic attachment.

My first impression of Ali is one of a strong, resourceful, and emotionally intelligent young woman. Her anxiety and difficulties are not visible externally; she looks composed. Ali describes her difficulties in a detailed and insightful manner. She explains that she tends to think and reflect a lot. It feels like she had therapy before in the way she expresses her feelings and understands what happens to her, even though this is not the case. Ali is clearly very insightful.

Ali also appeared to be a creative young woman. She had always dreamed of being a famous writer since her childhood; it was that dream that kept her hoping for a better future in the neglectful environment she grew up in. Her mother seemed to lack maturity and the emotional resources to support her daughter in a healthy way, preoccupied as she was by her own issues. Ali had to be an adult very early on and tried to regulate her mother. This controlling strategy, described in disorganised children in Chapter 3, enables them to create more order and predictability and thereby protect them from the terror they experienced earlier on in their lives. She described their relationship as "very close when she was little and then a love/hate relationship"; it was probably a fusional relationship that later became too intense and toxic; her mother would have cherished the fusional relationship she had with her baby as she was yearning for the love and care she probably didn't receive.

Her mother would want her as her best friend or would boss her around, she told me. How confusing and disorganising that must have been for little Ali. She considers her mum as rather "egocentric and manipulative". Regarding her childhood dream, Ali still wanted to be a writer but suffered from a disabling fear of being exposed.

I also noticed that Ali somatises a lot; for example, she would often have palpitations and had had many odd illnesses and allergies since she was a child. She also dreamt a lot and had suffered from night terrors since childhood. Her body seemed to be saying what she couldn't say with words.

Ali seldom mentioned her father; at first she described him as absent, constantly working and travelling, and then, with time, she said he was authoritarian and distant. We later worked on episodes of educational violence that happened with him. She perceived her parents as having a love/hate relationship and her mother as very jealous.

Ali is the second child of two, after an older brother. She describes him as the favourite child; they would always say "yes" to him and he was difficult and would constantly bully her. At present Ali doesn't feel very close to her family and lives in a different country. Nevertheless, she is on good terms with them and visits them occasionally.

To focus on our work together, we started by clarifying her therapy goals which were to work on her anxiety and relationships. She also wanted to get rid of her fear of darkness and of being alone. Relationship-wise she believed in polyamorous love but had recently realised that it might have been an excuse to keep others at a distance. She mentioned having good friends. She said she tends to be dominant in her romantic relationships, taking decisions etc.

This echoes her need to control the attachment figure that children with a traumatic attachment manifest with their parents. Later in the therapy, she also expressed "self-esteem difficulties at work" resulting in her not being assertive, struggling to stand up for herself or to say no. Assertiveness issues tend to have their root in staying stuck in child-like scared reactions from the past, that are still dissociated and active in the psychological system in the present.

As Pace says:

> Our neurological systems are designed to alert us and protect us from perceived danger. The defensive systems we create in childhood stay with us, whether needed or not. Repeated journeys through the timeline of memories and images enable the client's neural system to bypass outmoded defensive neurological networks while creating new networks which are more useful and adaptive … Lifespan Integration is extremely efficient in its ability to track directly to the archaic defensive strategy, insert new and current information, and connect the associated ego states (neural network) to the current operating system, the adult self of the client. (Pace, 2015, pp. v–vi)

Ali used both avoidant and anxious/ambivalent attachment strategies when we started the therapy, but also some characteristic controlling behaviours associated with the *traumatic attachment*.

First part of the therapy using Lifespan Integration

Ali's anxiety symptoms and relationship difficulties were signs of profound lack of internal security, coming from her early childhood. It felt like some of her foundations had been made from a fragile material due to her parents' emotional limitations. At the start of the therapy, I asked her to do a timeline of memories, one per year, from her first memories to the present. This timeline is necessary to work with LI therapy as it is its main tool to process childhood trauma and show the body's ANS and limbic system that time has passed, that she is an adult now and not stuck in these past implicit memories or somatic memories. The emotional brain doesn't have a sense of time passing and isolated implicit or unconscious/body memories make one feeling like "it is happening now" through our body sensations.

In her timeline Ali had many memories that showed a lack of safety, such as being left alone at home at three or four years old, and a lack of attunement from her parents who could not understand or connect with her needs appropriately. She felt like they didn't know her, she was often afraid of her dad's violent reactions, and she adapted by being a "good girl".

After doing a bit of psychoeducation to help her to start understanding more of her symptoms and make sense of what happened to her, we started with the LI protocol sessions. Psychoeducation promotes consciousness, one of the nine domains of integration, according to Siegel (2010).

As deep insecurity felt like the key element, we started working with the full-life timeline directly to calm her system and show her emotional brain that time has passed and that she is now safe. I repeated Ali's timeline many times during the session, while being very attuned to her, regulating the rhythm and memories to maintain her in the "window of tolerance" (Siegel, 1999).

That exercise of repeatedly hearing how her life went kept feeling different each time. It slowly restarted her brain's natural healing process through neural integration. For this work to take place, Ali needed to be living in a safe environment, which was the case, and to feel that her psychotherapist was attuned to her.

In the first few repetitions of the timeline, she noticed that when I described how she grew up from being a small newborn baby to her first memories, it felt negative and at three or four years old the memories of being alone at home were very disagreeable.

We did more than ten sessions of repetitions of the timeline which led her to noticing that she kept remembering new memories in between sessions (sign of integration between sessions).

With the timeline we also worked on her deep belief patterns created in the past:

- "I have to save others," since her mother couldn't mother her but needed her instead.
- "Without me they die," since both her mother and ex-husband would both act as victims to get her care and attention.
- "I have to be perfect to be loved," due to Ali having to adapt so much during her childhood that she couldn't be herself. She had to be perfect for her mother to be well and to get her love.

As mentioned earlier, the emotional brain does not to have a sense of time passing and doesn't make the distinction between imagined events and real experiences. In LI therapy we use these very upsetting events to intervene as therapists by imagining visiting the Child Self and giving him or her what is so desperately needed at that point in time.

Seven months into therapy, I used the words "abuse" and "neglect" regarding Ali's childhood. She could hear them but was surprised as the way she grew up felt normal to her.

Gradually, she realised the effects of her childhood, how she adapted to keep on functioning. She also realised the link between the death of her mother and her recent divorce. Living abroad with her previous husband had been the unconscious way she had found to protect herself from her immature intrusive mother. That unconscious shield became more vital when her mother was ill as she was expected to deal with it a lot more than the rest of the family. When her mother died, Ali realised she had not been fully herself during the last few years, when her mother was ill.

The integration that was taking place for a few months enabled her to begin to see her life in a more coherent and chronological manner.

After a couple of months of therapy Ali noticed she cried less and slept a bit better. She also fell in love with a man and started a real relationship with him. Ali's early attachment relationships were slowly becoming more distant, and she was accessing her adult resources more often.

She came to realise through her LI therapy that her mother's expectations of her daughter were impossible to meet and that she had done the best she could: this was an important step in our work together.

Just as she had to become an adult too early, her mother also had an unstable mother and being the eldest daughter, she had looked after her many siblings from a very young age. As a result, she didn't seem to have had a childhood and was still very young emotionally. Ali often felt she bothered her parents and was a burden. She would play a lot in her room by herself. Her mother used her to unload emotionally and tell her how unhappy she was with her father. As we saw in Chapter 3, the *traumatic attachment* is often transmitted by mothers that were neglected and/or abused.

After nine months in therapy, Ali reported that she was "very well, but would still like to be surer of herself at work and be more at ease if at home alone at night". She reported being less anxious, experiencing insomnia only once every five nights, and not feeling sad anymore. She could "understand her past better and felt that it affected her less". That summer Ali published a book!

At this point in time, some memories came up relating to the time when she felt very frightened of her dad. She started remembering this aspect of her relationship with him and processing these fearful memories. It was interesting to notice that not only was she frightened of losing Mum but that her father could be also scary. These fears had made her even more terrified of losing her mother and contributed to her developing a traumatic attachment.

Second stage of LI therapy

After all this work to prove to her system that time has passed, by restarting integration and processing past events connecting them into a coherent narrative of her life; we started working with her imagined "baby self", looking after her in an attuned manner when she was a two-week-old baby, just arrived at home, giving her what she needed then and making her experience one that she could then internalise.

When we did this work by using the LI attunement protocol, Ali imagined being baby-Ali and she experienced feeling tense, trying not to fall, with the tension located in her belly and a feeling that she was transparent. These implicit memories had been stuck in her body, unprocessed and disconnected since she was a baby when no adult was available then to help her regulate herself.

After looking after her baby self, I brought her to the present and looked after her attentively and in a very attuned way, Ali felt very relaxed. After three of those sessions she felt "more conscious of her emotions" and noticed that she used to keep many things to herself "out of fear of being screamed at".

When Ali decided to stop therapy, we did a final session in January 2020, fifteen months after starting her therapy. She felt less of a people-pleaser at work, she had managed to sleep when alone at home for the first time, she was not so afraid of darkness, and felt much more relaxed, more sociable and extroverted. Her mood was more stable (described as nine out of ten). She also noticed that she would defend herself, that she didn't need as much approval from others, and that professionally she didn't feel so much of a failure.

> The more we can shine the light of mindsight on the free floating puzzle pieces of the past—
> the implicit memories—and allow them to become explicit, the more we can free ourselves
> to live fully in the present and have new choices about how we live our lives. (Siegel, 2021)

Integration is blocked by "impairments to linkage, as in an unresolved trauma", "impairment from differentiation", or from learning disabilities and developmental difficulties. The "Sense of interconnection seems to be at the heart of living a life of meaning and purpose" (Siegel, 2021).

One year later in January 2021 (one year into Covid), when we thought of using the TAIP

Ali came back a year later (online) because of a blockage in her artistic projects even though she felt well in general. She feels exposed and judged when she writes and would like to be more productive. She often feels a failure professionally.

Through the sessions we realised together that writing was a dream she clung to, in order to survive, and that her creativity was her safeguard in times of loneliness and anguish. Another conflicting childhood emotional belief came up: "Being anonymous protects me"; not showing her true self at home had protected her and she felt in danger of exposing herself. We worked at integrating her Child Self that had helped her survive with her big dream.

Ali was reactivated about the loss of her mother as her friend went through the same experience and we did the timeline of her mother's illness and death to help her process this time of her life. Through this work we noticed again the *traumatic attachment* to her mother, as we noticed that she hadn't been able to grieve her loss.

I mentioned the TAIP, and we filled in the DES. Ali scored and her result was 20.7. This score is usually found in those who suffer from PTSD.

In the next session we worked on her mother's illness as it was our priority, and we didn't have the opportunity to carry out the TAIP. Ali expressed how she thought that her mother wanted to use her illness to get Ali back under her control, but Ali didn't allow that to happen. "Going abroad saved me from my mother but it destroyed my career." Ali felt anger at her mum for that. She added that her mother thought they were one and the same person, she said. That tells us they had a toxic relationship, and that the mother wanted a fusional relationship. It was hard to say this, but the death of her mother had been a relief for her.

When Ali turned forty in the summer, she was in the process of accepting more of what she had managed to do professionally, taking into consideration the childhood she had had. "It's time to accept reality and adjust my expectations." Ali still felt very nostalgic, dissatisfied, and disappointed, sometimes acknowledging that her life was "not how I wanted it to be and that won't happen anymore". She often felt jealousy at that time.

But then she would say that "her actual life is better than it has ever been" as she realised she had never been satisfied.

We continued working with her Child Self, each week going to look after her, repairing, showing her how unique and what a wonderful little baby she was, reassuring her. Through feeling looked after with unconditional love, Ali could rebuild a better sensation of herself, of what to expect from the other and of how a relationship felt.

When Ali started feeling safe in a deeper way, some memories of being humiliated and ridiculed at five years old arose, so we worked to repair them. We also strengthened the new belief that "now I can defend myself" and anger started to come up.

When in survival mode, the system can't process or externalise anger in an appropriate way when we feel wronged, so it accumulates unprocessed. When we finally feel safe enough, it can be hard to deal with so much anger emerging so suddenly. For a few sessions we repeated the timeline while she expressed anger in her imagination to be able to process past anger. A few sessions later Ali had a revelation that "she is satisfied with her life now!"

It has been a slow path, she said. She is now nicer to herself when she thinks of the past. She also notices that her father is a different person since her mother's death, more present, affectionate, sensitive, more relaxed. She is finally happy with her job as it gives her financial security, and she knows she needs that stability.

We went back to looking after her Child Self, and her Adult Self confronted her mother in her imagination to defend her Child Self. Following this experience, Ali reported that she felt less weight in the stomach, and she started feeling more and more relaxed.

This particular interaction between Ali's Adult Self and her imaginary mother is similar to the TAIP, so it is interesting that it leads to a similar initial result with the TAIP, that is, less weight in the stomach and feeling more relaxed. The TAIP, however, is designed to take the client much further in the course of integrating the Self, which we now know is split through dissociation.

We continued regularly looking after her baby or Child Self and she started realising that "I am good as I am even though I am not a writer. Writing is to express myself." She also remembered more of her relationship with her dad as a kid; he would read her stories, she used to connect with him, they are more similar, but mum was jealous. We often have more room to remember positive memories when we have processed the negative ones, and it allows us to see a fuller picture of what happened.

Another very important realisation was when we spotted a "depending is dangerous" pattern that she learnt from her parents. It had affected her intimate relationships for years.

We decided to do another DES to check where we were at and one year after the first one her perceived level of dissociation was reduced by half, to 9.6. We were thinking of doing a TAIP.

The TAIP session at the end

Ali had announced her first pregnancy in the previous session, and she informs me that she had a miscarriage that week but that she would like to stop therapy, as she doesn't feel it's helping her that much anymore; she had been thinking about this for a little while now. I was torn between the information of her miscarriage and the fact that she was much better and had resources now to deal with things.

Having expressed her desire to stop the therapy, we decided to do the TAIP with her mother halfway into the session in order to close the loop. It is not the common way to do it, but it felt right for her as we had worked so much on her attachment to her mother. TAIP would help us measure the changes and get rid of any remaining evidence of the *traumatic attachment*.

As we are working online, I ask Ali if she could find a place where she could imagine her mother could come and sit in her room and I add "and then I am going to say some words that you are going to say out loud to her and notice what happens in your body."

I feel the need to justify this approach by giving more explanations about the TAIP: "It allows us to see a little bit where we are in relation to her, and it can sometimes 'unlock' difficulties in the relationship … Even though she is not alive anymore, it may make you feel more at peace with her."

I then ask Ali to think about the things that she is "proud of" that she has done in her life. "For example, 'Mum I am … years old, I'm an adult, I've achieved this and that …' This will allow you to be your Adult Self. Do you have things you want to say that you're proud of?"

At first Ali finds it difficult to name anything she is proud of. I help her find achievements by giving her more examples, like the fact she is independent now, and she then finds more things she is proud of. She mentions this during this exercise, saying one of the things she is proud of. We then continued:

(A is the client; T is the therapist)

T: OK, you can imagine … you can close your eyes if you want, whatever helps you to imagine … and you can imagine that your mother comes, sits in that chair …
A: OK (Ali closes her eyes)

T: I propose that you say … (try to close your eyes), if you want, I say it once and then you repeat it: "Mum, I'm an adult, I'm forty years old, I'm independent, I have a stable job that I like, a stable relationship in which I'm happy and I'm proud of this ability to adapt to work with younger people …" You can say it with your words if you want, and "I don't need you anymore in the same way that I needed you when I was little". OK?

A: Yes.

T: You can say that out loud and notice what happens in your body.

A: OK (closes eyes), Mama I am forty years old, I have a stable job, I am financially independent, I am in a relationship where I am happy, and I am proud of my ability to adapt at work, to keep up with people much younger than me, and I don't need you like I used to need you when I was a child.

T: Do you notice in your body if something happening there, do you notice something?

A: In the belly, the pit of the stomach, a little bit of nausea.

T: Yes … you have nausea (says yes with head) if you want to open your eyes, whatever you feel is good for you. You say you feel nauseous … is that feeling familiar?

A: No

T: No? Is the tension in the stomach familiar?

A: (she nods)

T: The nausea is not, but the tension in the stomach is … OK … and what does that feeling make you think of? What do you feel that this feeling expresses here?

The nausea sensation usually links with fear, the other sensation is linked to some implicit memories with her mum.

A: I think it's the feeling that really, all this … what I just said to my mother, I can't really tell her, it's the feeling of "be careful what you're saying". It's a familiar feeling: "you better shut up", "watch what you're saying", "don't say what they don't want to hear" basically.

T: Today we are here for you, you know, and you can express it in your Adult Self, and see what comes up and, if necessary, we can say it again to get it out.

A: Aah (big expiration to help her relax) …

We explore together if this sensation is familiar and at what age she felt this? Thirteen years old came up, when she started having her own life and needed space but couldn't say it to her Mum. Here the TAIP brought up the reality of Ali's childhood, that she couldn't say what she wanted to Mum, that she was often scared, that Mum needed her.

I continue using the TAIP, adapting it more and more to help integrate more and more, to notice her Adult Self taking over now that she has grown up.

T: You notice that maybe this thirteen-year-old girl, if I understand correctly, that she needed to tell her those things. If she needed to tell her more things like that, we can use today to get it out, to say it … Knowing that you're an adult, you're no longer dependent on her in that way …

T: I suggest you say to her: "Mum, I'm forty years old and I've been needing space from you for years, let me grow up, let me be me. I need you to give me my space, you are weighing me down, your problems are not my problems …" something like that?

A: (hand on throat)

T: Do you want to try?

A: It's hard for me to talk … (laughs)

T: Try it if you can out loud because it's more powerful although it's more difficult.

A: (nods)

T: but then we adapt … I'm here with you!

A: Mum, I'm forty years old and I've needed for a long time that you give me my own space, that you let me grow, that I'm not you, I'm me, we're not the same person. I need my space and you need yours. (She speaks in an affirmed tone of voice, smiles, looks happy to be able to say it at last.)

T: Yes … What's going on inside you?

A: I still have this feeling. (She moves her hand around the area indicating it), it's like a tension now from my stomach to my throat … and when I say that it's difficult to speak, I feel almost as if my throat is closing up.

T: No wonder, it's very difficult, there is a reason this exercise is difficult (empathetic face) your Child Self feels in "danger" and your Adult Self does it because it knows that you are safe but there is a part of you that doesn't know yet. Maybe that part of you that doesn't know it can be told?

(… we keep discussing this)

T: How do you feel now?

A: Mm, similar, there is still this strange feeling between the mouth, the stomach and the throat. A bit better I think … there's like an excitement, in the sense of an enthusiasm, almost like when you're on a funfair ride, about to come out, it's scary but there's that excitement!

(We realise that to overcome that fear, repeating it is useful and so we continue with the exercise.)

A: (exhales loudly and launches herself with a little excited smile) Mum I'm forty, mm … I'm independent, I don't need you for anything anymore like I did when I was a kid and I haven't needed you for a long time. You needed me more than I needed you, and I found a way to be able to get away and get the space that I needed. And I'm sorry that that bothered you but that was your problem, it was you that had a problem and not me. And you should have worked on your problem and not made it my problem. But deep down, even though it was hard, I'm glad I did what I had to do to get away from you (looks at me proud and happy).

T: Phew! (I have happy and supportive big smile). It gives me goose bumps, I'm here with you full on! How are you feeling?

A: Fine, still this same excitement and at the same time weird stomach.

T: I have the feeling that it's very special that you tell me this today (nodding yes), when you're just saying that maybe you don't need me so much anymore. And all of a sudden to be able to say that to your mum, ouch that's strong! (she keeps nodding her head: yes). You know, everything we've been working on about feeling strong now, it's like "by the way" we're going to get it out of the way, you know what I mean?

A: Yeah ...

T: And how is the knot going?

A: (showing her mouth) I've got, you know, the feeling in my mouth again too, tingling ... I'm having like a lot of sensations but I don't feel it's bad.

(she shows her mouth and chest)

A: I don't know if there is still a sense of vertigo there.

T: OK, and if you ask "that feeling" what it needs, what happens?

(moment of silence)

A: (laughs after a silence) It comes to me as aggression towards my mother, like wanting to hit her.

T: OK, so it's the anger that's coming out?

A: (nods yes with the head)

T: OK, maybe we have to say something louder to get the anger out? There are times when anger has to come out and then sadness sometimes, to be able to really get things out, do you know what I mean?

(Accumulated anger can only start to appear when fear is not present anymore. It is then important to get it out as this old, accumulated anger pollutes the present if we don't. Ali then answers: yes.)

T: What does that part need? Saying strong words, gestures? Strong words would be enough for you to have to imagine that you are going to destroy the house or ...

A: (she pulls out a cushion with a naughty face, and we laugh)

A: I can hit the cushion (she smiles gleefully).

T: I think that through imagination we need to get (stuck) things out of here (and I gesture showing the brain). How do you feel about that?

A: Good, surprisingly good ... (and she laughs nervously. Then with an expression of satisfaction as she gets angry) Mum, I'm forty years old I don't need you anymore, and I haven't needed you for a long time, because it was you who needed me and you took advantage of me (hits the cushion regularly) leave me alone, leave me alone, give me my space and don't bother me anymore with your problems. I need you to solve them, you to look for the solution, you are the adult, not me! And that I'm fine the way I am and I'm happy. I feel much better! (she laughs)

T: I'm so proud, I can't stand it! Proud of you! That I feel that it's very special.

(and I add with warmth) How is the feeling in your body going?

A: It's going down, it's still there, but it's going down.

T: Do you feel that you need something else? (closes eyes, short silence)

A: I notice my mum right now is like surprised, maybe to tell her I don't care …

T: OK.

A: Mom, I don't care if you feel offended, if you don't like what I'm telling you, but it's the truth! And I don't care if you don't want to hear it.

T: And now how do you feel?

A: Well, there's still a kind of tingling between my mouth and throat … even the tension in my stomach has relaxed quite a lot.

T: Yes, that's the one you've known all your life, isn't it

A: Yes.

(we both smile)

T: Do you also feel proud to be able to say all that?

A: Yes, because it's really nothing new, I already knew all this, but of course I hadn't told her.

T: How do you feel now in your body?

A: I feel good, quite relaxed as if a weight has been lifted off my shoulders, although I still have this tingling in my mouth, I don't know if it has to do with the fact of verbalising everything I have said. Yes, it is coherent … when I unblock myself, when I can communicate …

T: I understand, it makes sense. Well, what a nice way to close this cycle! If you like I'm going to stop the video.

Both therapist and client ended this treatment very satisfied with the result of the TAIP. The second DES had indicated that despite a lot of progress through the use of LI, dissociation still remained. We now know from the work outlined in Chapter 6 that this means that the *traumatic attachment* is still operating, thereby reducing the brain's ability to process grief and many other psychological disorders.

Adjusting the TAIP and LI to the client's specific situation

The first time Jules came to see me, I met an amiable forty-five-year-old man, with a calm composure and a soft and kind gaze. He had waited a few months to start this therapy with me. Jules explained to me that he had had extensive therapy before. He had gained an understanding of his childhood story, his traumas and blockages. He explains that he is aware of his baggage but still needs some changes in his life and had heard through his colleague about me and LI therapy.

He comes to therapy because he burnt out at work a year ago, left his job and was not able to do anything for two months after that. Overall, he has been unemployed for a year, longer that he has ever been before, and he finds it very difficult as he is a very active man. He is keeping busy, starting a business with his brother, and meanwhile working on his artistic projects as a photographer.

When we clarify his goals and expectations, he expresses that he would like to change his negative perception of himself, as he believes that he is no good, struggles with compliments, and finds it hard to believe in the value of his artistic work. He would like to be able to affirm himself and say no to demands made on him, but also to affirm his needs and desires in his relationships; he tends to over-adapt, putting others' needs before his. He also mentions feeling others' emotions too much and would like to have more of a filter.

Jules is the third of three children, all three of them live abroad away from their parents. He has a good relationship with his eldest brother even though he describes him as a bit rigid, bossy, and harsh at times. He lives near his sister with whom he has a good relationship as well, although he also describes her as bossy. He is close to his nephews and nieces.

At first Jules described his relationship with his mother as having an "emotional aspect as I was last in her womb". He carries on telling me that she had lost her sister when she was eighteen and had never managed to grieve to this day. Later, he was able to express that his mother has a strong grip/influence on him, and that she is extremely bossy and controlling. When he tries to say to her that he wants something or prefers something, she would say: "No you don't, this is better for you" repeatedly until he would give in and has done ever since he was a young boy.

His father is described as very submissive to his wife, but also a real daredevil, never seeing danger. He would push himself into situations that were excessively dangerous while doing sports. His father's family was simple, working class, composed of many "naughty" brothers, also "daredevils". His father was "a disaster" at school, but his wife has made him work hard and succeed professionally. He loves handiwork but doesn't let Jules do anything and he keeps doing it for him, as he is not able to trust his son. Both parents seem to constantly tell him not do things his way, only their way or they end up doing everything for him.

This behaviour would have prevented Jules from developing a healthy self-esteem as one needs to struggle and manage to do things by oneself to believe in one's own capabilities. This is particularly important from the age of two when the toddler tries to learn new things by himself but needs the loving support of his attachment figures next to him.

When he was a child Jules was doing poorly at school and he repeated several years, which is what happens in France when you are not good enough to move into the next class. This was probably related to his parent's negativity about his abilities and the fear of change.

He was an active young boy and his parents realised he needed physical activity and took him to play many sports which he enjoyed and got very involved in; he became a black belt in judo at eighteen years old! He describes how judo is where he "can express rage, nothing stops him there". He worked to buy himself drums and he would also get his anger out in this way. Later in life, he started learning photography, an activity which he carries out with a lot of patience as he takes long shots in beautiful, calm places. Photography became his peaceful place. Jules developed resilience through these activities. Having discovered that he is prone to addiction, he also decided early on that he didn't want to drink or do drugs for fear of losing control.

Jules's love life has been full of relationships that often started and ended in a similar way. Usually women would approach him first, as he felt too shy to approach women he was attracted to, and they would start a relationship. He would not assert himself and the partner would become bossier and mistreat him repeatedly; he would be very compliant, until one day he would explode and end the relationship. He also noticed he was sometimes being passed over by friends or colleagues. His last boss had harassed him until he got burnt out; she didn't do that to his other colleagues as they set boundaries. He recently realised that he defends himself better with men than with women.

After treating the relationship with the bullying boss, the burnout, and the Covid period with LI, working with the timeline over the last two years, we did four sessions of timeline work on his whole life.

Seeing the huge role of his mother's extreme controlling behaviours in relation to his present problems, and realising the amount of fear stuck in him, we decided to explore and work on his traumatic attachment to his mother with the TAIP. When he filled in the DES, he scored 7.5, indicating a low level of dissociation.

The use of TAIP

Having explained what the TAIP is used for and the importance of recording the session, I noticed that Jules seemed tense, so I did a bit of grounding and stretching exercises to relax him. He still is not at ease with the video, and I wonder whether he really is happy with being recorded. I mention this to him, but he is keen to continue.

I then asked Jules to think of what achievements he is proud of in the present and Jules's first reaction was to wince and say: "I haven't done anything exceptional in my life", while laughing. He struggles to come out with anything that he is proud of but can share some of goals he has achieved: "getting my black belt at eighteen", getting his second Dan, being able to become a graphic designer which was his dream, receiving awards for his pictures. He also managed to buy his own house.

I then ask him to look around and tell me if there is a chair or a place where his mother could come and sit and to imagine her being there. He smiles slightly nervously but still looking calm, and I invite him to repeat the following words: "Mum, I am now forty-six, I am an adult, I got a black belt at eighteen, then my second Dan, I am in the job of my dreams, I have photo awards, I have my house now and I don't need you anymore as I needed you when I was a child."

Jules chuckles and raises his eyebrows when he hears the last bit.

"These exact words?" he asks.

(J is the client; T is the therapist)

T: Kind of, you can say it your way, but you need to repeat the end, yes.

J: (he keeps a little smile) Mum, I have managed to achieve some goals like getting my black belt, up to eighth Dan, doing photography to a good level and getting awards for it, and I got my own house and I don't need you as I needed you when I was little (his voice gets slightly mechanical and a bit jokey at the very end).

T: (smiling back at him) What happens in your body when you say that?

J: Hum … (his eyes shift from right to left and then right again) A kind of discomfort or embarrassment … (he smiles broadly) … yes, as I shouldn't have to tell her that, but I have to do it … in order to deal with a few problems.

T: A discomfort towards yourself or towards her?

J: Uhmm … A bit of both. Especially at the end, when I say I don't need her now, I have the feeling that I am shocking her a bit, in any case it will shake her up.

T: Yes, and what happens in your body?

J: Uhmm … Well, this discomfort, embarrassment in fact.

T: Where is it in your body? Can you show me?

J: In the area of the diaphragm.

T: Diaphragm, is it a familiar sensation?

J: Yes, it reminds me of my anxiety attacks. (He chuckles then he explains to me that when he has anxiety attacks the sensation starts in the same area and develops over many hours.)

T: Is it related to a fear of shocking your mum?

J: Yes. Discomfort and fear, this is why I have never dared mention certain aspects, as I was apprehensive of her reaction.

T And now, as an adult?

J: Still not. No, not very at ease or capable. I try with some physical distance. She doesn't want to hear, or she flees, she goes into another the room or pretends she doesn't understand.

T: It seems this anxiety is coming … something you would have felt when you needed her, somehow?

J: When I was little?

T: When you depended on her.

J: (His eyes move from left to right while he thinks.) I had her support for quite a few things. She always supported me in my studies. Somehow, she liked it, fine arts, what I like doing. Whereas she didn't support my brother or sister. On the contrary, she practically told them what they should do. Not me, but later there were other things emotionally. Then she turned her attention on me and I was supposed to be her … not her thing … not a scapegoat, but my opinion didn't count much, or not at all … the way she saw things was the only way to act.

(Jules gives me a clear example of a memory when mum would insist and make him do what she wanted.)

T: So if I don't want to lose my mother's love I need to?

J: Yes, exactly

T: If you try, as an exercise, to see what goes on in your body if you say to her: "Mum I am an adult, I don't need to obey your decisions, to accept your vision, I can defend myself, I am an adult." Do you want to try to say something like that?

J: (Chuckles then a little embarrassed) It's funny … well, it's not funny. Mum, I don't have to obey your decisions, I am an adult, capable of making my own decisions, I have good reasons, my choices are justified, as good as yours.

(Jules then describes the same sensation that he had earlier.)

J: Same as when I wanted to ask for something specific and it wasn't going to work. "This won't go well" …

(When I ask him what he needs, he mentions how all of his siblings and him live abroad away from his mum.)

J: Mum, I always had to over-adapt to your decisions that were not always good. Now I don't even know what I like sometimes, I am so happy to please others, to be accepted; you have to say yes, as yes avoids conflict.

We then speak to his Child Self, at around eight years old to reassure him and do some timelines from the age of eight onwards.

After this TAIP session, Jules felt overwhelmed and shattered for two days and had agitated dreams that would wake him up. A couple of weeks later, he explained that doing the TAIP felt like it was hard but necessary, like putting the finger in the wound and "what I had never been able to tell her I told her! It came out!" He realised how afraid of the consequences he was when telling her that.

He said that now he tells her more what he thinks even though she can't hear it. He is starting to feel angry that "she criticises a lot but then she won't listen to anything, you can't say things to her". When anger appears it is a good sign as it means he is not in survival mode anymore; he understands he is not in the same level of danger or dependence on her and he can allow himself to be angry.

A few weeks later Jules started mentioning his father who had seldom been mentioned before. Working on his *traumatic attachment* with his mother had left room for the issues in his relationship with his father to arise. His father is described as a perfectionist who tells him off constantly and won't let him do anything by himself without correcting him, but also as a "daredevil" that doesn't know when to stop.

Later in the therapy, Jules also noticed a pattern with the girls who he had dated; they had all chosen him and not the other way, and all of them had been abused, had trauma, and he would over-adapt to try and avoid triggering them. "In the family women are the boss, they rule."

A couple of months after the TAIP and working with LI, Jules notices that he finds it easier to present his work to galleries, a task he found very difficult before and avoided. He also notices he can express his needs and set his limits more easily in his everyday life. He doesn't accept any more how his parents treat him if he stays with them, not letting him even express himself or how he feels.

My combined approach using LI and the TAIP enabled Jules to find the courage to stand up for himself, develop his art, and to achieve what appears to be a more secure attachment in relation to his parents and his girlfriends.

I would now measure his levels of dissociation at the end of therapy to confirm that the *traumatic attachment* has been resolved.

* * *

What a pair! Integration and attachment repair are complementary and function together. The TAIP works especially on integration and melting the structural dissociation, which then allows the attachment system to get out of its old patterns in terms of attachment. It is impressive to see the difference after therapy and the TAIP, how a person can get into healthier relationships naturally, free of any toxic repetition pattern.

There is little doubt that combining the TAIP with most individual therapies when treating people who suffer the effects of the disorganised attachment, and the resulting *traumatic attachment*, could finally offer them the possibility of a normal life and psychological well-being. It is well worth the short time spent training and learning how to maximise the TAIP's effects.

Dissociation: the neglected portal to ill health

There was no reference to dissociation during my years of psychiatric training at the Maudsley Hospital and when it did come up, it was far from promising. I was sharing a recent experience with a senior colleague at the Institute of Psychiatry, telling him that I had recently met a psychotic young Englishman who suffered from a bipolar disorder on the locked ward where I worked. He was a linguist and, having worked out that I was of Spanish origin because of my name, he picked up the phone on my desk and started to talk to me in Spanish. Having said a few words, he put the phone down and then repeated the same action. The third time he spoke to me more directly in Spanish and said: "Isn't this strange doctor, when I speak to you in English, I am completely mad and, when I speak in Spanish, I am completely sane!" We both agreed that it was strange and I was very keen to find out the reason for this unusual phenomenon, having established that English was his mother tongue.

Having listened to my story, the eminent professor looked bemused and then said in a contemptuous voice: " I smell dissociation". He clearly felt it was not a subject worth pursuing. Fortunately, I had an altogether different response when I shared my story with Professor Lishman, a neuropsychiatrist, who told me that I had twenty years of research into bilingualism ahead of me (Zulueta, 1984, 1990, 1995; Zulueta, Gené-Cos, & Grachev, 2001). It proved to be a fascinating subject and very relevant to me as I speak four languages. However, when it came to carrying out a research project on this phenomenon backed by very senior figures in the Institute of Psychiatry, the Medical Research Council turned it down at the second round: the idea that a person could be "mad" in one language and "sane" in another was perhaps too much of a threat to the psychiatric establishment. Did it "smell" of dissociation? I will never know.

However, by this time I had heard Bessel van der Kolk speaking about trauma in his inimitable way: it made so much sense of what I had already learnt from my patients up to then and, of course, dissociation is also inherent to PTSD. There may also have been an unconscious thread in my mind running between the subject of dissociation and languages as I was to find out several years later.

I was on my return flight to England from a lovely holiday in Cuba, when I suddenly found myself weeping uncontrollably on the plane. My husband and teenage son did their best to console me, but I did not know why I was overcome with what felt like grief. I had noticed that I was very distracted a few hours before our journey and that I had "butterflies" in my stomach in the airport but nothing else.

Back in our home in the English village where we live, I felt like a lost child in the midst of strangers. I noticed that I wanted to speak in Spanish. As I spoke to my husband who speaks that language, I realised why I was so upset: I was the four-year-old child whose parents tore me away from my home life in Colombia to escape from "La Violencia", the civil war that had reached our home the day my father was whisked away by the local police. He was seen as dangerous by the government because of the nature of his work as a doctor. Fortunately, he was immediately released, thanks to a famous lawyer who happened to be a guest in our house. My father went into hiding and I personally witnessed the effects of La Violencia when I woke up one morning to find the floor of the house where my mother and I were staying covered with glass from the broken windows. My mother told me that *hombres malos* (bad men) had come in the night and thrown stones over the garden wall. What she did not tell me is that she drove them away by firing a pistol for the first time in her life and nearly shot her foot in the process.

So, in 1952, we left Colombia and sailed to the UK. My parents decided to leave me in London with my grandparents as they went to Spain with my baby sister to see my father's family. My English grandparents were kind and well-meaning, but they did not speak a word of Spanish and I did not speak a word of English, as my mother had always spoken to me in Spanish.

And here I was, in my forties, crying my heart out on the plane, having had to leave the island of Cuba where I had felt so much at home because the people spoke and acted as they did in Colombia; they also lived in something akin to a time warp, driving cars from the late 1950s, in part cut off from the West since the time of Fidel Castro. I had literally gone back in time, only this time I could cry and feel the grief of losing a home and way of life that my parents never mentioned when we settled next in Borneo, especially as they dealt with their own traumas and loss by switching to speaking English.

As I returned to my adult professional Self-state, I concluded that switching languages can be a dissociative linguistic defence that enables traumatised people to dissociate their past traumas (Zulueta, 1995). Whether, it is linked to an earlier *traumatic attachment*, I don't yet know.

The eminent professor at the Institute of Psychiatry was probably right to smell "dissociation", but it certainly does not have a bad smell. On the contrary, if by identifying its origin in the *traumatic attachment* we could give so many people a new lease of life, it is worth every minute spent in resolving its mysteries.

What we know so far

Whilst it has been known for many years that early childhood trauma and neglect has a severe and long-standing negative effect on the individual's future development, researchers in mental health have not been able to identify what mediates this distressing outcome.

> That there is unambiguous evidence from both human and nonhuman animal research that neglect and abuse are detrimental to brain development … Additionally, the specific enduring effects of the trauma are dependent on the age and type of trauma received … Identifying and helping these children is especially difficult if there are no bruises or physical injuries. The effects of early attachment can lie dormant in the brain until later life. The impact of these hidden events is that by adolescence 80% of abused children will be diagnosed with a major psychiatric disorder. Imaging studies of abuse survivors often show that brain areas controlling emotion and cognition are abnormal and underlie these psychiatric disorders and difficulties in functioning as a productive citizen. (Sullivan, 2012)

As a result of clinical research accomplished over several years, we can now identify the cause of so much long-term suffering and frustration: it is due to the development of the *traumatic attachment* during the human child's early development because of neglect and abuse.

Eliciting the traumatic attachment and restoring the fractured self

Much of the research on human attachment has been based on using Ainsworth's Strange Situation because it enables researchers to determine the type of attachment that children develop in relation to different parenting experiences.

It is not altogether surprising that, by using the TAIP, which is similar to the Strange Situation used by Main, we have been able to identify the same disorganised type of attachment in our adult clients that she identified in the infant survivors of abuse and neglect as well as in the infants whose mothers suffered from PTSD or recent grief (Main & Solomon, 1989; Main & Hesse, 1990).

Repeating the words "Mum, I am an adult now and have achieved many things [to be defined], I don't need you like I needed you as a child" whilst the clients imagine their mother sitting in front of them, elicits the same separation reaction that the Strange Situation elicited in the disorganised infants in Main's experiment.

However, in carrying out the TAIP, the disorganised adult clients are not aware of their embodied Child Self's *traumatic attachment* until they experience fear in their stomach, their chest, their throat, and feel their heart racing as they attempt to separate from their idealised mother (or their abusive mother, as sometimes happens). At this point, the clients do recognise these embodied responses as belonging to their childhood experiences.

Detecting the traumatic attachment and its internal working models by using the TAIP

We can conclude, even from our limited number of cases, that our therapeutic work using the TAIP demonstrates that the *traumatic attachment is the responsible agent for mediating the long-standing negative effects of child abuse and neglect.*

To provide the child with an idealised protective mother, the Self needs to undergo a dissociative split to protect the IWM of the good mother from the dysregulating terrifying IWMs of his or her abuser, as Schore described (2011, p. 240).

Because of this dissociative act, the *traumatic attachment* does, in fact, turn the open system of the mind, as defined by Siegel, into a closed system. "Lack of resolution implies a blockage in the flow of information both within the mind and between minds. One example of the failure to achieve integration is in the varied forms of dissociation that may accompany lack of resolution (of trauma or grief)" (2001, p. 88). This ensures the Child Self's survival, but it prevents the normal process of integration of the brain taking place for the rest of the child's development resulting in a less well integrated brain and poor emotional regulation.

Our case-by-case therapeutic work shows how the TAIP identifies the same *traumatic attachment* operating in several "difficult to treat disorders" that we have treated, such as complex PTSD, DAD or BPD, alcohol and other substance addictions, unresolved grief, anxiety disorders, and violence.

If the TAIP can demonstrate this effect with certain "difficult-to-treat disorders", it is more than likely to apply to many more such disorders because, as Şar states:

> Dissociation may accompany almost every psychiatric disorder and may influence their phenomenology as well as their response to treatment. (Şar, 2014, p. 172)

Lyssenko and her colleagues confirm this view when they end their review by concluding:

> In summary, our meta-analysis confirms the prevalence of dissociative symptoms not only in dissociative disorders, PTSD, and BPD, but in nearly all mental disorders. Research on the distinct diagnostic categories suggest a variety of mechanisms linking dissociative experiences to a higher burden of illness and detrimental effects on treatment. An evaluation of dissociation should therefore be part of every careful psychopathological assessment, and future studies should engage in a transdiagnostic perspective to enhance the development of treatment modules to deal with dissociative symptoms. (Lyssenko et al., 2018, p. 44)

However, what no one expected, least of all the authors of this book, is the positive outcome that can also be achieved by using the TAIP.

Healing "difficult-to-treat disorders" by reversing the dissociation with the TAIP

We gradually discovered, by noticing changes in the way certain clients spoke and behaved in the video-recordings following the use of the TAIP, that something quite unexpected seemed to be occurring, which we concluded must be the result of the dissolution or the "melting" as Johnson (2018) referred to it, of the dissociation that divided the Self. When this happened, it preceded the time when the clients began to realise that they had changed.

a. In order to achieve this, the TAIP needs to be carried out in two very different ways to the original Strange Situation because the clients are no longer infants but competent adults. This is why we ask our clients to recognise their achievements as adults and to enumerate them when speaking to their imaginary mother.

b. They also need to decide whether to give consent to the use of the TAIP and sign the consent form for the video-recording before it is actually carried out.

c. Another major difference with the TAIP, compared to the Strange Situation, lies in the role of the psychotherapist who carries out the procedure.

d. Unlike the abusive parent, the therapist must be felt to be safe and attuned to the client's emotional needs, both in terms of his or her Adult Self's potential feelings of shame, and in terms of the embodied Child Self's terror. These feelings need to be empathically acknowledged before the terror-induced dissociation can melt away in an attuned therapeutic context.

One could describe this healing process as enacting a triangle of love, as opposed to a triangle of abuse. By metaphorically holding both aspects of the client's divided Self, the psychotherapist facilitates their integration into a single Self. The TAIP becomes a compassionate version of the Strange Situation which enables the melting of the dissociation to take place to produce an integrated Self and a gradual return to normal functioning.

We can imagine that the TAIP acts as a metaphorical zipper which can be used to un-zip the *traumatic attachment* to reveal the hitherto unconscious IWM of idealised attachment to mother and, in so doing, it offers the therapist the opportunity to facilitate the zipping-up or the integration of the client's dissociated Self. The following are examples of this.

The "un-zipping" and exposure of the traumatic attachment in the case of a female client

During this procedure the individual's Adult Self is invited to imagine her mother, sitting there, in the room, and then to verbally attempt to express her emotional independence by telling this parent that, as an adult, she has achieved many things and that she no longer needs her mother anymore as she did when she was a little girl.

It is then that the hitherto unconscious and traumatically attached embodied Child Self experiences the deep fear of losing the support of this idealised protective mother who saved her life so long ago.

The use of the TAIP has the potential to elicit the *traumatic attachment* with its IWM as this unconscious attachment is expressed by our clients when we encourage them to carry out this imaginary separation from either their idealised, or, at times, their abusive parent, as happened to Emma who literally believed her mother would open the door of our office and beat her up. Such negative reactions are rare, whilst the clinging to the mother whom they still feel they need is the most common response to the TAIP in the men and women that we have worked with so far.

When expressing words such as "Mum, I am now an adult and do not need you as I needed you when I was little," the embodied experiences of fear and its associated emotional memories do occur regularly and are recognised by the Adult Self of our client as belonging to his or her childhood life and its terrors.

The zipping-up of the split Self through dissolution of the traumatic attachment and integration of the dissociated Self in a male client

As the attuned and gentle therapist supports the Adult Self in acknowledging the presence of the Child Self by reminding him that he is now a competent adult, the client is helped by the therapist to feel compassionate towards his Child Self; it is during this warm interaction between the "three of them", that the terror-induced dissociation between the two Selves can begin to dissolve.

At such times, the therapist can often witness a mixing of past emotions and allied thoughts, like the mixing of two streams that come together as a new integrated Self begins to develop. This process can vary in terms of time. It can be obvious within the same session or following the original TAIP session.

The length of therapy required to develop integration and attend to other remaining issues will depend on many factors, such as the level of dissociation involved, but, once both therapist and client take up the TAIP, the end of long-term suffering appears to be in sight as you may have witnessed in our work. However, we do not know yet how it will evolve with clients with very high levels of dissociation and different psychiatric conditions.

Therapeutic implications of our findings

Liotti (2006), and now Şar (2014) and Van der Hart (2018), recommend attending to the structural dissociation of the Self before carrying out any other work with people who suffer from the many conditions now found to show dissociative features and/or who score positively on the DES (Bernstein & Putnam, 1986). This means achieving attachment security first because attempts to do trauma work before dealing with the dissociation may be very difficult since "dissociation can disrupt one or more than one mental functions, affecting consciousness, memory and/or identity but also thinking, emotions, sensorimotor functioning and/or behaviour" (Liotti in Şar, 2014, p. 172).

The TAIP and other embodied therapies

The use of the TAIP has many similarities with recent embodied approaches to the healing of trauma: these have been very successful, such as Levine's "Somatic Experiencing", described in his book *Waking the Tiger* (1997) as well as the Sensorimotor Psychotherapy developed by Dr Pat Ogden, a body-centred approach that aims to treat the somatic symptoms of unresolved trauma (Ogden & Fisher, 2015). In one of her chapters, she describes the therapeutic need for the patient to develop a dual awareness of both the Child Self's past and the Adult's Self in the "here and now" engaged with the therapist (pp. 479–492). The TAIP takes the same approach but, by inducing the *traumatic attachment*, it deals with the origin of the client's disorder: the dissociation of the Self.

The social implications of our findings with the TAIP

We are also animals ...

The *traumatic attachment* is a natural mechanism developed through evolution to ensure the survival of the very vulnerable human infant in the early stages of development, a mechanism that we have inherited from our mammalian ancestors. Infant mammals, such as monkeys and rat pups, are also highly dependent on their mother in infancy, so this natural insurance policy helps them survive in those early days, as it is meant to help us.

The young "delinquent" adolescent elephants in the Pilanesberg Game Reserve were severely neglected because their mothers were killed early on in their lives, hence their subsequent chaotic and violent behaviour in adolescence. What is interesting is that their interaction with the two bull elephants clearly had a similar effect to that of the TAIP with our clients: it gave them a new lease of life, suggesting that in normal life, the *traumatic attachment* is healed through interactions with members of the same species.

However, both these young males and their female counterparts who were imported into the park in childhood missed out on the normal experiences that adolescent elephants normally have as they move into the second phase of socialisation with adult elephants. The females would have been involved in helping mother elephants deliver and bring up their young calves as well as gaining knowledge of the local area.

It is interesting that being deprived of this experience can lead, in elephants, to sexual reproduction at a young age as well as maternal neglect and high levels of stress, all of which are often apparent in young human mothers who have been neglected or abused in childhood.

The adolescent males would normally have left their original family to join other all-male groups where, under the influence of senior males, they would have learnt how to navigate the complex interactions that take place amongst them, as well as spar with younger males to establish their roles in the social hierarchy. Without this important experience, they can become troublesome and violent, as do so many human youngsters who have not had the experience of being lovingly cared for and steered through the complexities of adolescence.

We need to recognise how important adolescence is for our young and put much more effort into guiding them through this crucial time in their development.

Studies on the effects of social disruption on elephants caused by humans are also highly relevant for humans because many of us live in societies that bear the weight of past social disruptions due to war, political terror, and diseases:

> Understanding the impacts of disruption of social bonds can both provide crucial insights into processes central to social evolution and also throw light on the functioning of advanced animal societies that have been radically impacted by high levels of human disturbance. (Shannon et al., 2013)

Shannon et al.'s findings suggest that "both health and social functioning of wild populations of long-lived and highly social species, could be significantly impacted in the long term by elevated levels of anthropogenic (human induced) disturbance" which may compromise the ability of surviving individuals to respond appropriately to members of their own species and contribute to the abnormally aggressive behaviour in response to other species, such as the killing of humans by female elephant survivors of culls.

By studying elephants that had been separated from family members and translocated "decades previously", these authors found long-term severe impairment in their ability to process complex social information, such as the social identity of other members and age-related dominance: this led to disruption of their social groups.

This is very similar to the plight of the surviving Acholi children growing up in Northern Uganda described by Abe (1994) following the civil wars carried out by Idi Amin and then the NRA under Yoweri Museveni and the LRA.

Unfortunately, the effects of the man-made climate crisis are already affecting millions of people and in some cases, threatened communities are currently being translocated to safer places. I recently listened to a programme on the BBC about the need to move a community of Pacific Islanders from the island where they have lived for generations to a safer place on the mainland. Their community leader explained how much they had enjoyed their lives as islanders, having adapted their culture to be in tune with their environment, Mother Earth.

He emphasised the importance of keeping the community intact to survive and be able to adapt to their new environment on higher land. This would enable them to mourn their losses and give them the resilience not to succumb to trauma and depression. He was also trying to ensure that other Pacific Islanders, who also need rescuing, would be translocated to the same site, since they shared a similar culture. He did not seem to be finding it easy to convey the importance of his approach to those in charge because our Western socio-economic culture increasingly denies the value of attachment networks, both in terms of families and communities. As former British Prime Minister, Margaret Thatcher, who launched this individualistic competitive policy stated: "There is no such thing as society."

However, we know that the community leader was right in his request to translocate his community in its entirety: research evidence does show that closely knit communities provide their inhabitants with the resilience to resist developing PTSD and other mental health disorders. This is because humans are born to "connect" and to "cooperate", hence the need to belong to a network of attachments which enhance our natural inbuilt cognitive and emotional resources by keeping us, as much as possible, in the Green Zone.

For example, when an infant suffers from inadequate care and develops a *traumatic attachment* in a socially functioning indigenous village, like the Dayak villages of my childhood, the close family–community interactions will melt its potentially dissociative effects, as happened with the young elephants. Nature provides the remedy for this naturally induced dissociation.

We are such interconnected animals that our relationships to each other act as biological and psychological regulators: children who are close friends develop matching circadian rhythms which then give way to their parents' circadian rhythms when they join them at home (Field, 1985). The hand of an empathic loving partner can reduce the pain levels of his close companion and synchronise their brain activity (Goldstein, Weissman-Fogel, Dumas, & Shamay-Tsoory, 2018; Sahi et al., 2021).

Neuroscientists like Liebermann have carried out research that demonstrates again and again that "just as we have a basic need for food and shelter, we have a basic need to belong to a group and have relationships" (2013); attunement heals and rejection hurts.

Surviving indigenous people know that their sense of belonging and close contact to nature is to be treasured as they witness our Western societies flounder: listen to this interchange between an African villager and Dan Siegel on a visit to Namibia. He asked the villager through his translator: "There's horrible drought, famine and many endemic illnesses that are resistant to medications. And yet, the people in the village we've visited seem very happy. Why are they so happy?"

The villager replied, "We're happy because we belong. We belong to each other in our community, and we belong to Earth."

The villager then asked Dan, "Where you live, do you belong?" Dan was struck silent and realised how he could easily spend a whole day without meeting anyone he knows and that it takes an effort for him to be in contact with the earth. He wondered if that was why the people in the United States were some of the most unhappy on the planet (Siegel, 2017).

Liebermann (2013) also believes that the "Other" is essential for one's sense of Self which is why prolonged isolation can be so damaging and even kill, as we found out during the long pandemic lockdowns. Normally, in times of crisis, people band together to overcome their problems, as Londoners did during the Second World War and at the start of the Covid-19 pandemic until we had to isolate. Being alone to deal with anxieties, losses, and abuse is terrifying and can lead to mental illness and even suicide.

There is a famous Zulu Ubuntu saying: "umuntu ngumuntu ngabantu", which means "I am, because you are" or a person is a person through other people. It can be interpreted as "our sense of Self requires the Other to be". This is what Mead means when he defines the Self not as a structure but as a process of interactions between one's organism and others (Mead & Morris, 1934, p. 179), This view always made a lot of sense to me and is a view that appears intrinsic to many societies that resist the individualistic model of society.

There is an amusing short video online that illustrates how "ubuntu" also enhances cooperation and illustrates the destructiveness of our current political ideology: https://www.youtube.com/watch?v=GjVwsgL2i98.

So, what is this policy model that appears to be taking over our societies with such destructive consequences? A key contributor to this state of affairs is that when Ronald Reagan and Margaret Thatcher were in power in the 1980s, they endorsed the policy model of neoliberalism that promotes free and unfettered markets (Stiglitz, 2003). This approach eliminates price controls, deregulating capital markets, lowering trade barriers, and reducing, especially through privatisation of public services and subsequent austerity, state influence in the economy. Some refer to it as "market fundamentalism" because, to achieve its end, its proponents believe that its rules must apply to all people and to all areas of life, from education, health, and welfare to food and water supply and the wider environment. To achieve its end, it appears to know no limits to growth, not even the prospect of an environmental catastrophe or war without end.

As a result, the impact of these political, economic, and social changes means that people are suffering in many ways, both physically and mentally, because the system in which we live is no longer providing the social context in which we have evolved, particularly in terms of our attachment needs in relation to family and community life (Lanius et al., 2010).

A culture that promotes individualism and competition for power and money is not good for our physical health either:

> The decades of observation of the immigrant Italian village of Roseto in Pennsylvania by Wolf and Bruhn (1993) demonstrates a progressive rise in the incidence of coronary heart disease as family bonds, shared social values and the mutual affection of an initially vigorous Roman Catholic community eroded and, during the next two generations, increasingly joined the mainstream of American culture. Diet could be shown not to have played a part. (Henry, 1997, p. 27)

James Davies's book on *How Modern Capitalism Created Our Mental Health Crisis* (2022) describes how governments and big business blame the explosion in mental health illness on its victims instead of acknowledging that most mental distress is an understandable reaction to the unequal social conditions we are now facing.

His views have the backing of the UN's latest report calling for a "global paradigm shift in mental health care" (Pūras in Luiggi-Hernández, 2020). Pūras emphasises the need to abandon the biomedical model that individualises psychological distress and leads to institutionalisation and biological interventions (psychotropic medication) at the expense of human rights and social change.

An article in the *The Atlantic*, adapted from a forthcoming book entitled *The Injustice of Place: Uncovering the Legacy of Poverty in America*, summarises a very detailed account of poverty and its effects throughout cities and countryside in the United States. It concludes as follows:

> The lesson is that people seem to thrive—not always on high salaries but in health and life chances—when inequality is low; when land ownership is widespread; when social connection is high; when corruption and violence are rare. The social levelling that is characteristic of communities in the upper Midwest is more than just a quaint cultural feature. It is the foundation of a community's wellbeing. Until these regions' virtues are shared nationwide, poverty and disadvantage will continue to haunt America. (Edin, Schaefer, & Nelson, 2023)

A health crisis is a social crisis

It is important to remember the above findings regarding community well-being as we read the grim news about the state of the United States's health and that of the UK.

The Academy of Sciences reports rising mortality for adults, mainly for white adults with a secondary education or less. "The rise is largely attributable to 'deaths of despair' such as suicide and poisoning by alcohol and drugs with a strong contribution from the cardiovascular effects of rising obesity" (Harris, Woolf, & Gaskin, 2021). We cannot fail to notice that these are ACE-related and "difficult-to-treat" conditions which we have been describing and treating in this book. The Academy of Sciences report also notes that mortality is actually decreasing in a control group of sixteen wealthy countries (including countries in Western Europe, Canada, Australia, and Japan).

Sterling and Platt (2022) comment on these findings from an anthropological and neuroscientific perspective. Bearing in mind that human beings are constrained by their prolonged physical and emotional dependence and the need for communal support at all stages of the life-cycle:

> it is noticeable that these 16 wealthy nations provide communal assistance at every stage including education beyond adolescence for professional skills, thus facilitating diverse paths forward and protecting individuals and families from despair. The US could solve its health crisis by adopting the best practices of the 16-nation group.

For instance, in relation to single-parent families in the EU, most are employed, not at risk of poverty nor materially deprived. All the nations support prenatal and maternal care, mandate maternal leave for sixteen weeks with 74 per cent of their full salary. Thirteen of them provide pre-school care and pay 82 per cent of the cost. Public schools, which are government schools, are supported at national level and therefore the quality is less unequal. So, they conclude:

> From the onset of life across two decades of dependence, the 16 nations foster health by assisting children and parents to manage the intrinsic difficulties of the human life cycle. (Sterling & Platt, 2022)

I am sure that Professor Sir Michael Marmot, an eminent epidemiologist at University College London, would agree with their conclusion since life expectancy in the UK is falling down the global ranks (Hiam, Dorling, & McKee, 2023). He published "The Marmot Review 10 Years On" (Marmot, Allen, Boyce, Goldblatt, & Morrison, 2020), which explores changes in the UK since 2010 relating to his five policy objectives for England:

- giving every child the best start in life
- enabling all people to maximise their capabilities and have control over their lives
- ensuring a healthy standard of living for all
- creating fair employment and good work for all
- creating and developing healthy and sustainable places and communities.

It makes sad reading as he points out the inequalities that plague this country, predicting an increasing rise in poverty, even as four million children are already poor, decreased spending in childcare and in support for deprived families, as well as the closure of 500 children's centres, including Sure Start centres that were very helpful for young people. Food insecurity and food banks are to remain.

In the education system, he pointed out that though pupil numbers are going up, funding is going down with 66 per cent cuts in youth services from 2010 to 2016. Work quality is poor, and work is stressful and underpaid, with resulting wage and income inequalities forcing poor parents to both work, even when childcare is missing or very expensive. And, to top it all, his report clearly reveals that this government's tax and benefit policy has widened income and wealth inequalities, making the rich richer and the poor poorer. Marmot concludes that this "10 years on" report shows that, in England, health is getting worse for people living in more deprived districts and regions, health inequalities are increasing, and, for the population as a whole, health is also declining.

Of particular interest to us in relation to the importance of the *traumatic attachment* is that half a million children a year are recognised to suffer abuse in the UK according to a leading charity, the NSPCC (2022). In the US, 588,229 reported cases were recorded by the Statista Research Department (https://www.statista.com/topics/5910/child-abuse-in-the-united-states/#topic). In both countries the majority suffered from neglect.

The UN's recent report by Philip Alston on extreme poverty and human rights was also very critical of the UK government as he found that, as a consequence of austerity and increasing inequality, rates of health and social problems were higher, such as obesity, mental illness, suicides, homicides, teenage births, incarceration, child abuse, drug use (Alston, 2019). Many of these conditions we now know are directly related to the effects of the *traumatic attachment* on human development.

Two important conclusions emerge from these studies:

1. So many of these destructive aspects of our current societies are due to the long-term effects of families being unable to provide their children with the loving care and support that they need, thereby eliciting the *traumatic attachment*.
2. These destructive effects are preventable, as we have seen in other countries with different social policies.

There are movements afoot in the US and the UK to develop a different approach as we increasingly recognise our social needs and the enormous value to all of us of protecting and supporting parents in their incredibly difficult task of raising happy confident children. Their power could be significantly increased by integrating therapeutic approaches based on attunement, such as the TAIP and the following attunement-based treatments in programmes such as trauma-informed care.

From the cradle to the grave

Alternative therapeutic approaches to healing the divided Self

Our work so far has shown how the split Self of the disorganised attachment can be integrated and thereby healing can take place using the TAIP. However, this is a therapeutic modality designed for individual or group therapy as illustrated in the work with women who had suffered from child sexual abuse.

What is most urgently required, if we want to address the widespread need to improve the care of our infants and children, is a way of breaking the cycle of abuse that so many parents find themselves in and enable them to become more attuned and empathic with their children and with each other. This may sound like a miraculous cure, but the most surprising thing is that there are people out there who still manage to create miracles.

Video Interaction Guidance: a "turbo-charged" form of therapeutic attunement

A major development for me took place when I was invited to a conference on violence in Mexico in 2011, where I met the creator and founder of a new therapeutic modality called Video Interaction Guidance, or VIG, which is now spreading across many countries, enabling families to heal in a completely different way from what I had been taught.

Hilary Kennedy emanates positive energy. She introduced herself in the empty dining room of the conference and asked me who I was and what I did? As I had spent the previous few months being threatened and bullied by managers intent on implementing heavy cuts on the TSS, in line with the continuing downsizing of the NHS, I told her that I was contemplating retirement. Her response was uplifting: "I don't see you retiring." She said, "I think you will become a freelance consultant!" and with a warm smile and twinkling blue eyes, she invited me to attend her presentation, which I promptly did. It proved to be a revelation for me as I watched her work aimed at improving relationships between parents and children using video clips of recordings.

Fortunately, I knew that there are many ways of melting the dissociation that originally divides the Child's Self to ensure its integration and normal development: as Schore put it so simply: "attachment can provide both an attunement experience and the potential to repair the damage brought about by stressful experiences".

In my past experience as a family therapist, I had used video-recordings of sessions to notice the negative aspects of my clients' behaviours with the aim of changing them for the better. What I saw happening here was quite different: having obtained permission to record her client doing something she likes to do with her child, the "guide" (therapist) makes another appointment for a "review session". She uses the interim time to edit the video-recording of the first session by only selecting the "positive" moments in the relationship when the parent is observed attuning or connecting with her child. There may only be one or two such moments, but that is enough.

During the next session, the parent is naturally anxious, expecting the guide to criticise her parenting skills but, instead, she is presented with the happy face of her baby looking lovingly at her. Confused and delighted she comments: "Tommy is smiling"

"Yes," replies her guide, smiling with her, "and what did you do to make that happen?" She then rewinds the video to earlier moments which led to this happy outcome so that the mother can "be helped to become aware of the thoughts and feelings that underlie her behaviour, opening up new ways of being with her children" (Steele et al., 2014).

As I watched Hilary's work, I noted how her approach involved enabling her clients to attune with their child and that the review session was aimed at stimulating the parent's capacity to work out what was going on in her child's mind and her own, which is referred to as reflective-functioning or mentalizing, as we saw in Chapter 2: this involves the capacity to empathise, both emotionally and cognitively.

As we emerged from this remarkable session, we were approached by our host, Alison Lane, the director of the JUCONI Foundation in Mexico, which is involved in helping street children and their families. She told me that she wanted me to supervise the therapists who were having a hard time trying to treat the parents of these children, who were often drug addicts and violent.

I suddenly had a "light-bulb moment" as I realised that what Hilary had just shown me had the potential to heal such traumatised individuals by restoring or improving their capacity to both attune and mentalize. I then heard myself say, with conviction: "I think you need this person here." pointing at my companion Hilary Kennedy.

"But she is not a trauma specialist" was the immediate response.

"No," I replied, "but I think that what she does will actually heal your clients."

While I gave the team time to think about the idea, we returned to the UK and I shared my thoughts with Hilary regarding the possible role of VIG in treating the Mexican parents who were often addicted to drugs and violence because of their traumatic backgrounds.

I had come round to this view because, after so many years working in the TSS, what I observed was that those men and women who had endured the effects of childhood terror, war, torture, and other man-made horrors, suffered essentially from having lost their capacity to interconnect with others through the magical process of attunement. It is worth reminding ourselves here of how Siegel (2010) defines this process:

> When we attune with others, we allow our own internal state to shift, to come to resonate with the inner world of another. This resonance is at the heart of the important sense of "feeling felt" that emerges in close relationships. Children need attunement to feel secure and to develop well, and throughout our lives we need attunement to feel close and connected.

However, terror leads to the hijacking of the attachment system in favour of the defence system, making us ready to fight or flee at a moment's notice. This is the state our patients were in when I first met them in my office, sitting in fear, by the door, in a dark helpless world of their own.

I said to Hilary that I felt that her approach could heal those individuals with such backgrounds by working with their children, a powerful source of motivation which I believed had the potential to bring their parents back into the Green Zone of trust and love. Hilary was open to the idea of training the Mexicans in Puebla since many of her clients had suffered from domestic violence in all its forms. So, when Alison Lane invited her to train their team in the use of VIG with myself as guarantor, we both accepted.

Back in the Mexican town of Puebla, equipped with new iPads, the twelve members of the JUCONI team spent four days with Hilary learning how to use video clips of authentic moments of interaction to achieve better communication between parents and their children through the process of attunement. The VIG approach is based on the belief that every parent wants to do their best for their child and I add that, if they can't, it is because they are under the influence of their past IWMs developed during their own traumatic early life. VIG is also "client centred", which means that it moves at the client's pace with their individual goals in mind, not the therapist's. This is very empowering for the client.

In their review paper describing the study of the effects of the use of video-recordings in attachment-based interventions, the Steeles (Steele et al., 2014) recognised the "shared review session" as having the potential to stimulate reflective-functioning, the essential human capacity to understand behaviour in the light of underlying mental states and intentions. Looking at a study on insecure mothers who were treated with VIPP (video intervention to promote positive parenting), which is very similar to VIG, they noted that these insecure mothers had become more sensitive and fewer children had developed behavioural or emotional problems.

Basically, the use of VIG-like treatments is of great benefit to children as it increases the parent's capacity to both attune emotionally and understand their children's behaviour so as to meet their needs.

In addition, this approach also reduces parental stress and increases their self-confidence as well as inspiring hopefulness and joy, even in disadvantaged contexts. It also stimulates parents to solve their own problems, all manifestations of being in the Green Zone. For this reason, it is being used in communities with drug addicts in Ecuador, with street children in Tanzania, and in many community services across the UK with the support of the national clinical guidelines. It is even proving of benefit to psychotic mothers in mother–baby units.

If we go back to the initial review session involving the mother's response to her son's face, we can see what a powerful effect it was for her to see him beaming with happiness and love and then being told that she had some part to play in this. I found myself imagining a triangle of oxytocin flowing between her, her son, and her guide who joins her in sharing the delight of this moment: as Helen Gibson (2020), an experienced family therapist and VIG supervisor, writes: "a context of love is created" which naturally elicits the Green Zone via the mammalian vagus nerve. In so doing the activated attachment system overrides the "defence system" represented by the Yellow Zone mired in anxiety and self-recrimination, and the Red Zone of dissociation (see Figure 2.1 on p. 39)

At the beginning of treatment, such moments may only be momentary, yet long enough to enable Johnny's mother to find herself feeling calm and able to follow her guide as her brain function is optimised and she begins to attune and empathise with her child. Being in the Green Zone of attunement enables a neurobiological change to take place with the melting of the old terror-induced dissociation giving way to the integration of the Self. This process will be reinforced by many other such moving experiences in collaboration with her guide. Basically, the use of VIG results in the same psychobiological changes in the client that we induce with the TAIP.

However, with VIG the effect is two-fold: if the child has developed a disorganised attachment, which is likely with a disorganised mother, the same process will have healed his or her divided Self by making the *traumatic attachment* redundant, thereby enabling the child to develop a secure attachment. Therefore, VIG is a wonderful therapy for both disorganised children and their disorganised parents: it results in what is referred to as "an earned secure attachment" (Kennedy et al., 2017) for both of them (for more on VIG, visit their website: https://videoin-teractionguidance.net).

Last, but not least, is the fact that one can now treat individuals and families suffering from the effects of *complex trauma* without suffering from secondary traumatisation. On the contrary, their therapists also experience the benefits of being in the Green Zone and actually report feeling a "buzz" from the oxytocin they experience when doing this work, including Lupita when healing the violent Don Juan with his son Pablo.

For baby's sake

A new trauma-informed therapeutic programme called "For baby's sake" has been developed in the UK to prevent the abuse and neglect of infants by preventing domestic abuse. Their website and remarkable film point to the profound effects that child abuse can have on the rest of an infant's life and how babies are particularly affected, even in the womb. If left unresolved, as we have seen, these early wounds can lead to issues in later life that affect the whole of society, such as mental health issues, struggling at school, substance misuse, criminal behaviour, being a perpetrator or a victim of domestic violence, and many physical conditions, as we saw in Felitti's ACE study (2022).

The two-year long trauma-informed programme accepts couples before their baby is born and provides them with a strength-based therapeutic approach for each parent to work around their early life experience as well as a VIG approach for the couple in relation to their baby. It is the best therapeutic programme for the prevention of domestic violence that I have known in my many years of experience because it deals effectively with the roots of the problem and is backed by accompanying research (https://forbabyssake.org.uk).

"Where there is a will, there is a way"

We now know that the origin of most mental disorders and possibly many physical disorders, can be attributed to the development of the *traumatic attachment*, nature's way of protecting vulnerable mammalian infants exposed to a mother or substitute parent who is either terrifying or unavailable.

The above evidence shows that millions of children are being exposed in the UK and the United States to abuse and neglect which we know could be prevented by adopting social policies that foster social change in favour of parents' and children's well-being during their complex life-cycle. As long as such changes are avoided by those in government, a large proportion of infants will develop different mindsets in order to ensure their survival in a frightening world where others cannot be trusted.

Their survival is usually at the expense of their future and ours: those we meet in our consulting rooms or in hospital who are often labelled "as mentally ill" are those for whom the cost of these different ways of feeling, thinking, and behaving have outweighed their survival benefits. They suffer from many of the effects of addiction, unresolved grief, domestic and other forms of violence, BPD, complex trauma, and other mental disorders as well as associated medical conditions.

It is worth noting, however, that a few of these survivors have developed a "self-preservative" type of behaviour with its emphasis on "power and control", which, in our current neoliberal social context can be an asset and lead to positions of wealth and authority (Henry, 1997). Their decisions will be largely determined by the fact that their minds reflect the negative effects of their earlier life, which unfortunately tends to be at the expense of the "Other".

It is important to bear in mind Van der Kolk's statement regarding the effects of trauma:

> We have learned that trauma is not just an event that took place sometime in the past: it is also the imprint left by that experience on mind, brain and body. This imprint has ongoing consequences for how the human organism manages to survive the present. Trauma results in a fundamental re-organisation of the way mind and brain manage perceptions. (Van der Kolk, 2014)

A disorganised attachment leads to a different way of perceiving things, a different way of thinking, and a different way of behaving compared to those who are securely attached. It is highly sensitive to fear since it was born out of childhood terror.

Attunement and empathy are at the mercy of such states of mind which is why trauma must be reduced to enable the human "species-preservative behaviour" of love and cooperation to predominate.

What better way to do this than by making sure that human infants feel safe, loved, and supported throughout their development into adulthood. Such care depends on parents who have the time and the means to be both mentally and physically available for their children, backed up by a community network of relatives and friends as well as services that provide the extra guidance and support for those who need it.

With the development of the TAIP, therapists now have the means to both elicit and reverse the *traumatic attachment* which can offer so many sufferers the chance of a new lease of life and the possibility of developing secure attachments with their families and friends. Hilary Kennedy's admirable work is enabling thousands of families in different parts of the world to overcome their destructive relationships and, like the TAIP, melt the dissociative power of the *traumatic attachment*.

Both the TAIP and VIG can be learnt "on the job" and relatively quickly as well as being less expensive than most therapeutic training experiences. We hope that therapists of different modalities will join us in using and developing these approaches to thereby contribute to a reduction in mental suffering in individuals and families including vulnerable children.

These two new therapeutic approaches and others with similar positive outcomes can be integrated within the current "bio-social-ecological model" that defines resilience as those qualities of individuals and their social environments that help individuals adapt in the face of adversity. This summarises the new approach promoted in great part by Ungar (2013). It is an approach that is gaining ground in the United States as the Centres for Disease Control and Prevention is now promoting such an approach to prevent violence (Dahlberg & Krug, 2002).

This includes trauma-informed care aimed at reducing ACEs, which is being promoted in the United States as well as in Scotland and Wales. By providing the therapeutic potential for reducing mental illnesses and increasing resilience, TAIP therapies and VIG can be seen as an important step forward in healing our communities in these difficult times.

We hope that those who suffer from the painful and destructive effects of the *traumatic attachment* and their therapists will find hope and a means to end their suffering through this book and its therapeutic implications.

As Nelson Mandela (2000) said: "Our human compassion binds us the one to the other—not in pity or patronizingly, but as human beings who have learnt how to turn our common suffering into hope for the future."

References

Abe, E. L. (1994). The behavioural ecology of elephant survivors in Queen Elizabeth National Park, Uganda. [Doctoral thesis]. Available at: https://www.repository.cam.ac.uk/handle/1810/251890

Adshead, G., & Horne, E. (2021). *The Devil You Know: Encounters in Forensic Psychiatry*. London: Faber & Faber.

Ainsworth, M. D. S. (1967). *Infancy in Uganda: Infant Care and the Growth of Love*. Baltimore, MD: Johns Hopkins University Press.

Ainsworth, M. D. S., & Bowlby, J. (1954). Research strategy in the study of mother-child separation. *Courrier*, 4: 105–131.

Ainsworth, M. D. S., Blehar, M. C., Waters, E., & Wall, S. (1978). *Patterns of Attachment: A Psychological Study of the Strange Situation*. Mahwah, NJ: Lawrence Erlbaum Associates.

Aldridge, R. W., Lewer, D., Katikireddi, S. V., Mathur, R., Pathak, N., Burns, R., Fragaszy, E. B., Johnson, A. M., Devakumar, D., Abubakar, I., & Hayward, A. (2020). Black, Asian and minority ethnic groups in England are at increased risk of death from Covid-19: Indirect standardisation of NHS mortality data. *Wellcome Open Research*, 5: 88. doi: 10.12688/wellcomeopenres.15922.1

Alston, P. (2019). *Climate Change and Poverty: Report of the Special Rapporteur on Extreme Poverty and Human Rights, United Nations*. Available at: https://digitallibrary.un.org/record/3810720?ln=en#record-files-collapse-header [Accessed: 5/10/23].

American Psychiatric Association (2013). *Diagnostic and Statistical Manual of Mental Disorders: DSM-5* (5th edn). Washington, DC: American Psychiatric Publishing.

Anda, R. F., Felitti, V. J., Bremner, J. D., Walker, J. D., Whitfield, C., Perry, B. D., Dube, S. R., & Giles, W. H. (2006). The enduring effects of abuse and related adverse experiences in childhood: A convergence of evidence from neurobiology and epidemiology. *European Archives of Psychiatry and Clinical Neuroscience*, 256(3), 174–186. doi: 10.1007/s00406-005-0624-4neoli

Anderson, C. O., & Mason, W. A. (1978). Competitive social strategies in groups of deprived and experienced rhesus monkeys: *Macaca mulatta*. *Journal of Comparative and Physiological Psychology*, 87: 681–690.

Arntz, A., & Jacob, G. (2013). *Schema Therapy in Practice: An Introductory Guide to the Schema Mode Approach*. Chichester, West Sussex: John Wiley & Sons.

Bellis, M., Ashton, K., Hughes, K., Ford, K., Bishop, J., & Paranjothy, S. (2016). Adverse Childhood Experiences and their impact on health-harming behaviours in the Welsh adult population. doi: 10.13140/RG.2.1.4719.1122

Bernstein, E. M., & Putnam, F. W. (1986). Development, reliability, and validity of a dissociation scale. *Journal of Nervous & Mental Diseases, 174*(12): 727–735.

Bernstein, J. P. K., Fonda, J., Currao, A., Kim, S., Milberg, W. P., McGlinchey, R. E., & Fortier, C. B. (2022). Post-traumatic stress disorder and depression are uniquely associated with disability and life dissatisfaction in post-9/11 veterans. *Psychiatry Research, 313*: 114589. doi: 10.1016/j.psychres.2022.114589

Bloom, S. (2000). The grief that dare not speak its name part I: Dealing with the ravages of childhood abuse. *Psychotherapy Review, 2*(9): 1–9. SIEC No: 20140172. Part 11, Available at: https://www.academia.edu/2509660/THE_GRIEF_THAT_DARE_NOT_SPEAK_ITS_NAME_PART_II_DEALING_WITH_THE_RAVAGES_OF_CHILDHOOD_ABUSE [Accessed: 21/8/23].

Bonanno, G. A., Wortman, C. B., Lehman, D. R., Tweed, R. G., Haring, M., Sonnega, J., Carr, D., & Nesse, R. M. (2002). Resilience to loss and chronic grief: A prospective study from preloss to 18-months postloss. *Journal of Personality and Social Psychology, 83*(5), 1150–1164. doi: 10.1037//0022-3514.83.5.1150

Bowlby, J. (1944). Forty-four juvenile thieves: Their characters and home-life. *The International Journal of Psychoanalysis, 25*: 19–53.

Bowlby, J. (1951). Maternal Care and Mental Health. University of Oregon. Available at: https://darkwing.uoregon.edu/~eherman/teaching/texts/Bowlby%20Maternal%20Care%20and%20Mental%20Health.pdf [Accessed: 15/8/23].

Bowlby, J. (1969). *Attachment and Loss*. New York: Basic Books.

Bowlby, J. (1979). On knowing what you are not supposed to know and feeling what you are not supposed to feel. *Canadian Journal of Psychiatry, 24*(5): 403–408.

Bowlby, J. (1982). Attachment and loss: Retrospect and prospect. *American Journal of Orthopsychiatry, 52*(4): 664–667. doi: 10.1111/j.1939-0025.1982.tb01456.x

Bowlby, J. (1988). *A Secure Base: Clinical Applications of Attachment Theory*. London: Routledge.

Bradshaw, I. G. (2004) Not by bread alone: Symbolic loss, trauma, and recovery in elephant communities. *Society & Animals, 12*(2): 143–158. doi: 10.1163/1568530041446535

Bradshaw, G. A. (2005). Elephant trauma and recovery: From human violence to trans-species psychology. Dissertation: Pacifica Graduate Institute, Santa Barbara, California.

Bradshaw, G. A. (2015). Not by bread alone: Symbolic loss, trauma, and recovery in elephant communities. Available at: https://www.animalsandsociety.org/wp-content/uploads/2015/11/bradshaw.pdf (p. 23).

Bradshaw, G. A., & Schore, A. N. (2007). How elephants are opening doors: Developmental neuroethology, attachment and social context. *Ethology, 113*(5): 426–436. doi: 10.1111/j.1439-0310.2007.01333.x

Bresin, K., & Gordon, K. H. (2013). Endogenous opioids and nonsuicidal self-injury: A mechanism of affect regulation. *Neuroscience and Biobehavioral Reviews, 37*(3): 374–383. doi: 10.1016/j.neubiorev.2013.01.020

Bretherton, I. (1992). The origins of attachment theory: John Bowlby and Mary Ainsworth. *Developmental Psychology, 28*: 759–775.

Carlson, E. B., & Putnam, F. W. (1993). An update on the Dissociative Experience Scale. *Dissociation, 6*(1): 16–27. [Note: Dissociative Experiences Scale-II included in Appendix.]

Carter, C. S. (2017). The role of oxytocin and vasopressin in attachment. *Psychodynamic Psychiatry*, *45*(4): 499–517. doi: 10.1521/pdps.2017.45.4.499

CDC video. Center on the Developing Child at Harvard University (developingchild.harvard.edu). The following videos are available at http://www.youtube.com/HarvardCenter: Serve and return interaction shapes brain circuitry; Toxic stress derails healthy development; How resilience is built; The science of early childhood development; The impact of early adversity on children's development.

Cénat, J. M. (2023). Complex racial trauma: Evidence, theory, assessment, and treatment. *Perspectives on Psychological Science*, *18*(3): 675–687. doi: 10.1177/17456916221120428

Coe, C. L., Wiener, S. G., Rosenberg, L. T., & Levine, S. (1985). Endocrine and immune responses to separation and maternal loss in nonhuman primates. In: M. Reite & T. Field (Eds.), *The Psychobiology of Attachment and Separation*. London: Academic Press.

Cosgrove, L., & Krimsky, S. (2012). A comparison of DSM-IV and DSM-5 panel members' financial associations with industry: A pernicious problem persists. *PLoS Medicine*, *9*(3) e1001190. doi: 10.1371/journal.pmed.1001190

Clare, A. W. (1992). *In the Psychiatrist's Chair*. London: Random House.

Cloitre, M., Petkova, E., Wang, J., & Lassell, F. L. (2012). An examination of the influence of a sequential treatment on the course and impact of dissociation among women with PTSD related to childhood abuse. *Depression and Anxiety*, *29*(8): 709–717. doi: 10.1002/da.21920

Dahlberg, L. L., & Krug, E. G. (2002). Violence: A global public health problem. In: E. G. Krug, L. L. Dahlberg, J. A. Mercy, A. B. Zwi, & R. Lozano R. (Eds.), *World Report on Violence and Health* (pp. 1–21). Geneva, Switzerland: World Health Organization. Available at: https://www.cdc.gov/violenceprevention/about/social-ecologicalmodel.html

Davies, J. (2022). *Sedated: How Modern Capitalism Created Our Mental Health Crisis*. London: Atlantic Books.

Dobzhansky, T. (1962). *Mankind Evolving: The Evolution of the Human Species*. The Silliman Memorial Lecture Series. New Haven: Yale University Press.

Drummond, C. (2017). Cuts to addiction services are a false economy. *BMJ* 2017: 357.

DSM-5 (2022). *Diagnostic and Statistical Manual of Mental Disorders*. New York: American Psychiatric Association.

Edin, K. J., Shaefer, H. L., & Nelson, T. J. (2023). *The Injustice of Place: Uncovering the Legacy of Poverty in America*. New York: HarperCollins.

Ehlers, A., & Clark, D. M. (2000). A cognitive model of posttraumatic stress disorder. *Behaviour Research and Therapy*, *38*(4): 319–345. doi: 10.1016/s0005-7967(99)00123-0

Eisenberger, N. I., Lieberman, M. D., & Williams, K. D. (2003). Does rejection hurt? An fMRI study of Social Exclusion. *Science*, *302*(5643): pp. 290–292. doi: 10.1126/science.1089134

Equine-assisted therapy (2022). *Psychology Today*. Available at: https://www.psychologytoday.com/gb/therapy-types/equine-assisted-therapy [Accessed: 17/8/23].

Fairbairn, W. R. D. (1952). *Psychoanalytic Studies of the Personality*. London: Routledge & Kegan Paul.

Felitti, V. J. (2002). The relation between adverse childhood experiences and adult health: Turning gold into lead. *The Permanente Journal*. doi: 10.7812/tpp/02.994

Felitti, V. J. (2003). The origins of addiction: Evidence from the adverse childhood experiences study. *Praxis der Kinderpsychologie und Kinderpsychiatrie*, *52*: 547–559.

Ferenczi, S. (1988). Confusion of tongues between adults and the child (the language of tenderness and of passion). *Contemporary Psychoanalysis*, *24*: 196–206.

Field, T. (1985). Attachment as psychobiological attunement. In: M. Reite (Ed.), *The Psychobiology of Attachment and Separation*. New York: Academic Press. eBook ISBN: 9780323147217.

Fonagy, P., & Luyten, P. (2009). A developmental, mentalization-based approach to the understanding and treatment of borderline personality disorder. *Development and Psychopathology, 21*(4): 1355–1381. doi: 10.1017/s0954579409990198

Fonagy, P., & Target, M. (1997). Attachment and reflective function: Their role in self-organization. In: *Development and Psychopathology, 9*(4), pp. 679–700. doi: 10.1017/S0954579497001399

Freud, A., & Dann, S. (1951). An experiment in group upbringing. *The Psychoanalytic Study of the Child, 6*(1): 127–168. doi: 10.1080/00797308.1952.11822909

Freud, S. (1896c). The aetiology of hysteria. *S. E., 3*: 187–221. London: Hogarth.

Frewen, P., Zhu, J., & Lanius, R. (2019). Lifetime traumatic stressors and adverse childhood experiences uniquely predict concurrent PTSD, complex PTSD, and dissociative subtype of PTSD symptoms whereas recent adult non-traumatic stressors do not: results from an online survey study. *European Journal of Psychotraumatology, 10*(1): 1606625. doi: 10.1080/20008198.2019.1606625

Gallese, V. (2003). The roots of empathy: The shared manifold hypothesis and the neural basis of intersubjectivity. *Psychopathology, 36*(4): 171–180. doi: 10.1159/000072786

Gallese, V., & Sinigaglia, C. (2011). What is so special about embodied simulation? *Trends in Cognitive Sciences, 15*(11): 512–519. doi: 10.1016/j.tics.2011.09.003

Gallese, V., Keysers, C., & Rizzolatti, G. (2004). A unifying view of the basis of social cognition. *Trends in Cognitive Sciences, 8*(9): 396–403. doi: 10.1016/j.tics.2004.07.002

Gibson, H. (2020). Co-creating a "context of love". *Context, 172*: 10–12.

Gilligan, J. (1996). *Violence: Our Deadly Epidemic and its Causes*. New York: Putnam.

Gilligan, J. (2001). *Preventing Violence*. London: Thames & Hudson.

Goldstein, P., Weissman-Fogel, I., Dumas, G., & Shamay-Tsoory, S. G. (2018). Brain-to-brain coupling during handholding is associated with pain reduction. *Proceedings of the National Academy of Sciences, 115*(11). doi: 10.1073/pnas.1703643115

Goleman, D. (2006). *Social Intelligence: The New Science of Human Relationships*. New York: Bantam.

Goodall, J. (1990). *Through a Window: 30 Years with the Chimpanzees of Gombe*. London: Weidenfeld & Nicolson.

Gordon et al. (51 authors) (2023). A somatosensory-cognitive action network alternates with effector regions in motor cortex. *Nature, 617*: 351–359. doi: 10.1038/s41586-023-05964-2

Guardian (2017). Finland: The only country where fathers spend more time with kids than mothers. *The Guardian*. Available at: https://www.theguardian.com/lifeandstyle/2017/dec/04/finland-only-country-world-dad-more-time-kids-moms [Accessed: 15/8/23].

Guidano, V. F. (1987). *Complexity of the Self: A Developmental Approach to Psychopathology and Therapy*. New York: Guilford Press.

Harlow, H. F. (1974). *Learning to Love* (2nd edn). New York: Jason Aronson.

Harlow, H. F., & Mears, C. (1979). *Primate Perspectives*. New York: John Wiley.

Harlow, H. F., & Suomi, S. J. (1971). Social recovery by isolation-reared monkeys. *Proceedings of the National Academy of Sciences, 68*(7): 1534–1538. doi: 10.1073/pnas.68.7.1534

Harlow, H. F., Dodsworth, R. O., & Harlow, M. K. (1965). Total social isolation in monkeys. *Proceedings of the National Academy of Sciences, 54*(1): 90–97. doi: 10.1073/pnas.54.1.90

Harlow, H. F., Harlow, M. K., & Suomi, S. J. (1971). From thought to therapy: Lessons from a primate laboratory. *American Scientist, 59*(5): 538–549.

Harris, K. M., Woolf, S. H., & Gaskin, D. J. (2021). High and rising working-age mortality in the US: A Report from the National Academies of Sciences, Engineering, and Medicine. *JAMA*, 325(20): 2045–2046. doi: 10.1001/jama.2021.4073

Hebb, D. O. (1949). *The Organization of Behavior: A Neuropsychological Theory*. New York: John Wiley.

Henry, J. (1997). Psychological and physiological responses to stress: The right hemisphere and the hypothalamic-pituitary-adrenal axis, an inquiry into problems of human bonding. *Acta Physiologica Scandinavica*, 161: 10–25.

Herman, J. L. (1997). *Trauma and Recovery: The Aftermath of Violence—From Domestic Abuse to Political Terror*. New York: Basic Books.

Herman, J. L., & Hirschman, L. (2000). *Father-Daughter Incest*. Cambridge, MA: Harvard University Press.

Hesse, E., & Main, M. (2000). Disorganized infant, child, and adult attachment: Collapse in behavioral and attentional strategies. *Journal of the American Psychoanalytic Association*, 48(4): 1097–1127. doi: 10.1177/00030651000480041101

Hiam, L., Dorling, D., & McKee, M. (2023). Falling down the global ranks: Life expectancy in the UK, 1952–2021. *Journal of the Royal Society of Medicine*, 116(3): 89–92. doi: 10.1177/01410768231155637

Hofer, M. A. (1984). Relationships as regulators: A psychobiological perspective on bereavement. *Psychosomatic Medicine*, 46: 183–197.

Hofer, M. A. (1994). Hidden regulators in attachment, separation, and loss. *Monographs of the Society for Research in Child Development*, 59(2/3): 192. doi: 10.2307/1166146

Hofer, M. A. (2006). Psychobiological roots of early attachment. *Current Directions in Psychological Science*, 15(2): 84–88. doi: 10.1111/j.0963-7214.2006.00412.x

Hofer, M. A. (2014). The emerging synthesis of development and evolution: A new biology for psychoanalysis. *Neuropsychoanalysis*, 16(1): 3–22. doi: 10.1080/15294145.2014.901022

Jenson, G. D., Bobbitt, R. A., & Gordon, G. N. (1968). Effects of environment on the relationship between mother and infant pigtail monkeys. *Journal of Comparative Physiology and Psychology*, 66: 259–263.

Johnson, B. (1997). Narrative approaches with lifers. *The Therapist*, 4(3): 24–28. (Formerly the *Journal of the European Therapy Studies Institute*.)

Johnson, B. (2005). *Emotional Health: What Emotions Are and How They Cause Social and Mental Diseases*. New York: Trust Consent Publishing.

Johnson, B. (2018). *How Verbal Physiotherapy Works*. New York: Trust Consent Publishing.

Kahr, B. (2007). The infanticidal attachment. *New Directions in Relational Psychoanalysis and Psychotherapy*, 1(2): 117–132.

Kaplan, N. (1987). Internal representations of attachment in six-year-olds. ERIC. Available at: https://eric.ed.gov/?id=ED286590 [Accessed: 17/8/23].

Kaufman, I. C., & Rosenblum, L. A. (1967). The reaction to separation in infant monkeys: Anaclitic depression and conservation withdrawal. *Psychosomatic Medicine*, 29: 648–675.

Kearney, B. E., & Lanius, R. A. (2022). The brain-body disconnect: A somatic sensory basis for trauma-related disorders. *Frontiers in Neuroscience*, 16: 1015749. doi: 10.3389/fnins.2022.1015749

Kennedy, H., Ball, K., & Barlow, J. (2017). How does video interaction guidance contribute to infant and parental mental health and well-being? *Clinical Child Psychology and Psychiatry*, 22(3): 500–517. doi: 10.1177/1359104517704026

Klomek, A. B., Sourander, A., Neimela, S., Kumpulainen. K., Piha, J., Tamminen, T., …, & Gould, M. S. (2009). Childhood bullying behaviors as a risk for suicide attempts and completed suicides:

A population-based birth cohort study. *Journal of the American Academy of Child & Adolescent Psychiatry*, *48*(3): 254–261. doi: 10.1097/chi.0b013e318196b91f

Knutson, B., Adams, C. M., Fong, G. W., & Hommer, D. (2001). Anticipation of increasing monetary reward selectively recruits nucleus accumbens. *The Journal of Neuroscience*, *21*(16): RC159. doi: 10.1523/JNEUROSCI.21-16-j0002.2001

Lab, D., Santos, I., & Zulueta, F. de (2008). Treating post-traumatic stress disorder in the "real world": Evaluation of a specialist trauma service and adaptations to standard treatment approaches. *Psychiatric Bulletin*, *32*(1): 8–12. doi: 10.1192/pb.bp.105.008664

Lanius, R. A., Brand, B., Vermetten, E., Frewen, P. A., & Spiegel, D. (2012). The dissociative subtype of posttraumatic stress disorder: Rationale, clinical and neurobiological evidence, and implications. *Depression and Anxiety*, *29*(8): 701–708. doi: 10.1002/da.21889

Lanius, R. A., Vermetten, E., Loewenstein, R. J., Brand, B., Schmahl, C., Bremner, J. D., & Spiegel, D. (2010). Emotion modulation in PTSD: Clinical and neurobiological evidence for a dissociative subtype. *The American Journal of Psychiatry*, *167*(6): 640–647. doi: 10.1176/appi.ajp.2009.09081168

Levine, P. A. and Frederick, A. (1997). *Waking the Tiger: Healing Trauma: The Innate Capacity to Transform Overwhelming Experiences*. Berkeley, CA: North Atlantic Books.

Lieberman, M. D. (2013). *Social: Why Our Brains Are Wired to Connect*. New York: Penguin Random House.

Lifton, B. J. (1979). *Lost and Found: The Adoption Experience*. New York: The Dial Press.

Lindemann, E. (1944). Symptomatology and management of acute grief. *American Journal of Psychiatry*, *101*: 141–149.

Liotti, G. (2006). A model of dissociation based on attachment theory and research. *Journal of Trauma & Dissociation*, *7*(4): 55–73.

Liotti, G. (2011). Attachment disorganization and the controlling strategies: An illustration of the contributions of attachment theory to developmental psychopathology and to Psychotherapy Integration. *Journal of Psychotherapy Integration*, *21*(3): 232–252. doi: 10.1037/a0025422

Luiggi-Hernández, J. G. (2020). Latest UN report calls for Global Paradigm Shift in mental health care, Mad in America. Available at: https://www.madinamerica.com/2020/07/latest-un-report-calls-paradigm-shift-mental-health-care-globally/ [Accessed: 5/10/23].

Lyssenko, L., Schmahl, C., Bockhacker, L., Vonderlin, R., Bohus, M., & Kleindienst, N. (2018). Dissociation in psychiatric disorders: A meta-analysis of studies using the dissociative experiences scale. *The American Journal of Psychiatry*, *175*(1): 37–46. doi: 10.1176/appi.ajp.2017.17010025

Machin, A. (2018). *The Life of Dad: The Making of the Modern Father*. London: Simon & Schuster.

Main, M., & Hesse, E. (1990). Parents' unresolved traumatic experiences are related to infant disorganized attachment status: Is frightened/frightening parental behavior the linking mechanism? In: M. T. Greenberg, D. Cicchetti & E. M. Cummings (Eds.), *Attachment in the Preschool Years: Theory, Research, and Intervention* (pp. 161–182). Chicago, IL: University of Chicago Press.

Main, M., & Hesse, E. (1992). Disorganized/disoriented infant behavior in the Strange Situation, lapses in the monitoring of reasoning and discourse during the parent's Adult Attachment Interview, and dissociative states. In: M. Ammaniti & D. Stem (Eds.), *Attachment and Psychoanalysis* (pp. 86–140). Rome: Guis Laterza & Figli.

Main, M., & Solomon, J. (1986). Discovery of an insecure-disorganized/disoriented attachment pattern. In: T. B. Brazelton & M. W. Yogman (Eds.), *Affective Development in Infancy* (pp. 95–124). Westport, CT: Ablex.

Main, M., & Solomon, J. (1989). Procedures for identifying infants as disorganised/disoriented during the Ainsworth Strange Situation. In: M. Greenberg, D. Cicchetti & E. M. Cummings (Eds.), *Attachment During the Preschool Years*. Chicago: University of Chicago Press.

Mandela, N. (2000). Speech at Healing & Reconciliation Service dedicated to HIV/Aids sufferers and "The Healing of our Land", Johannesburg, 6 December 2000.

Mark, P., & Zulueta, F. de (2000). Attachment and Contained Splitting: A combined approach of group and individual therapy in the treatment of patients suffering from a borderline personality disorder. *Group Analysis, 33*: 486–500.

Marmot, M., Allen, J., Boyce, T., Goldblatt, P., & Morrison, J. (2020). *Health Equity in England: The Marmot Review 10 Years On*. Institute of Health Equity. Available at: health.org.uk/publications/reports/the-marmot-review-10-years-on

Maté, G. (2012). *Scattered Minds: The Origins and Healing of Attention Deficit Disorder*. Canada: Vintage, Canada.

Maté, G. (2018). *In the Realm of Hungry Ghosts: Close Encounters with Addictions*. London: Vermilion.

Maté, G. (2022). Available at: https://www.madinamerica.com/2022/03/the-power-of-addiction-and-the-addiction-to-power-gabor-mate-md

Mead, G. H., & Morris, C. W. (1934). *Mind, Self and Society: From the Standpoint of a Social Behaviorist*. Chicago, IL: University of Chicago.

Mosquera, D., Gonzalez, A., & Hart, O. (2011). Borderline personality disorder, childhood trauma and structural dissociation of the personality. *Revista Persona, 11*: 44–73.

Moss, C. (1988). *Elephant Memories: Thirteen Years in the Life of an Elephant Family*. Singapore: Elm Tree Books.

Moss, C. (1992). *Echo of the Elephants: The Story of an Elephant Family*. UK: Book Club Associates.

Murray, R. M. (2007). Obituary: Professor Anthony Clare. Published online by Cambridge University Press. Available at: https://www.cambridge.org/core/services/aop-cambridge-core/content/view/32F8A7D737E9BE63E366B13C93CC4B37/S0955603600035911a.pdf/professor-anthony-clare.pdf [Accessed: 12/11/2023].

National Institute for Health and Clinical Excellence (NICE) Guidance (UK). (2005). *Post-Traumatic Stress Disorder: The Management of PTSD in Adults and Children in Primary and Secondary Care*. UK: Gaskell.

Nemeroff, C. B. (2012). *Management of Treatment-resistant Major Psychiatric Disorders*. New York: Oxford University Press.

Ney, P. G., & Peters, A. (1995). *Ending the Cycle of Abuse: The Stories of Women Abused as Children and the Group Therapy Techniques That Helped Them Heal*. New York: Brunner/Mazel.

Ng, J., Sutherland, C., & Kolber, M. R. (2017). Does evidence support supervised injection sites?' *Canadian Family Physician Medecin de Famille Canadien, 63*(11): 866.

Nijenhuis, E. R., Spinhoven, P., Van Dyck, R., Van der Hart, O., & Vanderlinden, J. (1998). Degree of Somatoform and psychological dissociation in dissociative disorder is correlated with reported trauma. *Journal of Traumatic Stress, 11*(4): 711–730. doi: 10.1023/a:1024493332751

NSPCC (2022). Available at: https://www.nspcc.org.uk/about-us/news-opinion/2022/childhood-day

O'Connor, M. F., Wellisch, D. K., Stanton, A. L., Eisenberger, N. I., Irwin, M. R., & Lieberman, M. D. (2008). Craving love? Enduring grief activates brain's reward center. *NeuroImage, 42*(2): 969–972. doi: 10.1016/j.neuroimage.2008.04.256

OECD (2023). Available at: https://www.oecd.org/gender/FIN_OECD_Gender_Pay_Reporting_28092023.pdf

Ogden, P., & Fisher, J. (2015). *Sensorimotor Psychotherapy: Interventions for Trauma And Attachment.* London: W. W. Norton.

Opendak, M., Theisen, E., Blomkvist, A., Hollis, K., Lind, T., Sarro, E., Lundstrom, J. N., Tottenham, N., Dozier, M., Wilson, D. A., & Sullivan, R. M. (2020). Adverse caregiving in infancy blunts neural processing of the mother. *Nature Communications, 11*: 1119. doi: 10.1038/s41467-020-14801-3

Ott, C. H. Lueger, R. J., Kelber, S. T., & Prigerson, H. G. (2007). Spousal bereavement in older adults. *Journal of Nervous & Mental Disease, 195*(4): 332–341. doi: 10.1097/01.nmd.0000243890.93992.1e

Pace, P. (2003). *Lifespan Integration: Connecting Ego States Through Time.* Lifespanintegration.com

Papadopoulos, R. K. (2021). *Involuntary Dislocation: Home, Trauma, Resilience, and Adversity-activated Development.* London: Routledge.

Payne, K. (1998). *Silent Thunder: In the Presence of Elephants.* New York: Simon & Schuster.

Perry, B. D., Pollard, R. A., Blakley, T. L., Baker, W. L., & Vigilante, D. (1995). Childhood trauma, the neurobiology of adaptation, and "use-dependent" development of the brain: How "states" become "traits". *Infant Mental Health Journal, 16*(4): 271–291. doi: 10.1002/1097-0355(199524)16:4<271::AID-IMHJ2280160404>3.0.CO;2-B

Perry, R., & Sullivan, R. M. (2014). Neurobiology of attachment to an abusive caregiver: Short-term benefits and long-term costs. *Developmental Psychobiology, 56*(8): 1626–1634. doi: 10.1002/dev.21219

Pickersgill, M. D. (2014). Debating DSM-5: Diagnosis and the sociology of critique. *Journal of Medical Ethics, 40*(8): 521–525. doi: 10.1136/medethics-2013-101762

Plimpton, E., & Rosenblum, L. (1983). The ecological context of infant maltreatment in primates. In: M. Reite & N. G. Caine (Eds.), *Child Abuse: The Nonhuman Primate Data.* New York: Alan Liss.

Pols, H., & Oak, S. (2007). War and military mental health: The US psychiatric response in the 20th century. *American Journal of Public Health, 97*(12): 2132–2142. https://doi.org/10.2105/AJPH.2006.090910

Porges, S. W. (1997). Emotion: An evolutionary by-product of the Neural Regulation of the Autonomic Nervous System. *Annals of the New York Academy of Sciences, 807*(1 Integrative N): 62–77. doi: 10.1111/j.1749-6632.1997.tb51913.x

Porges, S. W. (2009). Reciprocal influences between body and brain in the perception and expression of affect: A polyvagal perspective. In: D. Fosha, D. J. Siegel, & M. F. Solomon (Eds.), *The Healing Power of Emotion: Affective Neuroscience, Development & Clinical Practice* (pp. 27–54). New York: W. W. Norton.

Porges, S. W. (2017). Vagal pathways. *Oxford Handbooks Online* [Preprint]. doi: 10.1093/oxfordhb/9780190464684.013.15

Rauch, S. L., Van der Kolk, B. A., Fisler, R. E., Alpert, N. M., Orr, S. P., Savage, C. R., Fischman, A. J., Jenike, M. A., & Pitman, R. K. (1996). A symptom provocation study of posttraumatic stress disorder using positron emission tomography and script-driven imagery. *Archives of General Psychiatry, 53*(5): 380–387. doi: 10.1001/archpsyc.1996.01830050014003

Reite, M., & Capitanio, J. P. (1985). On the nature of social separation and attachment. In: M. Reite & T. Field (Eds.), *The Psychobiology of Attachment and Separation* (pp. 223–255). London: Academic Press.

Ruiz, R. (2014). How childhood trauma could be mistaken for ADHD. *The Atlantic.* Available at: https://www.theatlantic.com/health/archive/2014/07/how-childhood-trauma-could-be-mistaken-for-adhd/373328/ [Accessed: 18/8/23].

Russell, M. J., Switz, G. M., & Thompson, K. (1980). Olfactory influences on the human menstrual cycle. *Pharmacology Biochemistry and Behavior, 13*(5): 737–738. doi: 10.1016/0091-3057(80)90020-9

Ryle, A. (1990). *Cognitive Analytic Therapy: Active Participation in Change.* Chichester: John Wiley & Sons.

Sadeghi, M., & Mazaheri, A. (2009). Comparison of attachment styles in mothers with and without a history of fetus abortion (intentional and spontaneous). *Fertility and Infertility Journal*, 8: 60–69.

Sahi, R. S., Dieffenbach, M. C., Gan, S., Lee, M., Hazlett, L. I., Burns, S. M., Lieberman, M. D., Shamay-Tsoory, S. G., & Eisenberger, N. I. (2021). The comfort in touch: Immediate and lasting effects of handholding on emotional pain. *PLOS ONE*, *16*(2). doi: 10.1371/journal.pone.0246753

Şar, V. (2014). The many faces of dissociation: Opportunities for innovative research in psychiatry. *Clinical Psychopharmacology and Neuroscience*, *12*(3): 171–179. doi: 10.9758/cpn.2014.12.3.171

Sawyer, S. M., Azzopardi, P. S., Wickremarathne, D., & Patton, G. C. (2018). The age of adolescence. *Lancet Child Adolescent Health*, *2*: 223–228. Published online 17 January 2018. http://dx.doi.org/10.1016/S2352-4642(18)30022-1

Schore, A. N. (1994). *Affect Regulation and the Origin of the Self: The Neurobiology of Emotional Development*. Hillsdale, NJ: Lawrence Erlbaum.

Schore, A. N. (1996). The experience-dependent maturation of a regulatory system in the orbital prefrontal cortex and the origin of Developmental Psychopathology. *Development and Psychopathology*, *8*(1): 59–87. doi: 10.1017/s0954579400006970

Schore, A. N. (2000). Attachment and the regulation of the right brain. *Attachment & Human Development*, *2*(1): 23–47. doi: 10.1080/146167300361309

Schore, A. N. (2001). The effects of early relational trauma on right brain development, affect regulation, and infant mental health. *Infant Mental Health Journal*, *22*: 201–269.

Schore, A. N. (2002). Dysregulation of the right brain: A fundamental mechanism of traumatic attachment and the psychopathogenesis of posttraumatic stress disorder. *Australian & New Zealand Journal of Psychiatry*, *36*: 9–30. doi: 10.1046/j.1440-1614.2002.00996.xJohnson

Schore, A. N. (2009). Attachment trauma and the developing right brain: Origins of pathological dissociation. In: P. F. Dell & J. A. O'Neill (Eds.), *Dissociation and the Dissociative Disorders* (pp. 107–141). New York: Routledge.

Schore, A. N. (2022). Right brain to right brain psychotherapy: recent scientific and clinical advances. *Annals of General Psychiatry*, *21*: 21–46. https://doi.org/10.1186/s12991-022-00420-3

Sheldrick, D., Moss, C., Bradshaw, G., & Schore, A. (2005). Elephant breakdown: Social trauma. *Nature*, *433*. Available at: www.nature.com/nature

Sheldrick Wildlife Trust (2021). Haven for Elephants & Rhinos, Sheldrick Wildlife Trust. Available at: https://www.sheldrickwildlifetrust.org/ [Accessed: 15/8/23].

Siebert, C. (2006). An elephant crackup? *The New York Times Magazine*, 42–35.

Siegel, D. J. (1999). *The Developing Mind: Toward a Neurobiology of Interpersonal Experience*. New York: Guilford Press.

Siegel, D. J. (2001). Toward an interpersonal neurobiology of the developing mind: Attachment relationships, "mindsight" and neural integration. *Infant Mental Health*, *22*: 67–94.

Siegel, D. J. (2006). The mind in psychotherapy: An interpersonal neurobiology framework for understanding and cultivating mental health. *Psychology and Psychotherapy: Theory, Research and Practice*, *92*(2): 224–237. doi: 10.1111/papt.12228. ISSN 1476-0835. PMID 31001926. S2CID 121658470

Siegel, D. J. (2010). *Mindsight: The New Science of Personal Transformation*. New York: Bantam.

Siegel, D. J. (2014). *Brainstorm: The Power and Purpose of the Teenage Brain*. London: Scribe.

Siegel, D. J. (2017). The science of consciousness and the future of psychotherapy. Available at: https://www.psychotherapynetworker.org/article/science-consciousness-and-future-psychotherapy [Accessed: 21/8/23].

Siegel, D. J. (2021). Available at: https://www.pesi.com/blog/details/1150/the-complexity-choir

Siegel, D. J., & Hartzell, M. (2003). *Parenting from the Inside Out: How a Deeper Self-Understanding Can Help You Raise Children Who Thrive*. New York: Penguin, 2004.

Silbersweig, D., Clarkin, J. F., Goldstein, M., Kernberg, O. F., Tuescher, O., Levy, K. N., Brendel, G., Pan, H., Beutel, M., Pavony, M. T., Epstein, J., Lenzenweger, M. F., Thomas, K. M., Posner, M. I., & Stern, E. (2007). Failure of frontolimbic inhibitory function in the context of negative emotion in borderline personality disorder. *The American Journal of Psychiatry*, *164*(12): 1832–1841. doi: 10.1176/appi.ajp.2007.06010126

Sinason, V. (1992). *Mental Handicap and the Human Condition*. London: Free Association.

Sinason, V. (1998). *Memory in Dispute*. London: Karnac.

Slotow, R., & Van Dyck, G. (2001) Role of delinquent young "orphan" male elephants in high mortality of white rhinoceros in Pilanesberg National Park. *Koedoe, 44*(2). doi: 10.4102/koedoe.v44i1.18

Sroufe, L. A. (2005). Attachment and development: A prospective, longitudinal study from birth to adulthood. *Attachment & Human Development*, *7*(4): 349–367. doi: 10.1080/14616730500365928

Steele, M., Steele, H., Bate, J., Knafo, H., Kinsey, M., Bonuck, K., Meisner, P., & Murphy, A. (2014). Looking from the outside in: The use of video in attachment-based interventions. *Attachment & Human Development*, *16*(4): 402–415. doi: 10.1080/14616734.2014.912491

Sterling, P., & Platt, M. L. (2022). Why deaths of despair are increasing in the us and not other industrial nations-insights from neuroscience and anthropology. *JAMA, 79*(4): 368–374. doi: 10.1001/jamapsychiatry.2021.4209

Stern, D. (1985). *The Interpersonal World of the Infant: A View from Psychoanalysis and Developmental Psychology*. New York: Basic Books.

Stevens, J. E. (2012). The Adverse Childhood Experiences Study—the largest, most important public health study you never heard of—began in an obesity clinic. Available at: https://www.mahena.org/images/Infolaegas/N%C3%B5ustajale/Artikkel-J-E-Stevens-The-Adverse-Childhood-Experiences-Study-2012.pdf [Updated: 6/12/17].

Stevens, J. E. (2022). Addiction doc says: It's not the drugs. it's The aces … adverse childhood experiences., ACEs Too High. Available at: https://acestoohigh.com/2017/05/02/addiction-doc-says-stop-chasing-the-drug-focus-on-aces-people-can-recover/ [Accessed: 3/10/23].

Stiglitz, J. E. (2003). *Globalization and its Discontents*. New York: W. W. Norton.

Stronach, E. P., Toth, S. L., Rogosch, F., Oshri, A., Manly, J. T., & Cicchetti, D. (2011). Child maltreatment, attachment security, and internal representations of mother and mother–child relationships. *Child Maltreatment*, *16*(2): 137–145. doi: 10.1177/1077559511398294

Sullivan, R. M. (2012). The neurobiology of attachment to nurturing and abusive caregivers. *The Hastings Law Journal*, *63*(6): 1553–1570.

Sumrok, D. (2017). Available at: https://www.socialjusticesolutions.org/2017/09/29/addiction-doc-says-not-drugs-adverse-childhood-experiences/

Suomi, S. J., Harlow, H. F. & Novak, M. A. (1974). Reversal of social deficits produced by isolation rearing in monkeys. *Journal of Human Evolution, 3*(6): 527–534. doi: 10.1016/0047-2484(74)90013-x

Transform (2019). Available at: https://transformdrugs.org/blog/if-canada-can-open-50-drug-consumption-rooms-to-save-lives-why-not-scotland

Trevarthen, C. (2011). What is it like to be a person who knows nothing? Defining the active intersubjective mind of a newborn human being. *Infant and Child Development, 20:* 119–135.

Tronick, E. Z., & Weinberg, M. K. (1997). Depressed mothers and infants: Failure to form dyadic states of consciousness. In: L. Murray & P. J. Cooper (Eds.), *Postpartum Depression and Child Development* (pp. 54–81). New York: Guilford Press.

Troy, M., & Sroufe, L. A. (1987). Victimization among preschoolers: Role of attachment relationship history. *Journal of the American Academy of Child & Adolescent Psychiatry, 26*(2): 166–172. doi: 10.1097/00004583-198703000-00007

Ungar, M. (2013). Resilience, trauma, context, and culture. *Trauma, Violence and Abuse, 14*(3): 255–266. doi: 10.1177/1524838013487805

Ustunsoz, A., Guvenc, G., Akyuz, A., & Oflaz, F. (2010). Comparison of maternal- and paternal-fetal attachment in Turkish couples. *Midwifery, 26*(2): e1–e9.

Vaillant, G. E., Sobowale, N. C., & McArthur. C. (1972). Some psychological vulnerabilities in physicians. *New England Journal of Medicine, 287*: 372–375.

Van der Hart, O. (2018). Understanding trauma-generated dissociation and disorganised attachment: Giovanni Liotti's lasting contributions. *Attachment: New Directions in Psychotherapy and Relational Psychoanalysis, 12*: 101–109.

Van der Kolk, B. A. (1989). the compulsion to repeat the trauma: Re-enactment, revictimization, and masochism. *Psychiatric Clinics of North America, 12*: 389–411.

Van der Kolk, B. A. (2005). Developmental trauma disorder: Toward a rational diagnosis for children with complex trauma histories. *Psychiatric Annals, 35*: 401–408. doi: 10.3928/00485713-20050501-06

Van der Kolk, B. A. (2014). *The Body Keeps the Score: Mind, Brain and Body in the Transformation of Trauma*. London: Penguin.

Van IJzendoorn, M. H., & Schüngel, C. (1996). The measurement of dissociation in normal and clinical populations: Meta-analytic validation of the Dissociative Experiences Scale (DES). *Clinical Psychology Review, 16*: 365–382.

Velasquez-Manoff, M. (2015). Before the trauma. *Scientific American Mind, 26*(4): 56–63.

Wang, S. (1997). Traumatic stress and attachment. *Acta Physiologica Scandinavica, 161*: 164–169.

Welldon, E. V. (1988). *Mother, Madonna, Whore: The Idealization and Denigration of Motherhood*. London: Free Association.

World Health Organization (2019/2021). *International Classification of Diseases, Eleventh Revision (ICD-11)*, https://icd.who.int/browse11

Yehuda, R. (1997). Sensitisation of the hypothalamic-pituitary axis in post traumatic stress disorder. In: R. Yehuda & A. C. McFarlane (Eds.), *Psychobiology of Post Traumatic Stress Disorder* (pp. 57–75). Annals of the New York Academy of Sciences, vol. 821. New York: New York Academy of Science.

Yehuda, R., Engel, S. M., Brand, S., Seckl, J., Marcus, S. M., & Berkowitz, G. S. (2005). Transgenerational effect of post traumatic stress disorder in babies of mothers exposed to the World Trade Center attacks during pregnancy. *Journal of Clinical Endocrinology and Metabolism, 90*(7), 4115–4118.

Young, J. E., Klosko, J. S., & Weishaar, M. E. (2003). *Schema Therapy: A Practitioner's Guide*. New York: Guilford Press.

Zimmerman, M., & Becker, L. (2022a). The hidden borderline patient: Patients with borderline personality disorder who do not engage in recurrent suicidal or self-injurious behavior. *Psychological Medicine*, 1–8. doi: 10.1017/s0033291722002197

Zimmerman, M., & Becker, L. (2022b). psychiatric patients who do not believe they deserve to get better. *The Journal of Clinical Psychiatry, 83*(4): 21br14314. doi: 10.4088/JCP.21br14314

Zulueta, F. de (1984). The implications of bilingualism in the study and treatment of psychiatric disorders: A review. *Psychological Medicine, 14*(3): 541–557. doi: 10.1017/S0033291700015154

Zulueta, F. de (1990). Bilingualism and family therapy. *Journal of Family Therapy, 12*(3): 225–265.

Zulueta, F. de (1995). Bilingualism and culture and identity. *Group Analysis, 28*(2): 179–190.

Zulueta, F. de (2006a). *From Pain to Violence: The Traumatic Roots of Destructiveness* (2nd edn). Chichester: Whurr.

Zulueta, F. de (2006b). Inducing traumatic attachment in adults with a history of child abuse: Forensic applications. *The British Journal of Forensic Practice*, 8(3): 4–15. doi: 10.1108/14636646200600015

Zulueta, F. de (2009). Post-traumatic stress disorder and attachment: Possible links with borderline personality disorder. *Advances in Psychiatric Treatment*, 15(3): 172–180. doi: 10.1192/apt.bp.106.003418

Zulueta, F. de (2010a). Post-traumatic stress disorder and dissociation: The Traumatic Stress Service in the Maudsley Hospital. In: V. Sinason (Ed.), *Attachment, Trauma and Multiplicity* (2nd edn). (pp. 96–109). London: Routledge.

Zulueta, F. de (2010b). Reflective practice using attachment therapy. In M. Webber & J. Nathan (Eds.), *Reflective Practice in Mental Health: Advanced Psychosocial Practice with Children, Adolescents and Adults*. London: Jessica Kingsley.

Zulueta, F. de (2015a). The perversion of the Professional Caring Relationship. *Psychotherapy Section Review*, 1(56): 71–75. doi: 10.53841/bpspsr.2015.1.56.71

Zulueta, F. de, Gené-Cos, N., & Grachev, S. (2001). Differential psychotic symptomatology in polyglot patients; case reports and their implications, *British Journal of Medical Psychology*, 74(3): 277–292.

Other types of references

Aviguk: Video Interaction Guidance Association for Video. Available at: https://www.videointeraction-guidance.net/ [Accessed: 18/8/23]. (See Chapters 6 and 10.)

For Baby's Sake: Break the Cycle (2023). Available at: https://www.forbabyssake.org.uk/ [Accessed: 5/10/23]. (See Chapter 10.)

Serve & Return Interaction Shapes Brain Circuitry (2011) *YouTube*. YouTube. Available at: https://www.youtube.com/watch?v=m_5u8-QSh6A [Accessed: 16/8/23]. (See Chapter 2.)

Zulueta, F. de (2015b). From pain to violence and how to break the cycle. TEDxEastEnd. YouTube. Available at: https://www.youtube.com/watch?v=8d2grzTn3M4 [Accessed: 18/8/23].

Index